Technology and Global Public Health

Padmini Murthy • Amy Ansehl
Editors

Technology and Global Public Health

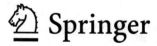 Springer

Editors
Padmini Murthy, MD, MPH, MS,
FAMWA, FRSPH
School of Health Sciences and Practice
New York Medical College
Valhalla, NY, USA

Amy Ansehl, RN, BSN, MSN,
FNP-BC, DNP
School of Health Sciences and Practice
New York Medical College
Valhalla, NY, USA

ISBN 978-3-030-46357-1   ISBN 978-3-030-46355-7   (eBook)
https://doi.org/10.1007/978-3-030-46355-7

This Springer imprint is published by the registered company Springer Nature Switzerland AG
The registered company address is: Gewerbestrasse 11, 6330 Cham, Switzerland

*To M.K. Kashinath and Krishna Kashinath –
my beloved parents – for instilling in me
values of global citizenship. I miss you!*

*To Sir M. Vishweshwariah – my grand-uncle,
a renowned trailblazer engineer and
technology pioneer*

–Padmini Murthy

*To Lawrence F. Cohen – my beloved father
for teaching me to value and enjoy all people*
–Amy Ansehl

Preface

Technology and health have been interconnected since ancient times, and as early as the sixth century BC, there is evidence that an Indian physician named Sushruta – who is considered as the father of surgery in India – was the author of one of the earliest works in the world on medicine and surgery. This scientific treatise, known as *The Sushruta Samhita*, described the etiology of more than 1100 diseases, the use of plants in treating diseases and the use of technology, and detailed surgical procedures including skin grafts and reconstructive procedures. This is an illustration of the use of technology in the practice of health [1].

The ancient Egyptians were known for their inventions and construction of edifices, as is evidenced in their pyramids and the burial chambers of the ancient kings and the nobles of Egypt. The culture of this country and the knowledge the ancient Egyptians had are fascinating, and there are several ancient monuments which were built using technology, such as the pyramids and the burial grounds. These monuments, especially the burial grounds, have provided us with a wealth of knowledge about examples of how culture and technology were intertwined in ancient Egypt. For example, one of the burial grounds where most probably a famous physician or surgeon (or an ancient healer) was buried, there are hieroglyphics that give an account of neurosurgical procedures. The Egyptians were well versed in preservation of dead bodies for centuries by a process known as mummification. It is amazing to learn about the link between health and technology since ancient times in different civilizations. The Incas in ancient Peru were known to have pioneered a surgical technique known as trepanation (trepanning), which involved removing small portions of the skull with instruments, that they designed to treat head injuries which were most probably sustained during armed conflict [2].

It is truly amazing and mind boggling to learn that our ancestors in so many civilizations had the knowledge which led to the development of innovative technology to improve the health of their fellow citizens.

Unfortunately, there were few or no means or ability to transfer this knowledge in ancient times, which existed centuries ago, from one region to another, and so to a great extent this knowledge and technology was more or less localized or regionalized.

At present when technology is advancing by leaps and bounds it is critical and essential that ancient knowledge and the technologies of bygone eras are shared to minimize their loss; and that current knowledge and technologies are shared to maximize their usage and effectiveness globally.

Some of the success stories in public health such as smallpox eradication, guinea worm, and the control of infectious diseases such as polio, measles, rubella, malaria, and neglected tropical diseases are the result of using technology. This knowledge depends on the use of various channels of communication including media, communications platforms, surveillance tools, optimal storage of vaccine, drugs, and reagents, and the production of low-cost diagnostic kits for detection and screening [3].

During outbreaks, the Global Outbreak Alert and Response Network (GOARN), which is overseen by the World Health Organization, works to "ensure the right technical expertise and skills are, on the ground where and when they are needed most." [4]

GOARN is an excellent undertaking built on the collaboration of various public health institutions and networks worldwide. The network is vital as the partners pool human and technical resources to confirm and respond to global outbreaks. In the past two decades, the GOARN has been of immense value in addressing threats such as SARS, Zika, Ebola, and the current COVID-19 crisis. Since 2000 The Global Outbreak Alert and Response Network has contributed towards global health security by "(1) Combating the international spread of outbreaks, (2) Ensuring that appropriate technical assistance reaches affected states rapidly, [and] (3) Contributing to long-term epidemic preparedness and capacity building." [4]

Technology can help to improve the health status of communities, enhance global security, and, when harnessed judiciously, can help the world achieve the targets of the 17 Sustainable Development Goals as adopted by the Member states of the United Nations in 2015.

During the past decade technology has been a driving force in disruptive innovations that have impacted the diverse fields of commerce, health care, education, pharmaceuticals, law, and social media across public and private sectors. Disruptive innovation refers to new organizations that are changing technologies to promote the evolution of that product or service over time [5].

This book aims to address the dynamic and pivotal role that the global community faces with unprecedented healthcare challenges and the impact that emerging technologies will have in the practice of global public health. These challenges are fueled by an aging population, rising rates of chronic disease, and persistent health disparities and inequities. New technologies have the potential to extend the reach of health professionals while improving the quality and efficiency of service delivery and reducing costs. The various technological advances that have contributed to improve the healthcare status of communities which are disadvantaged are discussed in depth in this book. Advances in technology as the result of new machines, treatments, and wearable devices, and applications for both smartphones and tablets have led to transformation across the sectors of commerce, social media, and health care. Cutting-edge developments and emerging trends in

Artificial Intelligence (AI) for disease surveillance and nanotechnology are disruptive innovators that have potential to produce equitable improvements in healthcare access and delivery on the global stage.

At present the existing technologies certainly hold the promise of equalizing health care throughout the world, but this will only happen if the global community unites to fight the digital divide and the ugly criminal element that technology currently fosters. As editors of this book, we hope to take our readers through a journey highlighting the tremendous role played by technology in improving health and transforming lives globally.

We begin this journey with reflections from five prominent players in the arena of global health and technology and empowerment of communities who have illustrated that technology on earth and in space has the power to strengthen the links between health and human rights for all by equalizing the playing field irrespective of the inequities caused by existing social determinants.

Valhalla, NY, USA
Padmini Murthy
Amy Ansehl

References

1. Columbia University. History of medicine: ancient Indian Nose Jobs & the Origins of plastic surgery. 1999–2019. https://columbiasurgery.org/news/2015/05/28/history-medicine-ancient-indian-nose-jobs-origins-plastic-surgery. Accessed 11 July 2019.
2. Norris, S. Science and Innovation. Inca Skull surgeons were 'Highly Skilled', study finds. 2008. https://www.nationalgeographic.com/science/2008/05/news-trepanation-inca-medicine-archaeology/. Accessed 9 July 2019.
3. Sabine institute Vaccine Institute. Smallpox Eradication continues to inspire innovations in Global Health. 2019. https://www.sabin.org/updates/pressreleases/smallpox-eradication-continues-inspire-innovations-global-health. Accessed 11 July 2019.
4. World Health Organization. Global outbreak alert and response network (GOARN) 2019. 2019. https://www.who.int/ihr/alert_and_response/outbreak-network/en/. Accessed 11 July 2019.
5. Hutt J. World Economic Forum. 2016. https://weforum.org/agenda/2016/what-is-disruptive-innovation. Accessed 12 July 2017.

Acknowledgments

My family especially my daughter Aishu, sister Apu for your continued support and encouragement throughout the years.

Thank you for friendship and support.

Amy (my partner in many adventures), Snehlata Champakalakshmi, Chantal Line Carpentier, Eliza Lo Chin, Coumba Coulibaly, Swati Dave, Norah A. Elgebreen, Cathey E. Falvo, Mamta Gautam, Falguni Gorti, Arun Gupta, Hawa M. Diallo, Ila Gupta, Renu Gupta, Vina Hulamm, Chyong-Huey Lai, Khatuna Kaladze, Anita Jindal, Satty Gill Keswani, Suhas Kirloskar, Nalini Krishnamoorthy, Sunita Marada, Mandakini Megh, Gertrude Ramanand, Raghu Ramakrishnan, Rukmini Ramakrishnan, Shelley Ross, Sonali Samarasinghe, Lalitha Sarabu, Mohan Sarabu, Usha Saraiya, Shanta Sista, Ginger Stillman, Saroja Subbaraman, Hary Suseelan, Meena Ugale, Gautami Veeragandham, Suba Vedula, Desiree Yap, and Winnie Yang

– *Padmini Murthy*

My family and Padmini (my co-conspirator)

– *Amy Ansehl*

We are grateful and highly appreciate our authors whose contributions have made this project a reality! We apologize for the numerous emails we sent to you all.

We wish to thank our students Jonathan V. Ogulnick, Alexander Boyer, Namrata Yadav, Chiamaka Agbasionwe, and Yaritzy Astudillo for their assistance in the preparation of the manuscript.

– *Padmini Murthy & Amy Ansehl*

November 2019, New York, USA

Endorsements

Technology and Global Public Health is a timely book addressing the health impact of technological and scientific advances globally. In order to provide cost-effective and quality healthcare services, innovations in AI, wearable devices, and early intervention methods must be implemented equitably to best serve the intended recipients in building healthier communities.

– Rupam Sarmah, *Computer scientist, musician, filmmaker, entrepreneur, and voting member of Grammy Awards*

With the advent of new technologies ranging from smartphones to mobile point-of-care diagnostic tools, the application and use of technology in the health sector has shifted beyond the field of medicine to public health, especially in limited-resource settings. This book provides a critical perspective to the key technological advancements in global health and the remaining challenges to achieve health equity globally. Edited by Dr. Murthy and Dr. Ansehl, this is an essential read for public health and global health students and practitioners. Particularly exciting is the inclusion of a range of global experts from space to youth to create a volume that provides new insights for all in this growing field.

– Roopa Dhatt, *Executive Director, Women in Global Health*

Contents

About the Contributors

Wale Idris Ajibade, MBA, PhD is the founder and elected executive director of African Views, a nonprofit research and multimedia organization in Hoboken, New Jersey, that focuses on improving African and African Diaspora communities and their relationships with the new world through cultural exchanges and collaborative projects. He started Foundation for Cultural Diversity and is the executive producer of World Cultural Diversity Day festivals. Wale is the architect of the African cultural exchange program for schoolchildren, which connects children in Africa by age group to schoolchildren in the United States through social media. He is the executive producer of the following African Views Radio programs on social and networking media: African Health Dialogues, Youth Initiatives, Millennium Development Goals, Green Africa, Culture Diplomats, New Deals, and The Future Women Want. Prior to joining the nonprofit sector, Wale was the director of research and marketing for International Investment Advisers (IIA) and has also worked for several distinguished financial firms such as Standard and Poor's, Reuters America, and Citibank Private Bank. He has a robust background in economics, research, data integration, variance and technical market analyses, and marketing, with 15 years' tenure in the financial market industry. Wale has an MBA from Columbus State University and a scholastic background in philosophy and economics from the University of Vienna. He is fluent in English, German, and Yoruba.

Arash Alaei, MD is co-founder and co-president of the Institute for International Health and Education (IIHE) in Albany, New York. He is a physician who bravely broke the silence on HIV/AIDS in the very conservative Muslim setting of Iran. Dr. Alaei has an established track record of cooperation with international scientists to foster medical diplomacy. He worked as the director of education and research for the National Research Institute of Tuberculosis and Lung Diseases at Shahid Beheshti University of Medical Sciences and the World Health Organization Collaborating Centre in Iran. Prior to establishing the IIHE, he and his brother Kamiar Alaei founded the Global Institute for Health and Human Rights (GIHHR) at the State University of New York (SUNY) at Albany in 2012, a university-wide research and education institute that focuses on developing interdisciplinary programs in the fields of health and human rights. Dr. Alaei was associate vice provost and clinical associate professor at SUNY Albany, vice chair of the School of Public Health Council, and a member of the admissions committee. He has extensive experience in clinical and non-clinical aspects of community-based care, HIV/AIDS, and addiction in the Middle East. His work has involved integrating HIV/AIDS prevention and treatment with addiction in primary healthcare services.

Kamiar Alaei, MD, MPH, MS, DrPH, Mst is chair and full professor in the Health Science Department at California State University, Long Beach. He is an award-winning human rights advocate and social entrepreneur, co-president of the Institute for International Health and Education (IIHE), and the founding director of the Global Institute for Health and Human Rights (GIHHR) at the State University of New York at Albany. Along with his brother Arash Alaei, he innovated the "Triangular Clinics" that offered medical care, counseling, and support for people living with HIV/AIDS, sexually transmitted infections (STIs), and injecting drug users (IDUs) – a first in the Middle East region that was documented by the United Nations/World Health Organization as a "Best Practice." Dr. Alaei is an internationally renowned expert on global health and teaches a course on Global Health Diplomacy in the Diplomatic Studies Program, Department of Continuing Education, at the University of Oxford in the United Kingdom. He is the recipient of several awards, including the Heinz R. Pagels Human Rights of Scientists Award, the Jonathan Mann Award for Global Health and Human Rights from the Global Health Council, the Inaugural Award for Leadership in Health and Human Rights from PAHO/WHO, the Inaugural Elizabeth Taylor Award in Recognition of Efforts to Advocate for Human Rights in the field of HIV, and the Ellis Island Medal of Honor.

David C. Alexander, BDS, MSc, MGDSRCS, DDPHRCS is a specialist in dental public health, having studied dentistry and community dental health in the United Kingdom and dental public health in a residency program at the US National Institute of Craniofacial Research, leading to board certification as a diplomate of the American Board of Dental Public Health. Through a diverse career in many settings in Europe, Asia, and North America. Dr. Alexander has developed an integrated approach to oral health and general health and the relationships between oral diseases and other noncommunicable diseases (NCDs). He follows a global view of health, its social and commercial determinants and inequalities, and is very concerned about the global burden of oral diseases and the long-standing separation of medicine and dentistry as a major contributing factor. Dr. Alexander has served as the chief executive of a Geneva-based NGO (World Dental Federation), liaising with the United Nations, World Health Organization, and global health civil society advocacy organizations. He is currently an adjunct professor in epidemiology and health promotion at New York University and an independent consultant in health communications and advocacy, translating science into actionable messaging. He is the principal founder of Appolonia Global Health Sciences in Green Brook, New Jersey. Dr. Alexander holds executive committee positions in the Academy of

Dentistry International, the Alliance for Oral Health Across Borders, and the Global Oral Health Inequalities Research Network of the International Association for Dental Research.

Camille Wardrop Alleyne, BSc, MSc, EdD is a rocket engineer, space scientist, internationally acclaimed speaker, writer, educational leader, and science ambassador. She has dedicated her 25-year career to advancing the areas of aerospace and space technology development, specifically in the fields of human and robotic space flight, space vehicle systems engineering, integration and testing, and space (microgravity) research. In the last several years, Dr. Alleyne has emerged as an expert in the areas of space, science, and technology application in international development, with a specific focus on developing countries. Her collective work has spanned many regions of the world including North America, the Caribbean, Europe, Asia, and Africa. In 2007, Dr. Alleyne founded the Brightest Stars Foundation, a 501(c)(3) non-governmental organization dedicated to educating, empowering, and inspiring young women to be future leaders through the study of science, math, and technology. The organization provides mentorship to young women from all across the world, providing them with the tools needed to select careers in science, technology, engineering, and mathematics (STEM) and to successfully matriculate through secondary and tertiary education in these fields. Dr. Alleyne has received numerous awards and commendations from national and international organizations including being awarded Outstanding Woman in Aerospace by the National Society of Black Engineers.

Amy Ansehl, RN, MSN, FNP-BC, DNP is a board-certified family nurse practitioner with significant experience in nursing and population health administration, leadership, interprofessional teaching, and community capacity building. She is a graduate of both Columbia University School of Nursing and the University of Pittsburgh School of Nursing, where she earned her doctorate. Amy is a founding member and an innovator of a healthcare startup in 2008 known as the Children's Environmental Health Center of the Hudson Valley (CEHCHV), which received a Westchester County distinguished public service award for addressing the needs of high-risk and underserved populations. It has been designated a Center of Excellence at New York Medical College (NYMC) and is part of the New York State Pediatric Environmental Health Specialty Units. Amy is associate professor in the Division of Environmental Health Sciences, School of Health Sciences and Practice, at New York Medical College in Valhalla. She is chairman of the foundation board of Westchester Visiting Nurse Services in New York. She is also the New York State representative to the Alliance of Nurses for Healthy Environments (ANHE). Amy is a fellow of the New Academy of Medicine.

Jessica Ansehl, MBA holds a Bachelor of Arts from the University of Chicago and a Master's in Business Administration from the Wharton School of the University of Pennsylvania. As an under-40 leader in the private sector, Jessica began her career as part of the Computer Sciences Corporation's Global Health Solutions consulting practice. She developed strategic partnerships and technology solutions with the world's leading hospitals, health insurance companies, and pharmaceutical organizations. Jessica is a board member of Visiting Nurse Services in Westchester and the University of Chicago New York Club, class representative of the Hackley School, and a member of the Family Advisory Council of New York University Langone Health.

Ramon Baez, DDS, MPH is adjunct professor in the School of Dentistry at the University of Texas Health Science Center at San Antonio and former director at the Office of Multicultural Affairs that included the Hispanic Center of Excellence–Dentistry and the World Health Organization (WHO) Collaborating Center. He is a consultant to the American Dental Association Council on Scientific Affairs, the WHO, and to several ministries of health, and is a member of the WHO Expert Advisory Panel on Oral Health. The Academy of Dentistry International (ADI) selected Dr. Baez as the International Dentist of the Year in 2001, the highest award granted by the academy to the dentist who best exemplifies international leadership. He has served on the ADI Executive Council as vice president for education, international affairs, finance, and administration; president-elect; president; and immediate past president.

Shewaye Belay, MSc first met Dr. Lewis Wall while working on a research project on obstetric fistula in the Tigray Region of Ethiopia. Since learning about nonprofit organization Dignity Period from Lewis and his wife, Helen, Shewaye has been dedicated to helping women and girls who lack menstrual hygiene management options. Shewaye holds an MSc in parasitology and immunology from Addis Ababa University and a BEd in biology from Mekelle University. He has contributed to studies on leishmaniosis, bed bug control, obstetric fistula, de-worming, and a number of other public health issues. Today, Shewaye is Dignity Period's go-to person on the ground. He is passionate about ensuring that young girls stay in school and that boys are educated to support them.

Christine C. Bennett, AO, MBBS, MPaed, FRACP was appointed professor and dean, School of Medicine, at the University of Notre Dame Australia, Sydney, in May 2011. Prior to this appointment, Dr. Bennett was the chief medical officer for Bupa Australia Group. Professor Bennett is a specialist pediatrician with over 30 years of health industry experience in clinical care, strategic planning, business operations, and senior management in the public, private, and not-for-profit sectors. She is a fellow of the Royal Australasian College of Physicians and has an active commitment to and involvement in medical professional issues, social policy, and medical research. Professor Bennett's professional experience has included being group executive and chief medical officer for MBF and the Bupa Health and Care Services, CEO of Research Australia, managing director of Total Health Enterprise Ltd, partner in health and life sciences for KPMG Australia, CEO of Westmead Hospital and Community Health Services, general manager for the Royal Hospital for Women, and head of planning in NSW Health. In February 2008, Professor

Bennett was appointed by the then Prime Minister Kevin Rudd to be chair of the National Health and Hospitals Reform Commission that provided advice to governments on a long-term blueprint for the future of the Australian health system and aged care. She is a consultant in the private and public sectors including the Digital Health Cooperative Research Centre in The Rocks, NSW, Australia. Professor Bennett was awarded Officer of the Order of Australia (AO) in the Australia Day 2014 Honours List.

Elvira Beracochea, MD, MPH is a global health expert with international experience in health systems improvement and project management, monitoring, and evaluation. She is the founder, president, and CEO of Realizing Global Health (RGH), a small woman-owned consulting business in Fairfax, Virginia. She founded RGH in 2005 to assist clients in developing stronger and sustainable health systems that achieve global health goals. Through RGH, she provides consulting, training, and professional coaching to clients who want to improve their professional performance and solve health system problems. She has developed innovative online training programs and a unique coaching approach to help health professionals deliver quality healthcare efficiently and consistently and improve their professional effectiveness. She has an MD from the Medical School at the University of the Republic of Uruguay and an MPH from the School of Public Health and Community Medicine at Hadassah Hebrew University in Jerusalem, Israel.

Nirma D. Bustamante, MD, MPH is an officer with the Epidemic Intelligence Service at the Centers for Disease Control and Prevention (CDC). Currently, she is assigned to the CDC Center for Global Health, Division of Global Health Protection, and has been involved in the response to several global infectious disease outbreaks including the Ebola crisis in the Democratic Republic of the Congo. She is trained as an emergency physician and completed her residency at the Harvard-affiliated residency and fellowship in international emergency medicine at Brigham and Women's Hospital in Boston, Massachusetts. She has conducted research on pre-hospital first response and HIV-care access in Uganda, the use of emergency care services of the local internally displaced urban population and their access to emergency care in Colombia, and gender-based insecurity in urban slums in Bangladesh, Ethiopia, and Haiti.

Chih-Wei Chen, FRGS is a fellow of the Royal Geographical Society (RGS) with IBG in London, UK, as well as a member of the American Association of Geographers (AAG). Currently, Chih-Wei co-leads the research center along with the Faculty of Engineering Sciences at the University College London (UCL); since 2019, he has been a visiting scholar at the National Graduate Institute for Policy Studies (GRIPS) in Japan. Before joining UCL, Chih-Wei served as the research advisor to Taiwan Geographic Information Centre (TGIC). As a policy specialist, he was formally invited to be a member of the National Council for Sustainable Development (NCSD) of the Taiwan Government in 2018, followed by immediate appointment as the Political Advisor to the Premier. Chih-Wei has been serving as the secretary general for the Council of Asia Liberals and Democrats (CALD) since 2018. As scholar and policy professional, Chih-Wei is dedicated to science, technology, and innovation (STI) policy with the expectation to achieve Sustainable Development Goals (SDGs) for embracing a better future.

Shana De Caro, Esq. is a personal injury attorney and partner at the law firm of De Caro & Kaplen, LLP, in New York; secretary and member of the board of directors of the Brain Injury Association of America; and first vice president of the American Academy of Brain Injury Attorneys. She is past chair, past secretary, and past treasurer of the Traumatic Brain Injury Litigation Group of the American Association for Justice. Shana serves as an advisory board member of the Acquired Brain Injury Program, Graduate School of Education and Human Development, The George Washington University, Washington, D.C. Shana is a member of the board of directors, the Judicial Screening Committee, the Pattern Jury Instruction Committee, and Amicus Committee and Amicus Counsel of the New York State Academy of Trial Lawyers, and is editor of their *Monthly Law Update*. She is on the board of advisors of the Interstate Bus Litigation Group of the American Association for Justice. Shana is an elected fellow of the Melvin M. Belli Society and has been selected as a New York Super Lawyer.

Hebah ElGibreen, PhD is an assistant professor in the Department of Information Technology, College of Computer and Information Sciences, at King Saud University in Riyadh, Saudi Arabia. She is currently a research affiliate with the Department of Mechanical Engineering (MRL Lab) at the Massachusetts Institute of Technology (MIT) in Cambridge and is also the female branch director of the Center of Smart Robotics Research at her college. Dr. Hebah holds the position of deputy director for the Alumni Center at King Saud University and is also the delegated vice dean for the e-Transaction and Telecommunication Deanship. Dr. Hebah received her MSc and PhD degrees from King Saud University in 2009 and 2015, respectively. During her graduate studies, she developed a strong interest in artificial intelligence and machine learning. Through her master's studies, she developed an expert system that can detect errors in medical prescriptions using data mining techniques, and during her PhD studies, she developed a knowledge extraction system that can be used as the brain of a collaborative expert system.

Satoshi Ezoe, MD, MPH, MPA, PhD is Counsellor of the Permanent Mission of Japan to the United Nations covering health and development matters. He has facilitated the negotiations on the political declaration on tuberculosis for the UN General Assembly (UNGA) High-Level Meeting on Tuberculosis in 2018. He then initiated the Group of Friends of Universal Health Coverage (UHC) and Global Health towards the UNGA High-Level Meeting on UHC in 2019. Prior to his current position, he was a medical officer at the Ministry of Health, Labour and Welfare in Japan, responsible for a broad range of health policy including global health, pandemic influenza response, national health insurance reform, and noncommunicable diseases (NCDs) including cancer and mental health, as well as national delegation to WHO/UNAIDS/UNGA boards and assemblies. From 2009 to 2012, he was seconded to UNAIDS, Geneva. He is a Japanese national, a medical doctor, a PhD, and holder of public administration and public health degrees from Harvard University.

Radha Ramana Murthy Gokula, MD, CMD is board certified in both family medicine and geriatrics. He has been an invited speaker at several national and regional conferences and has written multiple publications about elderly patients. He started the geriatric medicine fellowship at the University of Toledo in Ohio. Dr. Gokula is a pioneer in the "Stay Home" model of care for the elderly in nursing homes, assisted living, and independent living facilities. STAYHOME IWILL Concierge Connected Care integrates medicine and technology to promote aging in place with a focus on improving function and quality of life. Dr. Gokula is a post-acute care consultant for local nursing homes and a QAPI consultant/telemedicine provider for the University of Pittsburgh Medical Center, Curavi Health, which offers telemedicine in nursing homes. He is also currently working as a hospitalist and post-acute medical director for clinically integrated network at Mercy Health in Ohio and helps reduce hospital readmissions from all clinical sites. Outside of the office, he enjoys spirituality, meditation, watching cricket matches, Indian karaoke, and, most importantly, spending time with family.

Amanuel Haile, MD, is chief executive director of the College of Health Sciences, Ayder Comprehensive Specialized Hospital, with the rank of vice president, and an assistant professor of internal medicine at Mekelle University in Ethiopia.

Diane E. Heck, PhD is an expert in pharmacology and toxicology and is professor and associate dean for research in the Division of Environmental Health Sciences, School of Health Sciences and Practice, at New York Medical College (NYMC) in Valhalla. At NYMC, Dr. Heck also served as chair of the Division of Environmental Health Sciences. As an educator, scientist, and administrator, she has devoted her career to higher education, rigorous scholarship, and excellence in teaching and scholarly research. Dr. Heck is an expert in intellectual property and technology transfer and is actively engaged in addressing issues in health disparities and community development. For more than two decades, her specific focus has been on research, education, training, and the pursuit of knowledge to foster excellence in healthcare delivery. Her research interests focus on understanding mechanisms underlying inflammation and chemical toxicity. Dr. Heck has authored more than 100 journal articles as well as numerous book chapters and review articles.

Yi-Hua Jan, PhD is an assistant professor in the Department of Environmental and Occupational Medicine at Rutgers University-Robert Wood Johnson Medical School in Piscataway, New Jersey. She received her doctorate in environmental sciences from Rutgers University in 2007. Her current research interests focus on cellular and biochemical mechanisms of chemical toxicity and developing countermeasures against organophosphate intoxication and sulfur mustard exposure.

Mariam Jashi, MD, MPH, MPA is chair of the Education, Science and Culture Committee and member of the Health and Social Affairs Committee of the Parliament of Georgia in Tbilisi since 2016. Dr. Jashi is President of the Leading Group on Innovative Financing hosted by the French Ministry of Europe and Foreign Affairs (2017–2018); co-founder and CEO of the Prime Minister's Initiative – Solidarity Fund of Georgia (2014–2016), the largest integrated national platform for public-private partnerships and innovative financing; and Deputy Minister of Labour, Health, and Social Affairs of Georgia (2012–2014) in charge of the public health portfolio, including universal health coverage, hepatitis C, primary healthcare, and penitentiary health. For 11 years (1999–2010), Dr. Jashi served at the United Nations in charge of UNICEF Health Sector and UNAIDS programs in Georgia, UNICEF Immunization Portfolio in the Occupied Palestinian Territory, and HIV Partnerships at UNICEF New York Headquarters. Dr. Jashi is a member of the Independent Review Committee of the Gavi Alliance and consultant to UN agencies, the Global Fund, the World Bank, and other development partners (2011–2016). Dr. Jashi is an author/co-author of national strategic plans and country applications to the Global Fund, USAID, Unitaid, Gavi, The Global Alliance for Improved Nutrition (GAIN), and Japan Government that mobilized over US$105 million in grants for 19 countries of sub-Saharan Africa, Asia, CEE/CIS, and Middle East. Dr. Jashi is an Edward S. Mason Fellow from the Harvard Kennedy School of Government, holds an MPA degree from Harvard University, an MD from AIETI Medical University, an MPH from Tbilisi State University, and postgraduate diplomas from Lund University and University College London. Dr. Jashi is the recipient of awards from WHO EURO and National Alliance for Improved Nutrition, Parliament of Georgia. Dr. Jashi is author/co-author of publications in the 2010 UN MDG Good Practices, 2011 Harvard Kennedy School Review, and Oxford University Press.

Laurie B. Joseph, PhD is an adjunct professor in the Division of Environmental Health Sciences, School of Health Sciences and Practice, at New York Medical College in Valhalla. She has over 35 years of experience in toxicology, having developed clinical and in vitro human models plus in vivo animal models to understand the fundamentals of cellular damage and their response to environmental toxins. She received a BS in geology from The George Washington University in Washington, D.C., and an MS and PhD from Ohio State University, with postdoctoral training at Yale University and the University of Connecticut Medical Center. Her present studies include skin and vascular tissue wound repair with over 20 years of experience in the personal care industry. She is a member of the Personal Care Products Council, Society of Cosmetic Chemists, Society of Toxicology, and American Academy of Dermatology. Prior to coming to the Ernest Mario School of Pharmacy at Rutgers University in Piscataway, New Jersey, as associate research professor, she was the senior skin biologist for Croda Inc.

Hong-Duck Kim, PhD received his doctorate in 1996 from the Department of Pharmaceutical Sciences at the University of Tokyo in Japan. He completed his postdoctoral fellowship training at both academic institutions as well as biotechnology and pharmaceutical companies in Japan, South Korea, and the United States. He has experience in the fields of molecular pharmacology, neurobiology, cancer pharmacology such as multidrug resistance in solid cancers, vaccine development for Alzheimer's Disease and infectious disease, and innate immunity in Alzheimer's Disease. Currently, he is associate professor in the Division of Environmental Health Sciences, School of Health Sciences and Practice, at New York Medical College in Valhalla. Since 2008, Dr. Kim participates as a researcher at the Rutgers University CounterACT Research Center of Excellence in New Jersey.

Sean M. Kivlehan, MD, MPH is the director of the International Emergency Medicine Fellowship at Brigham and Women's Hospital in Boston, Massachusetts, where he is also a practicing emergency physician. He is an instructor of emergency medicine at Harvard Medical School and affiliate faculty at the Harvard Humanitarian Initiative in Cambridge, Massachusetts. He has served as a consultant for the World Health Organization's Emergency, Trauma, and Acute Care Programme, is the Harvard representative to the Global Health Cluster, chair of the International Emergency Medicine Fellowship Consortium, assistant managing editor of the Global Emergency Medicine Literature Review, and editorial board member at EMS World. Prior to medical school, he spent 10 years as a paramedic in New York City, and his current work focuses on strengthening emergency care in low-resource settings with a particular focus on pre-hospital care. He completed his fellowship in international emergency medicine at Brigham and Women's Hospital, residency at the University of California San Francisco, and medical and graduate school at New York Medical College in Valhalla.

Melissa Jane Kronfeld, MS, PhD is founder of Passion for a Purpose, which is a social impact consultancy. She completed her doctorate at Rutgers University's Division of Global Affairs. She received a BA in international relations from The George Washington University in Washington, D.C., an MS in global affairs from New York University, and an MS in global affairs from Rutgers University in New Jersey. Melissa has lectured on American foreign policy and national security at Rutgers University, Syracuse University, and New York University. In 2012, Melissa was awarded first place in the Richard A. Clarke National Security Essay Competition, and in 2014, she received the Rutgers University Walter F. Weiker Scholarship, celebrating students who possess academic excellence and a commitment to exceptional contributions to society. Her research has been featured in published works from Princeton University Press, Oxford University Press, Taylor & Francis Group, Hachette Book Group, Fairleigh Dickinson University Press, B&H Publishing, and Springer. Currently she is based in Israel.

Timothy Leddy, MBA has served as president and CEO of the Westchester Visiting Nurse Services (WVNS) Group in White Plains, New York, since November 2015, and in his prior roles as the agency's interim president and chief financial officer. Tim has had great success in improving the long-term financial viability of the agency, while simultaneously enhancing its reputation for high-quality, patient-centered care. Through his leadership at WVNS Group, and his three decades serving in prominent positions in home care, Tim has garnered a wealth of industry expertise that has enabled him to successfully bridge the needs between operations and finance, offering innovative solutions to effectively manage both areas. Among his accomplishments at WVNS, Tim has negotiated key managed care contracts, increased the quality outcomes for the agency, and has implemented new and creative programs that enhance the services provided to the communities the agency serves. He has installed new quality control initiatives that have helped the agency increase their CMS star ratings and to maintain one of the lowest re-hospitalization rates in the Lower Hudson Valley. Tim received a BBA and MBA with a focus in financial management from Iona College and received a Master of Science in Health Policy Management from New York University. He currently serves on the board of the Home Care Association of New York State and is also on the board of the Westchester Public/Private Partnership.

Roya Mahboob, MBA founder of Digital Citizen Fund in New York City, is a businesswoman and entrepreneur from Afghanistan. She also founded and serves as CEO of the Afghan Citadel Software Company, a full-service software development company based in Herat, Afghanistan. She has received attention for being among the first IT female CEOs in Afghanistan, where it is still relatively rare for women to work outside the home. Roya Mahboob was named as one of TIME magazine's 100 Most Influential People in the World for 2013 for her work in building Internet classrooms in high schools in Afghanistan and for Women's Annex, a multilingual blog and video site hosted by Film Annex. This was the 10th anniversary of the TIME special edition. Women's Annex gives the women of Afghanistan and Central Asia a platform to tell their stories to the world. US Secretary of State John Kerry met with Roya Mahboob and other Afghan women entrepreneurs at the International Center for Afghan Women's Economic Development at the American University of Afghanistan. She is also known for her work with online film distribution platform and web television network Film Annex on the Afghan Development Project. She is currently an advisor at the Forbes School of Business & Technology at Ashford University in California.

Prasad Mavuduri, MSc, MBA is a technology professional with approximately 30 years of experience in process control, systems engineering, product development, business transformations, and business systems (IT infrastructure, ERPs, CRMs, Web applications, reporting, etc.), with a particular focus on Digital Transformations with big data engineering, data science, Internet of Things (IoT), and analytics for the last 6 years. Prasad is the chairman of the board of directors of the nonprofit American Institute of Big Data Professionals (AIBDP) advocating for "applied technologists" vs. pure technologists. Prasad is an alumni leader for Kellogg School of Management at Northwestern University and advisory board member for the Rutgers University Data Science program in San Francisco. Having lived and worked in nine different countries, Prasad has global experience and has managed global teams. Currently Prasad is CEO of Data Magnum, a company involved in software services, and is also involved in a few startups.

Freweini Mebrahtu, BSc was born and raised in a small town in rural Ethiopia. She is the seventh child and youngest daughter of a family of eight. As an adolescent, Freweini will never forget the experience of having her first period. She was shocked and confused; her mother and her four sisters had not told her anything about periods. They would use pieces of old clothing as pads and make sure to bring large scarves to cover themselves if they stained their clothes by accident. Then Freweini got an opportunity to go to the United States to study chemical engineering at Prairie View A&M University in Texas, earning her degree in 1992. She remembered her first visit to the drug store with its overwhelming choice of sanitary pads. From that moment on, month after month, she wondered about the girls back home. Were things changing for them, too? She started by questioning the women in the village about their experience with periods. The stories she heard were shocking – digging a hole and squatting over it for 3–5 days or wrapping themselves with strips of cloth. She also noticed that they were uncomfortable talking about periods – this is still a taboo subject. Freweini needed to figure out a solution. She wanted to develop a product that was affordable, reliable, and environmentally friendly. In 2005, Freweini developed a reusable sanitary pad and piloted the product in Kelkel Debri on the edge of Mekelle with a lot of success. As a result of her work, she founded Mariam Seba Sanitary Products Factory and was named the 2019 CNN Hero of the Year.

Padmini (Mini) Murthy, MD, MPH, MS, FAMWA, FRSPH is professor and global health director at New York Medical College, School of Health Sciences and Practice, in Valhalla. Dr. Murthy is a physician (a trained obstetrician and gynecologist) and an activist. She has practiced medicine and public health for the past 30 years in various countries, has been working in various arenas of the healthcare industry, and worked as a consultant for the United Nations Population Fund (UNFPA). She has an MPH and an MS in management from New York University.

Dr. Murthy serves as the Medical Women's International Association NGO representative to the United Nations, vice president of the Global NGO Executive Committee, and also has been elected as secretary general of the Medical Women's International Association (which has women physician members from 80 countries). She is the first Indian-born American in 100 years to be elected to this role. She has worked on various women's health projects with UN diplomats, government officials, and first ladies in several countries. She also serves as Global Health Lead of the American Medical Women's Association.

Dr. Murthy has made over 150 presentations nationally and internationally on various health-related topics. She has scripted and co-hosted a successful radio talk show on women's health issues. Her areas of expertise include women's health, human rights, global health diplomacy, and designing online education. Dr. Murthy is widely published; she is the author and editor of *Women's Global Health and Human Rights* (Jones & Bartlett), which is used as a textbook worldwide. She serves as a peer reviewer for several publications. Dr. Murthy is the recipient of several awards nationally and internationally; some of the noteworthy awards include the Elizabeth Blackwell Medal (the first Indian-born American physician to receive this award in 70 years), the Sojourner Truth Pin, the Marie Catchatoor Memorial Award, the Jhirad Oration Award, the Mid-Career Award in International Health from the American Public Health Association (APHA), and the Distinguished Leadership and Achievement Award from the National Council of Women of the United States. Dr. Murthy is an elected fellow of the New York Academy of Medicine.

Mahtab Naji, MD graduated from the University of Debrecen Medical School in Hungary in 2016. She is an American-certified doctor who has worked in emergency medicine, internal medicine, and neurology departments in New York, California, and Arizona, with an interest in continuing her medical training in internal medicine. In 2018, she joined the Institute for International Health and Education (IIHE) in Albany, New York, as a researcher. Mahtab considers herself as a peace-loving world citizen and is passionate about helping others. She is a children's class animator and volunteers to serve homeless people in California. Aside from medicine, her favorite activities are running, photography, cooking, and baking for family and friends.

Aishwarya Narasimhadevara, MA, PhD(c) is involved in youth advocacy-related projects and interested in the importance of education in the field of international development. She has been involved with various non-governmental organizations working in the fields of education, the environment, and culture. She has a master's degree in international development from the University of Kent-Brussels School of International Studies in Belgium and is currently enrolled in a PhD program in international development at Chulalongkorn University in Bangkok, Thailand. Aishwarya served as co-chair of the Youth Sub-committee of the UN Department of Global Communications (DGC) NGO Conference in Salt Lake City, Utah in 2019. She has moderated and presented at conferences at the United Nations, nationally, and internationally. She is the recipient of the Exceptional Women of Excellence Award at the Women Economic Forum. Travelling is a passion of hers and she enjoys seeing new places. She also enjoys learning, taking photos, and practicing karate.

Erica L. Nelson, MD, PhM is an emergency medicine physician who conducts research on critical geography and the use of geospatial analysis for public health and humanitarian response. She completed her PhM in international peace studies and development at Trinity College Dublin in Ireland; her MAS in geospatial analysis for public health at Johns Hopkins University in Baltimore, Maryland; her MD at the University of Washington School of Medicine; and residency training at the Harvard-affiliated Emergency Medicine Residency Program in Boston, Massachusetts. She has worked as a researcher and policy consultant on the contextualization of medicine in conflict-affected populations including Nepal, Indonesia, the Balkans, Jamaica, Ethiopia, and Sudan, as well as on geospatial analyses of early warning indicators in Kenyan urban slum populations and the Palestinian/ Israeli Health Referral Program. Currently, she is a physician at South Shore Hospital in South Weymouth, Massachusetts; an instructor within the Division of International Emergency Medicine and Humanitarian Programs at Brigham and Women's Hospital of Harvard Medical School; and the co-founder of the Harvard Humanitarian Geospatial Analysis Program at the Harvard Humanitarian Initiative in Cambridge, Massachusetts.

Jonathan Ogulnick, BA, MusB is a member of New York Medical College (NYMC) School of Medicine Class of 2022. Originally from Newburgh, New York, he comes to medicine from a background of diverse interests, including his double majors of piano and chemistry from SUNY at Purchase College. Since starting at NYMC, he has been involved in numerous groups and activities, such as clinical research with the Department of Neurosurgery and participation in the Medical Education Concentration, which he is pursuing out of dedication to passing on medical knowledge to both patients and future generations of physicians. In his free time, Jonathan enjoys playing the piano, reading and writing fiction, and hiking.

Prathip Phantumvanit, DDS, MSc is currently dean, Faculty of Dentistry, at Thammasat University in Bangkok, Thailand. He has served on the WHO Expert Advisory Panel on Oral Health since 1988 and is past vice chair of the Public Health Committee of the FDI World Dental Federation. He is former dean of the Faculty of Dentistry at Khon Kaen University and founder-dean at Thammasat University Dental School in Thailand. Dr. Prathip Phantumvanit was the recipient of the Special Merit Award for Outstanding Achievement in Community Dentistry – International – from the American Association of Public Health Dentistry in 2005 and the Distinguished Service Award from the International Association for Dental Research in 2012. He was the inventor of the household water defluoridation device and co-developer of the Atraumatic Restorative Treatment (ART) for caries control. His research interests include the role of fluoride for caries prevention as well as appropriate restorative and preventive care for dental caries in the primary dentition.

Aaron Pied, MPM has more than 18 years of experience in education and global health, providing administrative and operational support to schools, community-based organizations, and international development organizations. Aaron began his career as a secondary education teacher and has taught in schools and conducted various trainings while living in the United States, Burkina Faso, and Thailand. Aaron currently works at Abt Associates in Boston, Massachusetts, on the PMI VectorLink Project as the lead project operations analyst supporting Burkina Faso, Cote d'Ivoire, Cameroon, Mali, Rwanda, and Zambia. He previously worked as a program analyst supporting USAID's Rapid Staff Support Services (RS3), providing budgetary and administrative support to US Personal Services Contractors and USAID staff, and as the director of operations for Realizing Global Health (RGH), where he managed the finance, communications, human resource, and marketing activities for RGH while providing support to select projects. Aaron currently holds a Master of Public Management (MPM) from the University of Maryland.

Renuka Rambhatla (née Pantulu), MPH, is a senior management professional who has worked across the health and community services sector for over 13 years. Her work has focused primarily on enabling employment and social engagement for people with disabilities and is guided by the professional qualifications obtained: Bachelor's in Health Science from the University of Western Australia (2011), complemented by a Master's in Public Health from the University of Sydney (2017). She is interested in solving public health issues through education and technology. This philosophy has led her to undertake volunteer roles at the Australian Red Cross, the Rotaract Club of Perth, and the Rotary Club of Perth. These activities have had a strong focus on international humanitarian support, public health, and the pursuit of the United Nations Sustainable Development Goals (SDGs).

Anindo Roy, PhD is an associate professor of neurology at the University of Maryland School of Medicine in Baltimore; adjunct associate professor of mechanical engineering at the A. James Clark School of Engineering, University of Maryland; and faculty at the Maryland Robotics Center, Institute for Systems Research, University of Maryland, College Park. In addition, he serves as the chief technology officer (CTO) for Next Step Robotics, Inc., an emergent company that manufactures low-cost portable ankle exoskeleton technology to rehabilitate walking function in persons with neurologic injuries such as stroke. Prior to his current positions, Dr. Roy held prestigious postdoctoral fellowships at Georgia Institute of Technology and the Massachusetts Institute of Technology (MIT). Dr. Roy conducts research in rehabilitation robotics, specifically in the development and clinical testing of ankle robotic technology for rehabilitation of gait and mobility function in neurologically disabled populations.

Gopal Sankaran, MD, DrPH, MNAMS, CHES is a tenured professor of public health at West Chester University (WCU) of Pennsylvania, which he joined in spring 1989. Dr. Sankaran's education, training, and experience span medicine, public health, and health promotion. He has consulted with the World Health Organization (WHO) on the National Smallpox Eradication Programme in India and the Global Programme on AIDS in Switzerland. He has worked with Plan International/Childreach on international HIV/AIDS prevention and control, child survival, and reproductive health projects in program design, implementation, and evaluation. He has trained family practice residents from Pennsylvania and Delaware in epidemiology and community-oriented primary care. He serves as guest faculty in epidemiology for graduate physician assistant students and previously for medical students at the Philadelphia College of Osteopathic Medicine (PCOM).

Denise Scotto, Esq. an international policy advisor, has represented law firms, governments, businesses, nonprofits, NGOs, and individual clients during her distinguished career. She is admitted to practice law in the courts of the State of New

York and the District of Columbia and advises clients on a wide range of matters, from legal analysis to advocacy strategy, policy development, conflict resolution, the United Nations System, and cross-cultural cooperation. Ms. Scotto is known for her thought leadership in communicating complex concepts easily through her dynamic presentations. As a trial specialist handling cases related to civil rights, labor and employment law, and negligence, Ms. Scotto started her career as an attorney in the Office of the Corporation Counsel of the City of New York. She represented the City of New York, its various agencies including the Board of Education, the Health and Hospitals Corporation, as well as City employees at all phases of trial and at the appellate level.

Anne Sebert Kuhlmann, PhD, MPH joined the College for Public Health and Social Justice at Saint Louis University (SLU) in Missouri in 2015 as an assistant professor of behavioral science and health education. She has an array of international experience in public health intervention development and program evaluation, and a well-established record of peer-reviewed publication in maternal and reproductive health. She currently collaborates on maternal health research with indigenous populations in the Andean Highlands of Ecuador and on the evaluation of community mobilization interventions to improve maternal health outcomes in Malawi. Locally, Dr. Sebert Kuhlmann works with St. Louis-based organizations involved in global health work, including Dignity Period and Microfinancing Partners in Africa. In addition, she supports SLU's partnership with the National Autonomous University of Honduras. Currently, she teaches Introduction to Global Health and Global Health Assessment and Evaluation, two required courses for the MPH concentration in global health.

Uma Srinivasan, PhD is a Senior Research Scientist at the Digital Health Cooperative Research Centre in Sydney, Australia; mentors PhD students in health informatics; and provides advice to research and product development for the health sector. Dr. Srinivasan was one of the early researchers who helped shape Health Insurance Analytics suite of solutions that went on to win the Excellence in Innovation award for a spin-off company, which now employs over 60 people in Australia. Dr. Srinivasan's vast experience in the health sector coupled with her research interests in data integration, analytics, and network theory has led to several international publications and a patent for Capital Markets Cooperative Research Centre (CMCRC). Her recent *Flying Blind* series of publications describing the Australian health sector are cited extensively and used all over Australia. Uma holds a PhD in computer science and formerly served as principal research scientist at Commonwealth Scientific and Industrial Research Organisation (CSIRO). Currently, she serves as an adjunct professor in the School of Business at Western Sydney University in Australia.

Tamar Tchelidze, MD, MPH is senior policy fellow at the Forum for Collaborative Research at UC Berkeley School of Public Health in California. She has over 22 years of progressive professional experience in public health, in-depth understanding of the opportunities and challenges of Global Health related to the 2030 Sustainable Development Goals (SDGs), hands-on experience in public-private partnerships and innovations for health, and senior-level policy advice at country and international levels. Dr. Tchelidze was one of the co-leads with Thailand on the historic process of the Universal Health Coverage (UHC) Political Declaration at the United Nations. Entrusted by the President of the UN General Assembly, Dr. Tchelidze leads drafting and negotiation rounds of the UHC Declaration among 150 UN member states, public and private sector partners, civil society, and academia. The UHC Political Declaration was launched at the UN General Assembly High-Level Meeting in September 2019. Prior to this appointment, Dr. Tchelidze was appointed as a counselor at the Embassy of Georgia to the United States in Washington, D.C. Dr. Tchelidze has established an esteemed reputation for her ability to galvanize international partners to plan and implement public health initiatives in Georgia. The projects that she designed and implemented have been recognized as models of efficient and effective healthcare and have made original contributions of major significance to the international healthcare community. Dr. Tchelidze's career goal is to play a principal role in policy, regulatory, and capacity-building interventions for ensuring equitable access to high-quality care both in public health and clinical interventions. Dr. Tchelidze is currently pursuing a Doctor of Public Health degree at Johns Hopkins Bloomberg School of Public Health in Baltimore, Maryland.

Gabriella Composto Wahler, PhD earned a doctoral degree in toxicology, specializing in dermal toxicology, from the Ernest Mario School of Pharmacy at Rutgers University in Piscataway, New Jersey. She received her BS in biology at Rider University in Lawrenceville, New Jersey, where she studied the tumor microenvironment. During her graduate training, she worked on in vitro and in vivo modeling to determine the degree of skin damage and wound repair for the development of countermeasures to mitigate chemical-induced injuries. She is a member of the Society of Toxicology (SOT) and American College of Toxicology. Gabriella has won many awards for her research including the SOT Dermal Toxicology Specialty Section's Paper of the Year Award (2017), the Charles River Student Travel Award (2017), and the Battelle Student Research Award (2018). She also received first place for the Student Travel Award in 2018 from the Comparative Toxicology, Pathology, and Veterinary Specialty Section of SOT. Gabriella also had the opportunity to study at Columbia University after receiving the Supplemental Training for Education Program (STEP) Award from SOT in 2018. In 2019, she was also awarded an educational grant for Countermeasures Against Chemical Threats by the New York Society of Cosmetic Chemists.

L. Lewis Wall, MD, DPhil, MBioeth professor of obstetrics and gynecology at Washington University in St. Louis, Missouri, is being honored for his work as a tireless advocate for African women with vesicovaginal fistulas, a devastating childbirth injury caused by obstructed labor in parts of the world where cesarean section is not available. In many poor countries, labor may last for days without relief, in the process destroying the tissues that separate the bladder from the vagina. Women who suffer this injury become totally incontinent and end up as outcasts. Estimates suggest that nearly 4 million African women currently have a vesicovaginal fistula. In 1995, Wall founded the Worldwide Fistula Fund, a charity that provides clinical care for fistula patients and supports public advocacy, surgical training, and medical research on the fistula problem. Wall has traveled extensively to perform fistula surgery, give lectures, conduct research, organize international meetings, and advocate on behalf of these women.

Joyce Tsung-Hsi Wang, MD, MPH, PhD holds a medical degree from National Yang-Ming University School of Medicine in Taipei, Taiwan, a master's degree in healthcare organization and administration, an EMBA (Executive Master of Business Administration), and a PhD degree in occupational medicine and industrial hygiene from National Taiwan University. She is also a gynecologist and specialized in healthcare administration and management, healthcare industry development, crisis communication and response, healthcare quality and patient safety, and occupational medicine. Dr. Wang currently is the director of the Hsinchu City Public Health Bureau in Taiwan, R.O.C. She was formerly senior advisor/director of the Health Division, Taipei Economic and Cultural Representative Office (TECRO) in the United States. She has worked extensively on policy planning, coordination, promotion of bilateral (America) health, and welfare cooperation. As the first female secretary general of the Ministry of Health and Welfare from 2016 to 2018, she supervised and oversaw important documents and policies in the ministry.

Irene M. Wohlman, PhD earned her doctorate in toxicology from Rutgers University in Piscataway, New Jersey. While working as a financial/marketing assistant with Velankani Communications Technologies, Inc. during her graduate school years, she developed an interest in the public health aspect of telecommunications and connecting the world to improve health outcomes. In keeping with her interest in using technology in a public health forum, she currently teaches toxicology-based online public health courses for New York Medical College.

About the Editors

Padmini Murthy, MD, MPH, MS, FAMWA, FRSPH, is professor and global health director at New York Medical College, School of Health Sciences and Practice, in Valhalla, New York, USA. Dr. Murthy is Medical Women's International Associations Secretary - General and NGO representative to the United Nations. She is also Global Health lead of American Medical Women's Association and a Fellow of the New York Academy of Medicine.

Amy Ansehl, DNP, RN, MSN, FNP-BC, is associate dean for Student Experience at New York Medical College, School of Health Sciences and Practice, in Valhalla, New York, USA. She is a Fellow of the New York Academy of Medicine and Chairperson of the Visiting Nurse Service Westchester Foundation.

Part I
Reflections

Space and Global Health

Camille Wardrop Alleyne

Introduction

In the twenty-first century, when vulnerable populations around the world are faced with the most challenging issues surrounding diseases, epidemics, and high mortality rates in children and mothers, there is an increasing awareness of the role that technology plays in the advancement of public and global health. Beyond this, space-based technology and the environment of space itself are advancing our knowledge in the public health sphere, bringing the notion of a relatively new use for space to the conversation. There is a push to use and apply these technologies as innovative solutions for promoting socioeconomic and sustainable development in developing countries and the United Nations system as a whole. Throughout this introduction, we go beyond traditional terrestrial methods and focus on the use of satellites and other spacecraft, such as the International Space Station, as "out-of-this-world" platforms for advancing our scientific knowledge in health while also producing benefits from space research that improves the quality of lives here on Earth.

Uniqueness of the Space Environment

The International Space Station is the largest and most complex human-tended space vehicle ever built. Since 1999, when the first few elements of the ISS were launched, scientists and researchers from around the world have had access to this world-class space facility. It has served as a platform for cutting-edge research in a

C. W. Alleyne (✉)
Brightest Stars Foundation, Houston, TX, USA
e-mail: cwalleyne@yahoo.com

© Springer Nature Switzerland AG 2020
P. Murthy, A. Ansehl (eds.), *Technology and Global Public Health*,
https://doi.org/10.1007/978-3-030-46355-7_1

variety of scientific disciplines, including but not limited to biological and human health research. The environment of space, or more specifically the environment of microgravity that space provides, affords many benefits to research in the life sciences. We often don't realize how gravitational forces mask everything we know about how things behave here on Earth. Every biological, chemical, and physical process is impacted by the forces of gravity. However, in a micro- or almost zero-gravity environment, such as that on the International Space Station or Low Earth Orbit small satellite platforms, the influence of this force diminishes greatly. Various terrestrial physical phenomena that are driven by gravitational forces are no longer factors. One example of this is buoyancy-driven convection, a gravity-dependent phenomenon that affects both liquids and gases. This phenomenon allows hot air balloons to rise and soar into Earth's atmosphere. But this is not possible in space. Another gravity-driven phenomenon is the process of sedimentation, the act of heavier particles in suspension falling and settling at the bottom of a container. This process is not present in a microgravity environment. Finally, fluids in space have low-shear fluid dynamic forces and move very differently than they do when they are under a gravitational influence. With this knowledge, you may ask how this is important to human health systems. We can easily answer this question because when flown in the space environment, biological systems behave differently than they do on Earth, which gives us the potential to uncover alternative mechanisms that can be the basis for treatments and cures.

Types of Research Conducted

The absence of gravitational forces in space has led to discoveries and breakthroughs in the life sciences fields of cellular biology, macromolecular protein crystallography, and nanofluidics, for example. Organisms from bacteria to viruses, in addition to human physiology, are often altered in this unique environment. The human body undergoes space adaptation effects that lead to health conditions such as bone density loss, muscle atrophy, immune system dysfunction, and cardiovascular deconditioning. These effects often mimic the aging process of human beings and model conditions such as osteoporosis and other degenerative and chronic diseases found here on Earth. Some of the countermeasures developed to keep astronauts safe and healthy during extended space missions, such as those used to minimize the loss of bone density, have been adapted as protocols for elderly patients here on Earth.

As mentioned earlier, the microgravity environment has yielded results in medical technology in the area of protein crystallography. Protein crystals – the fundamental building blocks of life – grown in space have been found to be bigger, more highly ordered, and of higher quality than terrestrial-grown crystals. Once returned to Earth, the crystals, which are mostly imaged using x-ray diffraction, often reveal previously unknown three-dimensional structural details of how the proteins function. An example of a protein that was successfully crystallized in space is hematopoietic prostaglandin D synthase (H-PGDS), which is expressed in the muscular fibers of patients with Duchenne's Muscular Dystrophy (DMD) – a muscular degenerative disease that debilitates one in three thousand boys by the age of 9 years old, often leaving them unable to walk. The space-grown protein-inhibitor complex led to the design of a more effective drug treatment to combat this disease. Over the last couple of decades, hundreds of proteins have been crystallized in space. Not all yield the type of results shown in the fight against DMD, but every success gained by this area of research represents a step toward improving health outcomes here on Earth.

In the field of cell biology, the fluid dynamic effects in this unique environment lead to the three-dimensional aggregation of cells that alter the cell division process, gene expression, and cell shape. The cell behavior in space mimics that of the human body in a 1-g environment. As a result, numerous studies have been conducted examining the effects of microgravity on the regenerative process of stem cells in living organisms, the function of T-cells that affect the human immune system, and the growth of tumor cells, for example. These investigations not only advance our scientific knowledge of diseases but also provide a better understanding of the mechanisms that control cellular functions that can lead to new drug therapies.

The Value of Space-Based Technology

It is, however, not just the research that is conducted in space that holds potential benefits for human health, but also the technologies developed and used for space exploration that have been adapted for terrestrial applications. For example, the ISS is home to a crew of astronauts who live and work 400 km (250 miles) above the Earth's surface for 6-month durations. Because of the remoteness of the ISS there was a need for rapid and accurate diagnosis of crewmembers for routine medical operations and in the event of an emergency. This need led to the adaptation of ultrasound technology for space use in addition to the development of innovative imaging techniques that equipped astronauts with skills to perform self-imaging with support from teams on the ground. As a result of the effectiveness of the innovative solutions for addressing remote medical care, space ultrasound diagnostic technology and telemedicine techniques were adapted to monitor vulnerable populations with little or no access to medical services, providing remote care to thousands of people worldwide.

Additionally, besides human-tended platforms such as the ISS, free-flying space technologies are becoming increasingly valuable in Earth applications and in supporting global health and development. Satellites that have remote sensing capabilities can be used to track disease epidemics on Earth. Remote sensing is a process of obtaining information on the physical properties of an area from a distance. Satellites outfitted with imagers or cameras can detect and monitor trends across geographical distances. Geospatial data obtained from such platforms are analyzed by researchers and used to identify trends and patterns during disease outbreaks. They can also be used to study the effects and impact of the environment to the extent that it contributes to the spread of diseases, as well as assess risks to vulnerable populations.

The outcome of such analysis provides decision makers with tools and information to develop countermeasures to combat epidemiological challenges. This is a growing area called tele-epidemiology.

Finally, in the almost 25 years working in the space industry, I have had the opportunity to oversee and be a part of numerous groundbreaking projects. Of these projects, the space technology development that has occurred in human space flight and microgravity research on the ISS has been among the most rewarding to watch due to its countless advancements and the speed at which these advancements are being made. Many may ask why space research is important. My answer is not just that it is fascinating, cutting-edge, and truly out of this world, but it is about the innovative technological developments and applications that arise as a result, that continue to help us solve some of the most challenging issues we face on Earth. The research we conduct in space is most widely known to be in the business of exploration, but with these breakthroughs and advances in human health, as mentioned throughout this chapter, it is clear that space research is also in the business of changing lives and improving human health. The intersection between space and health is not only about the health effects of our astronauts and countermeasures that keep them safe for long-duration spaceflight, but it is also about improving the health of the general public down here on Earth.

Universal Health Coverage in Japan: Leveraging Technologies to Ensure Equitable, Affordable, and Quality Health Care for All

Satoshi Ezoe

Introduction

There is a growing global momentum towards achieving universal health coverage (UHC), defined by the World Health Organization (WHO) as the ability of "all people and communities [to] use the promotive, preventive, curative, rehabilitative and palliative health services they need, of sufficient quality to be effective, while also ensuring that the use of these services does not expose the user to financial hardship" [1]. The goal of achieving UHC was adopted by the world's leaders at the United Nations (UN) General Assembly in 2015 under the framework of the Sustainable Development Goals (SDGs), which all countries of the world committed to achieving by the year 2030 [2].

Japan has been a vocal advocate in advancing the UHC agenda through various global forums, including the Group of Seven (G7), the Group of Twenty (G20), and UN [3–5], based on its experience of achieving and managing its own UHC system since 1961, as laid out in an article by Prime Minister Shinzo Abe, "Japan's Vision for a Peaceful and Healthier World" [6]. This chapter's aim is to provide a brief overview of Japan's UHC system, followed by its global contributions to achieving UHC by 2030.

Japan and UHC

Japan has been able to sustain its UHC system for more than half a century since launching universal coverage in 1961. The main characteristics of Japan's UHC system include (1) compulsory enrollment of all citizens in a national social

S. Ezoe (✉)
Counsellor, Permanent Mission of Japan to the United Nations, New York, NY, USA
e-mail: toshiezoe@gmail.com

© Springer Nature Switzerland AG 2020
P. Murthy, A. Ansehl (eds.), *Technology and Global Public Health*,
https://doi.org/10.1007/978-3-030-46355-7_2

insurance scheme that includes multiple insurers supplemented by public revenues, (2) open access to any generalist or specialist healthcare provider, which are mostly private not-for-profit entities, (3) generous financial risk protection including catastrophic health spending coverage, and (4) a nationwide comprehensive benefit package to manage new technologies and control overall health expenditures (see details from "Japan health system review." [7]). Under this scheme, Japan continuously adapts and upgrades its healthcare system by introducing new technologies, including medicines, vaccines, medical devices, diagnostics, and genomic medicines.

This UHC system, coupled with a series of public health interventions, including vaccination and immunization, safe water and sanitation, improved nutrition, and school health programs, has enabled Japan to become one of the world's healthiest nations, with leading health metrics including the world's lowest infant mortality rate and longest life expectancy [8]. Furthermore, Japan's UHC system ensures affordable access to quality basic healthcare without financial hardship and minimizes catastrophic out-of-pocket health spending, saving many Japanese people from impoverishment due to health conditions, even as health expenditures remain a major cause of impoverishment and bankruptcy in other parts of the world, including in the United States [9, 10].

It is important to note that the people and leaders of Japan made the political choice to introduce UHC at a time when Japan was still recovering from the devastation of World War II. In addition to fostering a healthier population, it was UHC that underpinned Japan's later rapid economic development, not the other way around.

However, achieving UHC is not the end of the story. A country also needs to ensure its health system's long-term sustainability in the context of the changing demographics and needs of its population while managing overall cost. This is particularly relevant for Japan, which is experiencing rising healthcare costs and the most aged population in the world. A sustainable healthcare system with the highest attainable outcomes must utilize limited resources as effectively and efficiently as possible and maximize patient value. To this end, Japan is further capitalizing on innovation for sustainable UHC including in the following areas.

UHC and Technology

One way to accomplish this is to promote data-driven healthcare. Japan is developing a first-of-its-kind large-scale national health data platform, which integrates health check-ups, medical care, and long-term care data, comprising over 10 billion health claims, to maximize value for patients. This platform will facilitate the creation of new medicines and innovative healthcare technologies by leveraging optimal clinical data linked with outcomes. This will also empower people to fully utilize their own health data to make better informed health decisions while minimizing unnecessary tests and procedures. Furthermore, health insurance payers are encouraged to play a key role in urging healthcare providers to improve the quality and efficiency of medical interventions and in motivating the insured to engage in disease prevention efforts [11].

Another way is to incorporate genomic medicine further into clinical practice to provide personalized medicine to meet individual patients' needs. For example, genomic medicine is one of the keys to tackling the burden of cancer. This is in line with Japan's national plan to end cancer and the establishment of a nationwide consortium for joint clinical data collection to facilitate genomic treatment by maximizing effectiveness while minimizing adverse effects. Big data analysis will also contribute to the development of new drugs and treatment [11].

Another promising area is the application of artificial intelligence (AI) analytics to big data, including biometric, medical, and insurance data, thereby promoting real-time diagnosis and optimized treatment. We are also looking into addressing access issues by utilizing information and communications technology (ICT) and drone technologies for remote consultation, diagnosis, and delivery. This is in line with the concept of "Society 5.0 for the SDGs" that Japan is promoting. "Society 5.0" refers to a guideline for facilitating science, technology, and innovation as a mechanism to fuse cyberspace and physical space in order to bring about a human-centered society that balances economic advancement with the resolution of social problems [12].

Role of Japan on Global Stage

Based on Japan's ongoing journey to pursue sustainable UHC, the core message is that UHC is not a luxury; it is a necessity. It is not just the right choice but a smart choice for countries to develop and prosper. At the same time, UHC is a continuous journey that must always adapt to changing needs and demographics. Every country will face population aging sooner or later; therefore, countries may wish to prepare sooner rather than later to establish their UHC with the vision of making it sustainable and leveraging the latest technologies.

Drawing on these experiences, Japan is committed to contributing to the global movement to advance global health and achieve UHC around the world. Prime Minister Abe articulated Japan's commitment in his article, writing that "Japan is determined to contribute further to galvanize renewed momentum for global health so that all people can receive the basic quality services they need, and are protected from health threats, without financial hardship" [6].

Under this vision, Japan has advocated for global health, including UHC in particular, at major global forums, including through hosting high-level conferences on UHC [13–16], the G7 presidency [3–5, 17, 18], the G20 presidency [19, 20], and by establishing the Group of Friends of UHC and Global Health in New York [21] in the lead-up to the UN General Assembly high-level meeting on UHC in 2019, at which the world leaders agreed to a landmark Political Declaration on UHC (A/RES/74/2), and beyond.

Conclusion

Japan's journey to achieve and sustain UHC provides good lessons for countries facing similar challenges. As articulated in Japan's long-term vision *Japan Vision: Health Care 2035* [22], which the author was involved in crafting, Japan is committed to contributing to the global community's efforts to tackle common challenges such as UHC, sharing lessons learned and policy evidence along the way, in the quest for a peaceful and healthier world.

References

1. What is universal coverage? World Health Organization. https://www.who.int/health_financing/universal_coverage_definition/en/. Published July 9, 2019. Accessed 16 July 2019.
2. United Nations Official Document. United Nations. https://www.un.org/ga/search/view_doc.asp?symbol=A/RES/70/1&Lang=E. Accessed 16 July 2019.
3. Sakamoto H, Ezoe S, Hara K, et al. Japan's contribution to making global health architecture a top political agenda by leveraging the G7 presidency. J Glob Health. 2018;8(2). https://doi.org/10.7189/jogh.08.020313.
4. The G7 presidency and universal health coverage, Japan's contribution. World Health Organization. https://www.who.int/bulletin/volumes/96/5/17-200402/en/. Published April 30, 2018. Accessed 16 July 2019.
5. Hara K, Ezoe S. Why does global health matter to diplomacy? Global health as a security and economic challenge and as an opportunity for world leaders, with a special focus on the G7 Ise-Shima Summit. https://www.shu.edu/. http://blogs.shu.edu/ghg/files/2019/06/Spring-2019-Issue.pdf#page=23. Accessed 16 July 2019.
6. Abe S. Japans vision for a peaceful and healthier world. Lancet. 2015;386(10011):2367–9. https://doi.org/10.1016/s0140-6736(15)01172-1.
7. Japan health system review. New Delhi: WHO Regional Office for South-East Asia; 2018.
8. Lancet T. Japan: universal health care at 50 years. Lancet. 2011;378(9796):1049. https://doi.org/10.1016/s0140-6736(11)61223-3.
9. Wagstaff A, Flores G, Smitz M-F, Hsu J, Chepynoga K, Eozenou P. Progress on impoverishing health spending in 122 countries: a retrospective observational study. Lancet Glob Health. 2018;6(2) https://doi.org/10.1016/s2214-109x(17)30486-2.
10. Myth and measurement – the case of medical bankruptcies. N Engl J Med. 2018;378(23):2245–7. https://doi.org/10.1056/nejmc1805444.
11. Shiozaki Y. "A conversation with Health Ministers" people at the centre: OECD policy forum on the future of health. Speech presented at the OECD Health Ministerial "A conversation with Health Ministers" people at the centre: OECD policy forum on the future of health. https://www.mhlw.go.jp/file/06-Seisakujouhou-10500000-Daijinkanboukokusaika/0000137631_1.pdf. Accessed 16 July 2019.
12. Realizing Society 5.0. The government of Japan. https://www.japan.go.jp/abenomics/_userdata/abenomics/pdf/society_5.0.pdf. Accessed 16 July 2019.
13. Japan-World Bank partnership program on universal health coverage global conference on universal health coverage for inclusive and sustainable growth. In: Global Conference on Universal Health Coverage for Inclusive and Sustainable Growth. Tokyo http://documents.worldbank.org/curated/en/888101468149093450/pdf/831410WP0JPP0U0Box0379884B00PUBLIC0.pdf. Accessed 16 July 2019.

14. Horton R. Offline: Japans daring gamble in an age of apprehension. Lancet. 2016;387(10013):13. https://doi.org/10.1016/s0140-6736(15)01310-0.
15. [Press Releases] UHC Forum 2017. Ministry of foreign affairs of Japan. https://www.mofa.go.jp/press/release/press4e_001823.html. Accessed 16 July 2019.
16. UHC2030. UHC Forum 2017: all together to accelerate progress towards UHC. UHC2030. https://www.uhc2030.org/news-events/uhc2030-news/uhc-forum-2017-all-together-to-accelerate-progress-towards-uhc-449822/. Published February 12, 2018. Accessed 16 July 2019.
17. G7 Ise-Shima Summit, 26–27 May 2016. In: G7 Ise-Shima leaders' declaration. Ministry of Foreign of Affairs of Japan. https://www.mofa.go.jp/files/000160266.pdf. Accessed 16 July 2019.
18. G7 Ise-Shima Summit. In: G7 Ise-Shima vision for global health. Ministry of Foreign Affairs of Japan. https://www.mofa.go.jp/files/000160273.pdf. Accessed 16 July 2019.
19. G20 Osaka. In: G20 Osaka leaders' declaration. G20 2019 Japan. https://www.g20.org/pdf/documents/en/FINAL_G20_Osaka_Leaders_Declaration.pdf. Accessed 16 July 2019.
20. G20 Osaka. In: G20 shared understanding on the importance of UHC financing in developing countries —towards sustainable and inclusive growth—. G20 2019 Japan. https://www.g20.org/pdf/documents/en/annex_05.pdf. Accessed 16 July 2019.
21. Ezoe S. Concept note group of friends of universal health coverage and Global Health. Permanent Mission of Japan to the United Nations. https://www.un.emb-japan.go.jp/files/000430434.pdf. Accessed 16 July 2019.
22. Miyata H, Ezoe S, Hori M, Inoue M, Oguro K, Okamoto T, Onishi K, Onozaki K, Sakakibara T, Takeuchi K, Tokuda Y, Yamamoto Y, Yamazaki M, Shibuya K. Japan's vision for health care in 2035. Lancet. 2015;385(9987):2549–50.

Georgia's Success Towards Universal Health Coverage

Mariam Jashi and Tamar Tchelidze

Overview of Universal Healthcare Development in Georgia

The year 2013 marked a turning point for the national healthcare system of Georgia. Six years ago, the country launched its flagship program of universal health coverage (UHC), thereby providing a basic package of emergency, in- and out-patient services for all its citizens and permanent residents. Over 90% of the population was covered by the state UHC program.

As of 2012, Georgia was ensuring state-subsidized medical insurance to only socially vulnerable groups of the population, including families living below the poverty line, pension-aged citizens, people living with disabilities, children, students, and teachers. Over 1.6 million beneficiaries were secured by targeted medical insurance programs funded by the Ministry of Labour, Health and Social Affairs (MLHSA). At the same time, more than 362,000 people were enrolled in private or company health plans [1]. Health coverage of 1.9 million individuals [2], or over 50% of the population, was already an important achievement for a newly independent Georgia, a country that has gone through a series of political and socioeconomic crises since the early 1990s.

However, as of 2012, more than half of families living in Georgia were still without any financial protection against catastrophic health expenditures. In fact, based on the 2011 National Health Accounts [3], out-of-pocket expenditures for health in the country exceeded 70%. In the same year a report on catastrophic health expenditures [4] indicated that 9% of Georgia's population had become impoverished due to health spending, and the lead causes of household impoverishment in the country

M. Jashi (✉)
Education, Science and Culture Committee, Parliament of Georgia, Tbilisi, Georgia
e-mail: mariam.jashi@gmail.com

T. Tchelidze
Forum for Collaborative Research, UC Berkeley, Berkeley, CA, USA

© Springer Nature Switzerland AG 2020
P. Murthy, A. Ansehl (eds.), *Technology and Global Public Health*,
https://doi.org/10.1007/978-3-030-46355-7_3

13

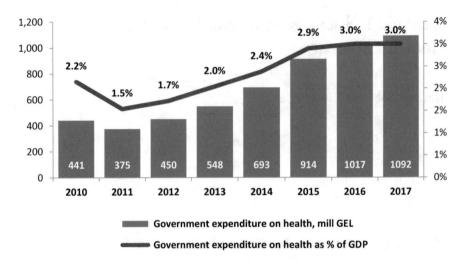

Fig. 1 Public health expenditures, Georgia. (Adapted from Results of National Health Accounts 2012–2017. Ministry of Labour, Health and Social Affairs of Georgia. Retrieved from https://www.moh.gov.ge/uploads/files/2019/Failebi/02.05.19-2012-2017-geo.pdf)

were costs related to hospitalization, management of chronic diseases, and acute health conditions. Later the United Nations Development Programme (UNDP) reported that in more than 80% of households not all family members had proper health insurance [5].

As noted, UHC became the flagship initiative of the government of Georgia in 2013, and the program's launch was made possible through unprecedented political commitment and financial investments. Overall in 2012–2017 government expenditures on health, in absolute figures and as a percentage of GDP, increased from GEL450 million to GEL1092 million and from 1.7% to 2.9%, respectively (cf. Fig. 1) [6].

Georgia's commitment to UHC was a timely response to the emerging global dialogue endorsed by the UN General Assembly and other high-level international forums. The December 2012 UN Resolution on Global Health and Foreign Policy [7] and the 66th General Assembly of the World Health Organization (WHO) positioned UHC among the top priorities for the 2030 sustainable development agenda.

In 2013, as part of its UHC program, Georgia started offering an expanded primary healthcare package, including visits to general practitioners and specialists and a series of evidence-based diagnostic tests to reduce the disease burden attributed to the leading noncommunicable and communicable diseases (e.g., cholesterol, international normalized ratio, chest X-rays). UHC also provided 100% coverage of emergency medical care both at ambulatory and hospital levels (GEL15,000 annual limit), 70%–100% funding for elective surgical care (GEL15,000 annual limit), oncology treatment (chemo- and radiotherapy with GEL12,000 annual limit), and maternity services (both vaginal delivery and C-section). Most importantly, patients were free to choose health service providers throughout the country, though health-care costs for specific clinical interventions might have varied.

In parallel to the UHC portfolio, targeted health programs or vertical programs were operating in the country, including for immunization, HIV/AIDS, tuberculosis and diabetes treatment, dialysis, organ transplantation (cofunding) with lifetime immunosuppression medications, and mental health, for example. The standalone vertical programs are being gradually integrated into the comprehensive UHC package in order to improve operational cost-effectiveness of the services.

The universal health program, similar to medical insurance plans in general, had its limitations. Some of the main interventions remaining beyond the UHC program included plastic surgery, spa and resort therapies, high-cost procedures and interventions with proven lower-cost alternatives, infertility, and dental care.

To improve the cost-effectiveness of the UHC program, in May 2017, the government introduced a differentiated approach for UHC eligibility criteria that excluded individuals with high annual incomes (exceeding GEL40,000).

Finally, in July 2017, the UHC program was expanded to include medications for chronic health conditions (cardiovascular, respiratory, diabetes, and thyroid diseases) [8] for socially vulnerable groups, while in July 2018 a similar drug affordability initiative was launched for pension-aged citizens and people living with disabilities.

Key Results of UHC

The UHC initiative in Georgia resulted in a major expansion of access to publicly financed health services for the population. More than 90% of citizens and permanent residents of the country became entitled to a defined package of state-funded benefits in 2013 vs. 45% in 2012 [9].

Based on the state health authority reports, since the commencement of the UHC initiative in 2013, over four million clinical interventions have been provided nationwide [10], including routine primary healthcare, maternity services, emergency care, elective surgery, and oncology care.

The improved access to health services was translated into increased numbers of primary healthcare visits per person per year and hospitalization rates per 100 population in the period 2012–2017 from 2.3 to 3.5 and from 11.3 to 14.2, respectively [8].

More importantly, the UHC program has significantly reduced out-of-pocket (OOP) payments and improved financial protection of the population from catastrophic health expenditures. Specifically, based on the data from the National Health Accounts, OOP spending declined from 73.4% in 2012 to 54.7% in 2017 (Fig. 2). [6]

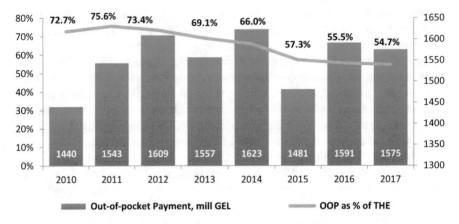

Fig. 2 Out-of-pocket payment as percentage of total health expenditure, Georgia. (Adapted from Results of National Health Accounts 2012–2017. Ministry of Labour, Health and Social Affairs of Georgia. Retrieved from https://www.moh.gov.ge/uploads/files/2019/Failebi/02.05.19-2012-2017-geo.pdf)

Health Management Information System and UHC

The Health Management Information System (HMIS) was instrumental to the successful operationalization of the universal healthcare program in Georgia. The project was launched in 2011 with technical assistance from Abt Associates Inc. and MDI Informatics within the scope of the U.S. Agency for International Development (USAID) Health System Strengthening Project (HSSP) [11]. However, with the commencement of the UHC program, the HMIS project became systematically integrated into the national health authority as the main eHealth portal of the ministry. To date the eHealth products and modules developed within the scope of the HMIS project ensure core digital/technological support for the management and monitoring of the UHC and other state health programs in Georgia https://www.abtassociates.com/projects/republic-of-georgia-health-system-strengthening-project.

The eHealth system currently gathers comprehensive information related to UHC and ensures transparent connections among the main stakeholders of the healthcare sector, including the Health Ministry, healthcare providers, private insurance companies, the pharmaceutical industry, and the general population. In addition, the system ensures interagency links of the health authority to other state agencies, including Civil Registry (CRA), Social Service Agency (SSA), National Agency of Public Registry (NAPR), and the revenue system of the Ministry of Finance.

Prior to the launch of the HMIS system, the collection, exchange, and analysis of health system–related information was largely fragmented. Today, eHealth ensures a unified platform for real-time information exchange, administration, monitoring, and analysis of state-supported health programs, including the flagship program of

UHC. Furthermore, the system ensures standardization of data based on internationally established indicators for comparative analysis at national and international levels.

Some of the main eHealth modules developed within the scope of the USAID-supported HMIS project include the following:

- *HMIS Portal*, the main website, a user-friendly platform for accessing different modules of the eHealth system.
- *Healthcare Facilities Licensing/Permitting module*, the central registry of healthcare facilities by legal and licensing status, services offered, ownership, and other characteristics.
- *Accounting and Financial Management* component, including the Case Registration Module and Healthcare Program Financing Module.
- *Pharmacy Module* covering information on legal/licensing status of pharmacies operating nationwide and bringing together modules on pharmaceutical products and E-subscriptions.
- *Immunopack*, centralized portal for the registration and monitoring of the vaccination status of children and adults per the national immunization schedule.
- *Analytical Tools* for integrated data visualization with graphic presentations to facilitate analysis and decision-making on different aspects of the state-supported health programs at the process, output, and outcome results levels.

While the HMIS project played a critical role in the daily management of the UHC program in Georgia, unfortunately, so far, no documented evidence is available on the contribution of the eHealth portal and its various modules on the transparency, data accessibility, analytical, and management capacities of the state health program in the country. State health authorities and public health practitioners should prioritize evidence generation on the impact of the eHealth system in Georgia on its UHC efforts. Further details on the HMIS modules may be accessed on the main portal of the state health authority: http://ehealth.moh.gov.ge/Hmis/Portal/Documents.aspx.

Remaining Challenges and the Way Forward

While Georgia has made historic progress toward the attainment of UHC goals, the country prioritizes further improvement of access to and quality of health services. Some of the strategic priorities for the future of the Georgian healthcare system include improvement of the quality assurance systems at both the primary and hospital levels, strengthening of human resources for health, a focus on preventive medicine by strengthening the gatekeeper role of the primary healthcare network, and improvement of the financial management of UHC through selective contracting and performance-based funding.

Despite historic improvements in the government's budget allocations to health in recent years, the current level of state health expenditures as a percentage of GDP (3.1% in 2016 [12] and 2.9% in 2017) remains considerably lower than resources allocated by EU countries (from the lowest 5% in Romania to the highest 12.3% in Switzerland [13]). Similarly, World Bank data indicate that Georgia's public health expenditures as a share of total state expenditures (6.9% of GDP) [14] are still low in comparison with other countries of Central and Eastern Europe and Central Asia.

Finally, although the UHC program has led to a reduction in OOP payments from 73.4% in 2012 to 54.7% in 2017 (Fig. 2), Georgia still has one of the highest shares of OOP costs in the European region in general and Central and Eastern Europe, in particular. By 2016, pharmaceuticals remained major cost drivers of OOP payments for health in the country [15]. In response to this situation, the government has initiated an affordable drug program for the most vulnerable groups.

Further monitoring and evaluation efforts are essential both for documenting the dynamics of OOP payments as well as the overall progress of Georgia toward quality UHC.

Georgia in the Global UHC Dialogue

Independent from the national UHC program, in 2019 Georgia, together with Thailand, was entrusted by the President of the UN General Assembly to cofacilitate the historic process of drafting and negotiating a UHC Political Declaration. The UHC declaration, which was launched in September 2019 at a UN General Assembly high-level meeting, will be the new global health agenda for UN member states, public and private partners, civil society, and academia to progressively increase UHC and ensure that no one is left behind.

References

1. Kankava K., Verulava T. Effects of the universal health programme on health service utilization in Georgia. Health Policy Econ Soc. https://heconomic.wordpress.com/2018/01/03/universal. Accessed 17 Aug 2019.
2. Richardson E, Gugeshashvili N. Voluntary health insurance in Europe: country experience. National Center for Biotechnology Information. https://www.ncbi.nlm.nih.gov/books/NBK447726. Accessed 19 Aug 2019.
3. National Health Accounts. Ministry of Labour, Health and Social Affairs of Georgia. 2011. https://www.moh.gov.ge/uploads/files/2017/angarishebi/en/2011-NHA.pdf. Accessed 11 July 2019.
4. Cylus J, Thomson S, Evetovits T. Catastrophic health spending in Europe: equity and policy implications of different calculation methods. Bull World Health Organ. 2018;96:599–609. https://doi.org/10.2471/BLT.18.209031.. Accessed 25 July 2019
5. Gassmann F, Berulava G, Tokmazishvili M. Economic and social vulnerability in Georgia. 2012. http://www.ge.undp.org/content/dam/georgia/docs/publications/GE_vnerability_eng.pdf. Accessed 19 Aug 2019.
6. Results of National Health Accounts 2012–2017. Ministry of Labour, Health and Social Affairs of Georgia. https://www.moh.gov.ge/uploads/files/2019/Failebi/02.05.19-2012-2017-geo.pdf. Accessed 11 July 2019.

7. Resolution adopted by the General Assembly on 12 December 2012. 67/81 Global health and foreign policy. A/RES/67/81. https://wwwunorg/en/ga/search/view_docasp?symbol=A/RES/67/81. Accessed 11 Aug 2019.
8. Health Care Statistical Yearbook, 2017. National Centre for Diseases Control and Public Health, Ministry of Internally Displaced Persons from the Occupied Territories, Labour, Health and Social Affairs of Georgia. http://ncdc.ge/Handlers/GetFile.ashx?ID=114b7ef6-0fa1-424a-9c01-6af08ffa63cc. Accessed 15 July 2019.
9. Richardson E, Berdzuli N. Georgia: health system review. Health Syst Transit. 2017;19(4):1–90. http://www.euro.who.int/__data/assets/pdf_file/0008/374615/hit-georgia-eng.pdf. Accessed 19 Aug 2019.
10. Report of the Ministry of Internally Displaced Persons from the Occupied Territories, Labour, Health and Social Affairs of Georgia. December 2018.
11. Health Management Information System (HMIS), Georgia, January 2013. USAID Health System Strengthening Project (HSSP), Ministry of Labour, Health and Social Affairs of Georgia. http://www.georgia-ccm.ge/wp-content/uploads/HMIS_Module_Descriptions_ENG.pdf. Accessed 17 Aug 2019.
12. Results of National Health Accounts 2011–2017. Ministry of Labour, Health and Social Affairs of Georgia. https://www.moh.gov.ge/uploads/files/2019/Failebi/02.05.19-2012-2017-geo.pdf. Accessed 11 July 2019.
13. Healthcare expenditure statistics, 2016. Eurostat. https://ec.europa.eu/eurostat/statistics-explained/index.php/Healthcare_expenditure_statistics#Health_care_expenditure. Accessed 19 Aug 2019.
14. Verulava T. Healthcare costs in line with the recommendations of the World Health Organization and the funding of Georgia's healthcare system. Institute for Development of Freedom of Information (IDFI). https://idfi.ge/en/health-care-expenditure-who-recommendations-georgia. Accessed 15 Aug 2019.
15. Georgia Public Expenditure Review. World Bank Group. 2017. http://documents.worldbank.org/curated/en/630321497350151165/pdf/114062-PERP156724-PUBLIC-PERFINAL.pdf. Accessed 19 Aug 2019.

Women, Girls, and STEM

Roya Mahboob

Introduction

My main purpose is to get tech into the hands of women, to make it accessible to them, and to make science, technology, engineering, and mathematics (STEM) and tech education a fundamental component of girls' education.

I am originally from Afghanistan, where I became one of the first female tech entrepreneurs in that country. It was an incredibly lonely field. Few women were in business, much less in the tech world. This was a contributing factor in my decision to dedicate my work to building a tech-friendly world in Afghanistan filled with women, starting first by educating girls in STEM fields.

In Afghanistan, girls are not raised and educated for the Fourth Industrial Revolution, which is so eagerly anticipated in the West. Girls are educated to keep the home. But Afghan girls want so much more. I founded Digital Citizen Fund to create platforms that enable women and girls to achieve their full potential. We build information technology (IT) classrooms and provide STEM education opportunities for thousands of girls in Afghanistan. We give them access to education and technology. Unfortunately, the Internet is accessible to only half the world. The other half lives in digital darkness, the majority being women and girls, mostly the working poor. Some of you may have heard of the Afghan Girls Robotics Team – the Afghan Dreamers. I am humbled and inspired to be their coach and mentor. These girls are utterly brilliant, but discrimination and ignorance nearly denied them their rightful place on the world stage.

From #MeToo to the Afghan Dreamers, technology and its benefits have been vital to changing the global conversation about the rights of girls and women. Because of the Afghan Dreamers and women in tech, women in Afghanistan are

R. Mahboob (✉)
Digital Citizen Fund, New York, NY, USA
e-mail: mahboob.roya@gmail.com

© Springer Nature Switzerland AG 2020
P. Murthy, A. Ansehl (eds.), *Technology and Global Public Health*,
https://doi.org/10.1007/978-3-030-46355-7_4

beginning to see themselves differently, with value and contributions beyond the home. In addition, the embedded views of men in society are slowly changing, too. Despite all the progress we see in the world, the gap between rich and poor, within countries and between countries, is still growing by the day.

Role of Technology

I am a champion of artificial intelligence, robotics, blockchain, and other exciting new technologies. But as tech entrepreneurs, we need to reexamine ourselves. We must evaluate the technology we build through the lens of how it enables stronger societies. It is crucial, however, that tech companies have a code of ethics.

If technology does not enhance lives or if it prevents people from participating in the economy, then we must question its investment potential and long-term return.

When we create jobs and opportunities for people, we give them hope. And hope powers future generations. When we create jobs and opportunities for girls and women, we build a new world for the benefit of generations now and those to come. It starts with education, and it thrives through gender equity.

People, both women and men, must move forward and achieve the dignity of working or having a job. We in the tech world have an obligation to enable that.

We also need a rules- and values-based system that keeps companies in check and encourages them to invest in training people from developing countries for the jobs of the future. Building such an ethical framework is the work of government, whose goal should be to create universal access to the web for all people, rich and poor. And finally, we all need to educate our children from the very beginning of their lives on how to be good digital citizens, to participate in and contribute to society.

Activism

I will continue to use my power to demand that we build technologies that enhance lives and do not eliminate jobs for girls and women. I will be even more vocal in asking world leaders: Are we investing in the lifelong needs of girls and women, so that, instead of staying poor, they gain access to quality education, economic opportunities, and leadership? And I will continue to fight incrementalism, insisting that we can do more.

The most exciting potential for tech is the pathway it provides for quality education, healthcare, and the ability to include women and girls in the economy. If we can achieve these three goals, we can finally say that women's voices are no longer silent.

Role of New Media in Advancing Gender Harmony (Gender Equality)

Wale Idris Ajibade

The Learning Curve

One of the most important areas of progress made in the last few decades is the advancement of women across cultures. This has happened with the power of social media, which made it possible to create a network of hundreds of thousands of followers and to communicate with them, regardless of technological knowledge, thorough blogs, and audio or video podcasts. Current technology makes it possible for an idea to spread very quickly ("go viral"). At the African Views organization, we use several types of new communication technology devices to connect and advocate for causes within our mandates. One of the goals of African Views has always been to establish a consensus on a sustainable strategic solution for effective localization of the universal agenda on Gender Equality in Africa with its Anti-Violence Against Women Act (AVAWA) advocacy.

African Views facilitates a collaborative global intelligence initiative for the advancement of women and girls. Together, and collaboratively, African Views works with several organizations in various countries and has formed satellite organizations to promote programs and services advancing the status of women. Many of our partners have traversed all the continents to attend the CSW conferences. The CSW (Commission on the Status of Women) is the principal global intergovernmental body exclusively dedicated to the promotion of gender equality and the empowerment of women. A functional commission of the Economic and Social Council (ECOSOC), was established by Council resolution 11(II) of 21 June 1946. The CSW is instrumental in promoting women's rights, documenting the reality of women's lives throughout the world, and shaping global standards on gender

W. I. Ajibade (✉)
Founder and Executive Director, African Views, Hoboken, NJ, USA
e-mail: wale.ajibade@africanviews.org

© Springer Nature Switzerland AG 2020
P. Murthy, A. Ansehl (eds.), *Technology and Global Public Health*,
https://doi.org/10.1007/978-3-030-46355-7_5

equality and the empowerment of women.African Views conducts annual parallel events as an ECOSOC-accredited non-governmental organization to support the agenda of the CSW in achieving its goals for improving the status of women ending violence against women. African Views promotes sustainable development strategies for effective localization of the universal agenda on gender equality in Africa, and other regions of advocacy such as the Caribbean and the US through its Anti Violence Against Women Act (AVAWA) advocacy.

From 2010 to 2014, African Views Organization has hosted more than 500 episodes of the AV Teleforum, of which 250 were dedicated to topics covering the advancement of women featuring experts on various aspects of the subject from around the world. AV Teleforum is a virtual forum that connects local individuals to global resources, overcoming barriers of distance, costs of travel, and resources by allowing people to take part in a professionally moderated and coordinated forum conducted by phone and compatible VOIP apps from the comfort of their private domain. The audience can listen live online, on social media platforms, smartphones, mobile devices, or the radio. Audiences can ask questions in writing and verbally; it is a platform to teach and learn, as well as merely share information about local-scale challenges and connect the global community to explore and find common interests and support worldwide in real time. All these experiences have prepared us all to engage with historical, contemporary, and future challenges on gender issues more objectively. We see the recent phenomenon with Zoom during the COVID-19 Pandemic. However, this has been going on for a long time and African Views Organization was at the forefront of this trend.

Role of Technology

The Teleforum is not just about talking. It is about consensus, action, intelligence gathering, surveys, education, capacity building, monitoring, and evaluation. Though the process has always been accompanied by dynamic technical challenges, the results and effectiveness achieved have exceeded all expectations. The Teleforum education, experiences, and presentations from various leaders in their fields are what led to the global call to support AVAWA as a sustainable strategy for peace and security in Africa.

Instead of relying on treaties that have no effect, we are considering another approach that can mobilize society through a more effective awareness and by effectuating attitudinal and behavioral changes from within. In order for the vision for ending violence against women to become a reality, countries must be morally and legally committed to controlling violence against women within their own domestic laws. The AVAWA provides a solution that some people have interpreted as the missing link and have agreed to support because they see it also as an effective and sustainable strategy for effective localization of the universal agenda on gender equality in Africa.

Advocacy

The AVAWA provides countries with the opportunity to formulate a detailed plan on how they will implement the existing legal provision for women in its constitution. The AVAWA is therefore a comprehensive national action plan that includes programs, policies, and procedures for fulfilling a country's mandate to protect and empower women as written in its constitution. For example, the constitution of Egypt states: "The state commits to the protection of women against all forms of violence and ensures women's empowerment to reconcile the duties of a woman toward her family and her work requirements." In this case, Egypt's AVAWA will be Egypt's national action plan, guiding policies, procedures, budget, and institutions responsible for meeting this constitutional mandate. The AVAWA also serves as an impetus for developing a comprehensive national strategy as well as for updating judicial, legislative, enforcement, and budgetary policies to address complex challenges of violence against women and other specific needs for healing with emphasis on the rehabilitation of victims and advancing gender equality measures. This detailed action plan is published for domestic and international review and updated annually.

AVAWA is essentially an "act" of accountability on the need to respect a country's obligation to the contract with its society. The AVAWA complements to CEDAW, Maputo Protocol, I-VAWA, DEVAW, and AWAVA. Its self-determination procedure makes it easily embraced in developing societies. AVAWA is original, nonintrusive initiative and adopting the process will improve women's condition dramatically without compromising the integrity of the country within the international community of nations.

The Power of the Constitution and the Importance of Gender-Sensitive Policies

Moreover, the constitutionality of every law and every act of the government is one of the most important political principles of democracies and universally accepted rule of legal norms. Because constitutions are understood to be the supreme law of the land, they must be respected, and their implementation must be prioritized. The parliamentary or congressional approval requirement and the harmonization of the implementation of the AVAWA with institutions designed to enforce it are not as complicated as if it were a bilateral or multilateral interventionist ratification agenda.

Milestones Reached

In the area of education for women, the AVAWA has helped create good models that governments could replicate and scale up. These include those piloted by international Civil Society Organizations (CSOs) and humanitarian agencies working collaboratively and connecting through African Views Teleforum. The African Views women's education model has been widely successful. A good example is the Learn as you Earn Advancement Program (LEAP) Uganda project. The LEAP model works in partnership with vocational schools and provides tremendous opportunities for adults and young people alike, and especially for individuals who otherwise would be hindered by a lack of money or daily childcare responsibilities, which today remains the main cause of dropping out of school in sub-Saharan Africa. Evidence from our research suggests a need for remedial, basic, informal, and technical education as well as vocational and formal reentry into formal education system. Remedial education programs would enable those who missed months or years of formal education to acquire an age-appropriate education to help them complete their primary or secondary education, rejoining their age cohort at an appropriate stage in the process. Basic and informal education would be targeted at those who had missed formal education and did not want to rejoin the formal school system, because of age or other issues. These individuals might nevertheless benefit from basic literacy and numeracy and basic computer skills and data entry. The added technology provided opportunities for data collection and resource allocation to beneficiries.

Since its inception, the AVAWA has been on a steady growth trajectory. The number of women signing up to join this local government area has grown exponentially, and membership currently stands at around 6000. This number continues to rise. Members meet regularly as we continue to emphasize the role of women and document the need for women's empowerment and advancement to protect women and girls in the region. We also developed an app that allows the women at risk to keep a journal or diary and share their various experiences with peers. The app also has an emergency prompt that enables them to send a direct alert to the police when in danger. Nevertheless, we have concluded that their problems are mostly rooted in financial abuse or poverty. We understand that poverty is more than just a lack of money, and we are putting in place structures for education, capacity building, and psychosocial programs. These women are registered with the organization, and each has been given an ID card. The digital identification system allows us to track subjects more easily and provides other benefits to members. We were able to negotiate with the United Bank of Africa (UBA) to accept this ID as valid for opening a bank account for each of the members. Several women who were previously committed to the old tradition of Susu are now registered bank account owners.

Conclusion

In conclusion, the AV Teleforum has helped to identify, survey, recommend and implement solutions to socioeconomic issues women face. New media and technology have also helped to formulate possible ways and means to address the local challenges. With access to global intelligence through technology and social media, women at-risk have access to immediate support to navigate or address through the abuses and other challenges they face locally.

Given these challenges, the Teleforum facilitated the formulation of specific solutions to each challenge; on the issues of lack of financial empowerment people suggested the establishment of vocational training programs for women and the inclusion of women in politics.

We were able to identify and provide effective solutions with the help of the Teleforum we conducted over the years. For example, to address financial difficulties, we provided access to bank loans, not micro-loans, but tailored loans to occupations within a cooperative, we the established vocational training programs, and we encouraged forming a voting block and participation in local politics. We also use the data collected to engage and advise relevant organs of government to provide counselling and support for victims as well as establish legal departments that focus mainly on advocating for legislation against social practices that harm women such as early child marriages, breast pressing, feet bidding, and female genital mutilation. Finally, we advocate for the dignity of rural women and we advocate to businesses operating locally to for uphold a global ethical standard and professionalism as enshrined in the policies established under the corporate social responsibility agenda.

African Views Organization stands on the principle that the society as a whole will improve and benefit if its institutions are used to support women's empowerment and advancement, which should be a central focus that includes protecting women and girls, fostering child development, and safeguarding society and its moral recovery, infrastructure development, cultural reconstruction, and economic sustainability. The AVAWA is guided by African Views and we hope to benefit from the development programs offered by UN Women and of the institution and civil society program on an international scale.

Part II
Technology in Advancing Health: Meeting Sustainable Development Goal (SDG) 3 Targets

Chapter 1: Role of Digital Health, mHealth, and Low-Cost Technologies in Advancing Universal Health Coverage in Emerging Economies

Padmini Murthy and Mahtab Naji

Introduction

The Sustainable Development Goals (SDGs) that were adopted by the United Nations (UN) member states in 2015 are closely linked to universal health coverage. To meet the targets of the SDGs, especially SDG 3, and to advance the global agenda for universal health coverage, UN agencies, member states, think tanks, foundations, nongovernmental organizations, and universities are working in partnership to incorporate technology into healthcare systems and improve service delivery to global communities. This chapter discusses examples of best practices, challenges, and existing barriers in healthcare systems with a special focus on how they affect low- and middle-income countries, as well as how mobile health (mHealth) technology, digital health, and other low-cost technologies can address and overcome these challenges and barriers and their impact in leveling the playing field for global citizens in meeting the targets of SDG 3, which is to ensure healthy lives and promote well-being for all at all ages. The ways in which these factors can function as a catalyst to achieve universal health coverage will also be discussed.

P. Murthy (✉)
New York Medical College School of Health Sciences and Practice, Valhalla, NY, USA

Medical Women's International Association and NGO Representative to United Nations, New York, NY, USA

American Medical Women's Association, Schaumburg, IL, USA
e-mail: padmini_murthy@nymc.edu

M. Naji
Institute for International Health and Education, Albany, NY, USA

© Springer Nature Switzerland AG 2020
P. Murthy, A. Ansehl (eds.), *Technology and Global Public Health*,
https://doi.org/10.1007/978-3-030-46355-7_6

Digital Health

In May 2018, the Seventy-First World Health Assembly (WHA) passed Resolution WHA71.7 on digital health. Among other items, the resolution requested the director-general "to develop, in close consultation with Member States and with inputs from stakeholders, a global strategy on digital health, identifying priority areas including where WHO should focus its efforts" [1].

The idea behind having member states forge ahead with a global strategy on digital health is so that they can meet the various targets of SDG 3.

Digital health has tremendous potential to meet the targets of the SDGs by providing support for health systems and strengthening them in health promotion and disease prevention [2]. The field of digital health is expanding by leaps and bounds and is dynamic in its rapid progress globally. Telemedicine, e health, mHealth, and digital informatics are some of the terms used to describe the various technologies used for the past 50 years. It is interesting to note that these terms have been used in different settings to describe the role and application of information and communications technology (ICT) in healthcare and other aspects of health, including service delivery [1].

According to the definition outlined in the World Health Organization (WHO) Document EB 142/120, "In the context of this Global Strategy, Digital Health is understood to mean 'the field of knowledge and practice associated with any aspect of adopting digital technologies to improve health, from inception to operation'" [3].

As the paradigm shifts from eHealth to digital health, it changes the focus by putting more emphasis on digital consumers and encompasses the use of a wider range of smart devices, its connectivity to technology, and other innovative concepts such as Internet of Things (IoT) and by increasing the use of artificial intelligence (AI) as well as big data platforms, such as cloud computing and analytics. To put it simply, digital health/eHealth/mHealth is changing the face of health systems and the delivery of healthcare globally [1].

Mobile Health

For the past few years, mobile devices such as smartphones, tablets, and other cost-effective technologies have been playing an important role in global societies, and their importance in public health is increasing. These devices are used for a variety of health-related activities, such as delivering health information, sending medication reminders, monitoring vital signs, and providing ease of access to information about disease prevention and treatment.

mHealth is a useful tool for delivering health information, especially to geographically hard-to-reach areas, and a cost-effective method for reaching and monitoring the health needs of a large population.

One of the most important advantages of mHealth is its ability to overcome the various barriers that exist in accessing healthcare services globally. Health education and health promotion strategies have been scaled up in recent years using mHealth so that it can reach a larger population to deliver information in comparison to other forms of healthcare delivery. Healthcare systems globally face a wide variety of barriers, and these barriers can differ based on the socially determined patterns of behavior in a given country, as well as other factors. In many countries, the most common healthcare barriers are financial, challenges in cultural beliefs and practices, health literacy level, access, geographical limitations, and limited human resources [4].

For more than two decades, the aim of all global health programs and projects has been to decrease the significant health disparities that exist between high-income countries and low- or middle-income countries. To address this problem, collaboration and coordination of multiple sectors at national and international levels are required, which makes it more challenging [4].

mHealth refers to the use of any mobile and wireless devices in practicing medicine. The introduction of mHealth represents a revolutionary approach in addressing health challenges in low- and middle-income countries, with several successful mHealth projects having been implemented in countries with emerging economies. According to a survey conducted by the WHO, out of 112 of its member states, mHealth initiatives were reported by 83% of them, and the majority of them reported 4 or more mHealth projects in their country. Of the low-income countries, 77% reported mHealth initiatives in comparison to 88% in high-income countries [5].

Technological Advances in the Past Decade [6, 7]

1. Increased use of electronic medical records in various settings.
2. Increased use of mHealth devices by physicians and other healthcare providers for writing prescriptions, providing documentation, and gaining access to more information when with patients.
3. Increased use of portal technology, which has increased patient empowerment.
4. Increased use of telemedicine/teleheath in rural settings.
5. Self-service kiosks for patient registration to expedite the registration process.
6. Increased use of remote monitoring tools, i.e., home monitoring.
7. **Increased use of sensors and wearable technology.**
8. **Wireless communication, which includes the use of platforms to send messages about lab tests and data.**
9. Use of **real-time locating services that use** data-monitoring tools and real-time locating services, which help hospitals focus on efficiency and instantly identifying problem areas.
10. **Pharmacogenomics/genome sequencing, which is advancing and laying the foundation for personalized medicine.**

11. **The use of virtual reality in medicine, which has been instrumental with its calming effects on patients before treatment and eliciting better response.**
12. **Inexpensive ways of detecting hepatitis B in developing countries (test called Treat-B).**
13. **Development of a fast-acting influenza pill in Japan that, when administered as a single dose, can treat influenza in 24 hours.**
14. **Increased use of big data collection, which is valuable in assisting patients with managing chronic diseases such as diabetes.**

Examples of Best Practices

Drone Technology

Modern technology has been harnessed to improve access to healthcare services and improve delivery. In April 2019, a drone service was launched in Ghana to make on-demand emergency deliveries, which included vaccines, blood products such as plasma, and life-saving medications when needed. The drone service for delivery was launched in Ghana by Silicon Valley-based company Zipline. Drones with products are dispatched from the drone center at Omenako and reduce the transport time of delivery from 40 minutes by road, which is often difficult to navigate in the rainy season, to 12 minutes when sent by drone. The central distribution center receives messages via text from the healthcare centers and the necessary supplies are sent by a drone. The service is scheduled to expand, and there is a proposal to open three additional centers in Ghana by the end of the year. Once these centers are operational, they will make over 600 flights every day to 2000 health facilities and deliver supplies to 12 million people in Ghana. This is a groundbreaking initiative that uses technology to provide access to healthcare and improve service delivery, strengthen healthcare systems, and meet the targets of SDG 3 and work toward achieving universal healthcare. In the short time the drones have been used from the sole existing service center in Omenako, many lives have been saved in Ghana at the four health centers [8].

Technology and Women's Health

In recent years, investors, venture capitalists, healthcare professionals, researchers, and technology gurus and developers have started focusing on using technology in the arena of women's health. This initiative/submarket is referred to as "femtech." This includes using specific software, diagnostic tools, and various online platforms and services that make use of digital technology to improve women's health. Frost and Sullivan, a well-known research firm, has stated that "female technology

(FemTech) is emerging as the next big disruptor in global health care market" [9]. The following are examples of technology used in addressing women's health:

1. Period-tracking apps and smart menstrual cups will help women address their menstrual health.
2. A Swedish company has become one of the earliest to obtain approval from the United States Food and Drug Administration and the European Union for its digital birth control app known as Natural Cycles, which at present has over half a million subscribers in 160 countries, including developing countries. It is a fertility tracking app and a tool to empower women to make decisions about birth control and pregnancy [9].
3. Apps and online platforms to support women during pregnancy and postpartum have been developed to provide medical information and emotional support when needed, and specifically to address postpartum depression.
4. Thermal imaging and digital mammography are examples of technology that have been instrumental in the early detection of breast cancer.
5. Telemedicine is being used by a Seattle-based company to provide community support for women to address menopausal health [9].

Technology can be a disruptor in addressing women's health, as illustrated by the aforementioned examples, which illustrate the different healthcare needs during a woman's lifetime.

Aviation Industry and Health

Project Orbis International was the brainchild of Dr. David Paton, U.S. ophthalmologist who was a faculty member at the Wilmer Eye Institute at Johns Hopkins Universtiy. His extensive overseas travels made him aware of the enormous number of visually impaired people living overseas. Unfortunately, more than 90% of the world's avoidable blindness occurs in the developing world, and Dr. Paton realized that the lack of access to preventive and treatment services and financial barriers prevented doctors and nurses in low-income countries from coming to the USA for training. Sustained efforts by a diverse group of people led to the launch of Project Orbis in 1973. It is interesting to note that "In Latin Orbis means 'Of the Eye' and in Greek it means 'around the world'" [10]. Project Orbis International took flight in 1992 with the launch of the Flying Eye Hospital, made possible by generous donations, a grant from the U.S. Agency for International Development (USAID), and a plane donated by United Airlines, Inc. In May 1982, the Orbis plane went on its pilot mission to Panama. In 2003, Orbis International launched a global telemedicine initiative called CyberSight, which has been at the forefront of providing follow-up ophthalmic education and real-time consultations between physicians in developed and developing nations about patient care. This resource is available for patients and providers around the clock. One of the landmark achievements of the country program initiatives introduced by Orbis is the distribution of more than 10.2 million doses of antibiotics in Ethiopia to prevent trachoma, a major cause of blindness [10].

Shipping Industry and Health

Don Stephens founded Mercy Ships in 1978 with the purchase of the *Anastasis*, which was fitted to provide healthcare access and healthcare delivery to socially disadvantaged populations worldwide. Mercy Ships Africa has transformed lives by using technology, and in March 2019 the repair of a young girl with a cleft lip was the 100,000th surgery performed by Mercy Ship volunteer health professionals [11]. According to a report published in *The Lancet*, 93% of the people living in sub-Saharan Africa cannot get the surgery they need [12]. Mercy Ships has been at the forefront of addressing this crisis by sending ships with international volunteers to parts of Africa, which has a shortage of surgeons. These volunteer healthcare professionals have helped to local healthcare professionals in the local areas they visit. This is an excellent illustration of strengthening healthcare systems and increasing access to healthcare services among the most vulnerable, and Mercy Ships have provided healthcare to over 2.7 million people since 1978 [11].

Types of mHealth in Use Globally

Different types of mHealth technologies are in use globally, including smartphone apps, wireless medical devices, text messages, voice calls, and electronic medical records systems; of these, smartphone apps are among the most widely used. There are many apps with a wide variety of health-related topics. Some apps provide information to healthcare providers when making clinical diagnoses and treatment suggestions; other types are remote monitoring apps, clinical reference apps, and healthy lifestyle apps, which are used by the general population [13].

According to a 2019 survey conducted by the Pew Research Center to assess the availability and accessibility of mobile phones in 11 different emerging market economies, the majority of people in these countries have access to mobile phones and more than 53% of them have access to a smartphone. This survey was conducted in middle-income countries as defined by the World Bank, including Mexico, Venezuela, and Colombia; South Africa and Kenya; India, Vietnam, and the Philippines; and Tunisia, Jordan, and Lebanon. Based on the same survey, most people found mobile phones to be a useful tool for education, understanding the economy, and connecting people [14]. Thus mHealth is an innovative way of using mobile technologies to deliver health information and services, and it has a great impact on public health. This is especially true in developing countries, where there is a shortage of healthcare infrastructures [15].

Data from the International Telecommunication Union (ITU) show widespread use of mobile-cellular devices worldwide, with more than 7 billion subscribers, 3.6 million people using mobile broadband [16], and the availability of more than 318,000 mHealth apps to consumers [14]. This suggests mHealth holds great potential in terms of global use for both individualized medical care and public health.

Barriers to Use of Technology

In countries with emerging economies, the most prominent challenges to the healthcare system are a lack of infrastructure, paper-based data collection and clinical information, and shortage of trained healthcare workers [16]. Other barriers include geography-related accessibility, low availability of services, high cost of medical services, cultural limitations, and myths and fear about using technology due to limited knowledge about its benefits in healthcare.

For more than two decades, the aim of all global health programs and projects has been to decrease the significant health disparities that exist between high-income countries and low- or middle-income countries. To address this problem, collaboration and coordination of multiple sectors at national and international levels are required, which makes the problem even more challenging [4].

Acceptance and Advantages of Technology

According to a WHO report published in 2011, the development of ICT and eHealth in the past few years has increased people's expectations globally regarding healthcare. This may result in the improvement of healthcare delivery around the world [5]. One of the advantages of mHealth is its transferability, a feature that can overcome some of the existing barriers and serve as a bridge to increase accessibility and allow for a reduction in healthcare inequalities and disparities among different countries. This would reduce the gap between countries, regardless of their level of income and lack of uniformity in infrastructure [5].

Currently, mHealth is widely used in high-income countries in comparison to low- and middle-income countries. In high-income countries, mHealth has been used to facilitate smoking-cessation programs, encourage changes in lifestyles to promote weight loss and prevent cardiovascular diseases, and raise awareness about general and public health. Fortunately, mHealth use is growing in low- and middle-income countries as well, and it has been used in connection with maternal and child health, to promote awareness about communicable diseases such as HIV/AIDS, malaria, and tuberculosis, and as a reminder for taking medication [17].

mHealth can be used for many different purposes in healthcare, but one of the unique and creative applications of mHealth is its use in mobile phones in combination with wearable sensors that can record different parameters that help to improve medical care.

One of the major impacts of mHealth/eHealth in developing countries is on improving public health services, especially where there is a shortage of clinical resources and poor healthcare infrastructure. In such countries, technology is of great value as a tool in both treatment and prevention. Currently, various technologies can be used to deliver health information to improve the health literacy of both patients and healthcare professionals.

Use of Technology in Healthcare in Developing Countries and Emerging Economies

Emerging economies like China and India hold great growth potential for mHealth. Financial support from both governmental and private organizations is key to developing mHealth projects that are beneficial in addressing the needs of healthcare systems. The high demand for low-cost technologies in emerging economies is fueling the need to change the face of healthcare and its link to technology in these regions. In emerging market economies, mHealth remains in its infancy, but high demand and better access to the Internet and mobile devices in recent years have resulted in considerable growth. Other factors that have spurred the rapid growth of mHealth technology are population aging, increases in the prevalence of chronic diseases, and the high cost of healthcare services. mHealth decreases the cost of healthcare services by reducing the need for regular check-ups, since mHealth enables physicians to monitor patients remotely [18].

Bangladesh

Many developing countries have taken advantage of mobile phones to raise awareness about healthcare and to improve health at both the individual and public levels. For example, in 2007, the Ministry of Health and Family Welfare of Bangladesh initiated a project to raise awareness about health campaigns by sending text messages to all mobile phone users in the country. The first text message was sent on National Immunization Day to encourage parents to bring their children in for vaccination. According to the second global survey on eHealth, Bangladesh's Ministry of Health has been able to broadcast SMS health messages to "an estimated 55 million mobile telephone users." It also reports that through "the SMS service directed to nearly 100,000 health staff members," the ministry has become much more streamlined with reductions in both time lag and paperwork "and the use of fixed line telephony." The number of subscribers to the Health SMS subscription service is forecasted to increase significantly as news of the service spreads. The ministry continued this project for other immunization campaigns and other national health programs such as National Vitamin A Week, National Breastfeeding Week, and National Safe Motherhood Day [5].

To expand the use of ICT in delivering health services, the Ministry of Health of Bangladesh has launched two other projects that also use text messages to promote health. In 2009, the ministry started a project that aimed to raise awareness and help healthcare professionals better coordinate their activities in emergency situations. This project also provided healthcare professionals with useful information about their responsibilities during and after natural disasters and communicable disease epidemics. The second project started by the ministry and mobile operators began in 2010. This project allowed mobile phone users to subscribe to a text message service at lower rates to receive messages about a variety of health-related topics. It also allowed healthcare professionals throughout the country to give advice to patients and receive information, all through their mobile phones. The ease of access to information about prenatal alerts, advice, and reminders through mobile phones has been of tremendous assistance to pregnant women who live in remote or rural regions to raise their awareness on what to expect during their pregnancy [5].

Currently, the mobile telephony network in Bangladesh covers about 98% of the population targeted by the Ministry of Health. The use of technology in this context has represented a novel approach to delivering health information and raising awareness about health campaigns [5].

One of the important factors that has facilitated the use of technology and SMS to deliver health information and promote public health in Bangladesh is the regulatory framework for telecommunications. The Bangladesh Telecommunication Regulatory Commission (BTRC) can direct mobile operators to send SMS text messages free of charge for mobile phone users. The main benefits of using SMS text messages are its low cost and its ability to reach a wide population sector [5].

Ghana

Ghana is a low-income country where the doctor-to-patient ratio is very low; there is an obvious disparity between the health services offered in rural regions and those offered in urban regions of the country [19]. This shortage of human resources in the healthcare system of Ghana called for a reliable means of communication that would allow healthcare professionals to communicate with patients, consult with colleagues in the network of healthcare professionals, and refer patients to the appropriate doctor or facility. The initiative, called Mobile Doctors Network (MDN), started in 2008 to facilitate the communication among doctors [5]. Over 95% of doctors in Ghana have registered to the MDNet program, where they can communicate with other registered doctors at no cost. This initiative was supported by New York University in collaboration with Ghana's mobile telephony provider, Switchboard 5, which is a US-based nonprofit organization, and the Ghana Medical Association (GMA) [20].

This initiative enables all doctors registered in the healthcare system of Ghana to communicate and consult through text and voice messages. GMA has also used this service to send information and announcements to doctors about meetings and emergency situations [5].

The MDNet initiative was the first telemedicine project that started in Africa and aims to facilitate doctor-to-doctor communication and enable doctors to consult and share information via mobile phone [5]. This project has been very successful, and the result has been very impressive. According to the survey conducted by Switchboard in 2009, doctors consider MDNet to be an important and useful communication tool among doctors in the healthcare network of Ghana; the implementation of MDNet facilitates both communication among doctors who live in rural regions and referrals to the appropriate facilities [20].

The initial idea behind the MDNet project was to develop an online platform that would enable doctors to communicate, but owing to limited or lack of access to computers and the Internet, especially in rural regions, mobile phones were used because of wider availability and accessibility [5]. Following successful implementation and the positive feedback on the MDNet project in Ghana, the project was expanded to Liberia, where almost 100% of doctors became connected [20].

Senegal

One of the most important challenges that the healthcare system faces in developing countries is the lack of accurate and up-to-date data. Accurate data are required to identify the needs of healthcare systems, to inform decision makers, and to enable improvements in the quality and accessibility of healthcare services [5]. Therefore, developing a data-collection program through mobile phones that is accessible to most of the people in a particular region can be an effective way to tackle this obstacle.

In addressing this problem, the Ministry of Health in Senegal, in collaboration with the WHO, started to use mobile technology to collect health data. They connected 20 healthcare workers within the community in 10 different districts via handheld devices called personal digital assistants (PDAs), which were provided by EpiSurveyor. EpiSurveyor also trained these individuals on how to use the devices [5].

When this project started as a pilot in 2008, in the first 6 months, healthcare workers made field visits to 90 health posts and collected data using the EpiSurveyor. EpiSurveyor has an 82-question survey. For the collected data to be analyzed, all the data must be sent to the district level electronically. The collected data helped health officials reallocate the budget to meet the needs and shortages of the healthcare system that had been revealed by the collected data [5].

EpiSurveyor is another successful example of the application of mHealth in developing countries. This program helped the healthcare system in Senegal to have a better and more efficient data-collection system and made it possible to meet the demands of the healthcare system. EpiSurveyor is accessible through both mobile phones and the Internet and is an efficient and effective approach to collecting data about public health and the needs of the healthcare system via mobile phones. One of the shortages revealed through the use EpiSurveyor was the low availability of a birthing tool that is used by midwives to assess the progress of labor and assure safe delivery called a partogram. It was known that partograms could decrease both maternal and fetal mortality, but according to data collected through EpiSurveyor, only 55% of districts have access to partograms. This shortage was addressed by the Ministry of Health in Senegal via the distribution of more partogram programs to encourage midwives to use partograms to decrease maternal and fetal mortality. After 5 months of this project, access to partograms in the regions involved in the project increased by 28% in comparison to a 1% increase in the areas that were not part of the project [5].

This program can expand further, and data collection can be supported by similar projects in other regions. The key to addressing the needs of the population is successful data collection. The systematic gathering of accurate data can also help identify how healthcare systems should allocate their budgets.

Bolivia

According to the WHO, noncommunicable diseases (NCDs) such as heart disease, cancer, stroke, chronic respiratory diseases, and diabetes are the number one cause of mortality worldwide. The main risk factors of contracting NCDs are modifiable, including tobacco use, excessive use of alcohol, unhealthy diet, low level of physical activity, high blood pressure, high blood glucose level, and high cholesterol. Educating people and promoting healthy lifestyle can play a key role in preventing these diseases. The prevention of NCDs is highly cost-effective and at the same time very effective, but it requires actions at both national and global levels [21]. Bolivia is not an exception, and according to the World Bank, Bolivia is a low- to middle-income country half of whose population lives at or under the poverty line [22].

Economic, cultural, social, and geographical barriers represent the major challenges that more than 75% of people face in accessing healthcare in Bolivia. The high rate of uninsured people (57% in 2009) spurred the development of an mHealth program for patients who suffer from NCDs such as diabetes and hypertension. The aim of this program was to enable patients to manage their diseases by using their mobile phones and by receiving tailor-made educational sessions on their phones [22].

In the summer of 2013, potential program participants were identified through surveys from six different hospitals at the time of their visit with a primary care physician. A total of 165 patients with diabetes or hypertension enrolled in the Interactive Voice Response (IVR) platform trial. Blood pressure monitors were provided to all participants with hypertension, who received training on how to use the machine and record their daily systolic blood pressure. Participants were contacted on their mobile phones or landline telephones on a weekly basis for 12 consecutive weeks. To assess their health status and symptoms, participants used the IVR platform, which allowed them to report their health status, symptoms, compliance with medication prescriptions, and so forth. Based on the data reported by the participants, they were able to self-manage, and, in the case of uncontrolled diseases, they were advised to contact their doctor [22].

The overall of results of this program, based on interviews with 20 participants, were that over 95% of participants were satisfied with the program and indicated that they would recommend it to their friends. About 70% were satisfied with help they received via the IVR platform [22].

As with any other programs, some areas required further improvement, such as adding languages other than Spanish since 37% of the participants were not Spanish speakers. Technical challenges were reported by some of the participants. Some of the elderly participants had hearing problems [22]. Mental health disorders, such as depression, are the top priorities requiring attention in this program [23].

Ukraine

According to the World Bank, Ukraine is a lower- to middle-income European country [24]. The healthcare system in Ukraine struggles with existing barriers. One of the barriers that has been addressed by many mHealth technologies is geography. In 2010, the first telecommunications network was established in Ukraine, and the aim of this initiative was to facilitate healthcare delivery, especially for patients living in rural areas. This network enabled physicians to send and receive the results of diagnostic tests online, consult with specialists when needed, and participate in conferences while at their office. This telemedicine network is an affordable approach to overcoming existing barriers to healthcare access and represents an effective strategy to improve the healthcare infrastructure [24].

This initiative was unique from two perspectives; even though the United Nations played a key role in this project, the Ministry of Health and private sector were the leaders at the forefront of this project. The other important component of this project was its capacity to better connect patients with their doctors and doctors with their peers [25].

India

In line with the Make in India movement and Digital India program, the Indian government, through the Ministry of Health & Family Welfare, established governance initiatives with the ambitious goal of digitalizing national healthcare sectors in order to increase access to affordable healthcare services, which are also standardized.

The Indian government launched the *Ayushman Bharat Yogana* scheme in 2018, which is the national health protection scheme and one of the largest government-funded schemes in the world. It aims to enroll and provide healthcare access and coverage for 100 million economically disadvantaged families. The initiative was designed to be paperless, cashless, and completely digital using IT platforms and data analysis to streamline services, which would make the services more efficient and allow for the detection of fraudulent insurance claims [26]. The partnership between the Biocon Foundation and the government led to the establishment of so-called eLAJ smart clinics. The name is derived from the official language of India, which is Hindi, in which *ilaj* means "cure" and *elaj* denotes using technology to provide healthcare. "These are preventive and primary health care centers based in rural areas in Karnataka and Rajasthan, which operate under the Public Private Partnership" [26]. These smart clinics have successfully incorporated technology by using various monitoring devices to facilitate running multiple diagnostic tests that contribute to the creation of electronic health records (EHRs), which are in turn linked to the national identification card (Aadhar) of each citizen in India, which has a unique identification number and enables tracking of the patient's health information [26]. Another interesting and cost-effective initiative is the creation of the MedTech Zone in Andhra Pradesh – one of the hubs of the IT industry in India. This initiative is funded by the Indian government to promote *techno-centric* domestic manufacture of medical devices such as low-cost Bluetooth and IoT-enabled glucometers for the detection and monitoring of chronic diseases such as diabetes. Linear accelerators will be produced for cancer care [26]. The aforementioned examples are an excellent illustration of the dynamic and beneficial role played by technology in changing the face of healthcare by making it more affordable and accessible to one of the most populous countries in the world.

Conclusion

The past few decades, especially the last two, have seen an explosion of different technological platforms and devices. As discussed in this chapter, technology has become an integral part of the global healthcare industry. One of the most revolutionary forms of technology is the *blockchain,* which, in simple terms, is an ingenious way of "passing information from A to B in a fully automated and safe manner. One party to a transaction initiates the process by creating a block. This block is verified by thousands, perhaps millions of computers distributed around the net. The verified block is added to a chain, which is stored across the net, creating not just a unique record, but a unique record with a unique history" [27]. The advantage of this technology is in its decentralization, transparency, and immutability, which are built into the technology. Inoperability has been a major challenge in the healthcare industry, and efforts to improve healthcare inoperability is an important priority for stakeholders in the global healthcare industry, which is virtually everyone in the world. Using the disruptive technology of blockchain in healthcare has the following advantages. An important feature of the blockchain is its immutability and traceability; as a result, patients can easily send records to anyone without the fear of data corruption or tampering. Similarly, a medical record that has been generated and added to the blockchain will be completely secure [28]. The patient can have some control over how their medical data get used and shared by institutes and organization. A third party looking to obtain a patient's medical data would have to check with the blockchain to get the necessary permission to obtain the information [28].

Tremendous sums of money are spent on healthcare, and global annual health spending surpassed USD7 trillion in 2015, and this figure is estimated to reach USD8.734 trillion. In addition, according to a report published by BIS reach, the healthcare industry has the potential to save USD100 billion per year if blockchain technology is incorporated into the system; this would reduce expenses associated with IT, operational, and personnel costs. It would also help reduce the tremendous costs associated with counterfeit and insurance-related fraud [29].

In the words of James Michiel, senior mHealth and informatics analyst at Emory University's Rollins School, "the future of mHealth is open — open access, open source, open data, and open innovation" [30].

In conclusion, the seamless incorporation of technology into healthcare has many advantages, as presented in the chapter. On the other hand, some of the challenges faced are a lack of uniformity in the availability of digital platforms owing to an absence of the necessary infrastructure, cultural acceptance, lack of budget allocation by governments, and a shortage of trained personnel, for example. The use of technology in healthcare has tremendous potential in helping to make universal health coverage a reality and in meeting the targets of SDG 3 by 2030.

References

1. World Health Organization. Global Strategy on Digital Health 2020–2024. 2019. Accessed 10 July 2019. Retrieved from https://extranet.who.int/dataform/upload/surveys/183439/files/Draft%20Global%20Strategy%20on%20Digital%20Health.pdf
2. World Health Organization. WHO/ITU National eHealth Strategy Toolkit, 2012. Accessed 10 July 2019. Retrieved from https://apps.who.int/iris/handle/10665/75211
3. World Health Organization. WHO EB142/20 mHealth Use of appropriate digital technologies for public health. 2017. Accessed 10 July 2019. Retrieved from http://apps.who.int/gb/ebwha/pdf_files/EB142/B142_20-en.pdf
4. Weiss B, Pollack AA. Barriers to global health development: an international quantitative survey. PLoS One. 2017;12(10):e0184846. https://doi.org/10.1371/journal.pone.0184846.
5. World Health Organization.|Global Observatory for eHealth series – Volume 3. 2011. Accessed 10 July 2019. Retrieved from https://www.who.int/goe/publications/ehealth_series_vol3/en/
6. Becker Hospital review. 10 Biggest Technological Advancements for Healthcare in the Last Decade. 2014. Accessed 10 July 2019. Retrieved from https://www.beckershospitalreview.com/healthcare-information-technology/10-biggest-technological-advancements-for-healthcare-in-the-last-decade.html
7. Continuum. Top 20 Health care advances in 2018. 2018. Accessed 10 July 2019. Retrieved from https://www.carecloud.com/continuum/top-20-healthcare-technology-advances/

8. Voice of America. Drones deliver medical supplies in Ghana. 2019. Accessed 10 July 2019. Retrieved from https://www.voanews.com/africa/drones-deliver-medical-supplies-ghana

9. Med Tech Impact on Wellness. 2019. Accessed 10 July 2019. Retrieved from https://www.medtechimpact.com/how-technology-is-transforming-womens-health/

10. Orbis International. Orbis. n.d. Accessed 10 July 2019. Retrieved from https://www.orbis.org/en/about-us/our-history

11. Mercy ships. Mercy ships volunteers perform 100,000th free surgical procedure. n.d. Accessed 10 July 2019. Retrieved from https://www.mercyships.org/blog/mercy-ships-volunteers-perform-100000th-free-surgical-procedure/

12. Meara JG, Leather AJ, Hagander L, Alkire BC, Alonso N, Ameh EA et al. Global surgery 2030, evidence and solutions for achieving health care, welfare and economic development – Lancet (2015) https://doi.org/10.1016/S0140-6736(15)60160-X. Accessed 10 July 2019. Retrieved from https://www.thelancet.com/journals/lancet/article/PIIS0140-6736(15)60160-X/fulltext

13. Piette JD, Valverde H, Marinec N, et al. Establishing an independent mobile health program for chronic disease self-management support in Bolivia. Front Public Health. 2014;2:95. Published 2014 Aug 13. https://doi.org/10.3389/fpubh.2014.00095.

14. Silver L, Smith A, Johnson C et al. Mobile connectivity in emerging economies. Pew Research Center: Internet, Science & Tech. 2019. Accessed 10 July 2019. Retrieved from https://www.pewinternet.org/2019/03/07/mobile-connectivity-in-emerging-economies/

15. Latif S, Rana R, Qadir J, Ali A, Imran M, Younis M. Mobile health in the developing world: review of literature and lessons from a case study. IEEE Access. 2017;5:11540–56. https://doi.org/10.1109/access.2017.2710800.

16. Wasden C, Weirz D. mHealth transforming healthcare in emerging markets. 2014. Accessed 10 July 2019. Retrieved from https://www.himss.org/mhealth-transforming-healthcare-emerging-markets

17. O'Shea C, McGavigan A, Clark R, Chew D, Ganesan A. Mobile health: an emerging technology with implications for global internal medicine. Intern Med J. 2017;47(6):616–9. https://doi.org/10.1111/imj.13440.

18. Research P. Digital health market to have huge growth potential in the emerging economies of the world: P&S market research. GlobeNewswire News Room. 2018. Accessed 10 July 2019. Retrieved from https://www.globenewswire.com/news-release/2018/05/30/1514144/0/en/Digital-Health-Market-to-Have-Huge-Growth-Potential-in-the-Emerging-Economies-of-the-World-P-S-Market-Research.html

19. UNICEF USA Patrick, Mensah & Sanka Laar, David. E-Health dedicated hybrid cloud: a solution to Ghana's health delivery problems. 2012. Accessed 10 July 2019. Retrieved from https://www.researchgate.net/publication/285926789_E-Health_Dedicated_Hybrid_Cloud_a_Solution_to_Ghana's_Health_Delivery_Problems

20. Woods E. 2010. Accessed 10 July 2019. Retrieved from http://wikisarvn.pbworks.com/f/Africa+Aid+MDNet+Physician+In-Network.pdf

21. World Bank. Bolivia I Data. 2018. Accessed 10 July 2019. Retrieved from https://data.worldbank.org/country/bolivia

22. Piette JD, Valverde H, Marinec N, et al. Establishing an independent mobile health program for chronic disease self-management support in Bolivia. Front Public Health. 2014;2:95. Published 2014 Aug 13. https://doi.org/10.3389/fpubh.2014.00095.

23. Francis M. 5 Types of Mobile Health Apps. Skedulo. 2018. Accessed 10 July 2019. Retrieved from https://www.skedulo.com/blog/5-types-mobile-health-apps/

24. World Bank. Ukraine I Data. 2018. Accessed 10 July 2019. Retrieved from https://data.worldbank.org/country/ukraine

25. Launch of the first telemedicine network in Ukraine – United Nations in Ukraine. 2010. Accessed 10 July 2019. Retrieved from http://www.un.org.ua/en/information-centre/news/1218-2010-07-28-10-54-15

26. Iyer S. Decision resource group. 11 unique tech solutions that are transforming India's healthcare. 2018. Accessed 10 July 2019. Retrieved from https://decisionresourcesgroup.com/blog/11-unique-tech-solutions-transforming-indias-healthcare/

27. Block Geeks. Rosic, A., What is Blockchain technology? A step-by-step guide for beginners. 2016. Accessed 10 July 2019. Retrieved from https://blockgeeks.com/guides/what-is-blockchain-technology/
28. Block Geeks. Blockchain in healthcare: The Ultimate use case? 2019. Accessed 10 July 2019. Retrieved from https://blockgeeks.com/guides/blockchain-in-healthcare/
29. BIS Research. Global Blockchain in healthcare market. Focus on Industry Analysis and Opportunity Matrix – Analysis and Forecast:2018–25. Accessed 10 July 2019.. Retrieved from https://bisresearch.com/industry-report/global-blockchain-in-healthcare-market-2025.html
30. Collier J. mHealth: What is it, and how can it help us? 2018. Accessed 10 July 2019. Retrieved from https://www.medicalnewstoday.com/articles/322865.php

Chapter 2: Social Media and the Practice of Public Health

Amy Ansehl and Jessica Ansehl

Introduction

What is social media? Why is it an important communication, education, and amplification platform for promoting global public health? Social media is a critical link for people with health concerns to find a community that enables information access, exchange, debate, and knowledge enrichment. Social media refers to an array of online tools that advance interaction among individuals, groups, and organizations. It includes social, professional, and career-building networks. Examples include Facebook, Instagram, Twitter, and LinkedIn. Informational platforms that provide medical and health-related forums for content, discussion, and commentary are also considered important components of social media. Social media, when used in a responsible manner, can enhance engagement, participation, and outcomes to meet the strategic goals of stakeholders, including public health practitioners and organizations [1].

Social media provides a platform to engage people and has become an integral part of the public health conversation worldwide. As a collection of digital channels and tools, Heldman et al. describe social media as enabling multiway conversation without requiring participants to be colocated. These tools, such as Facebook, Twitter, YouTube, Instagram, Flickr, WhatsApp, and Storify, have in common an ability to foster interaction and communication with a wide range of people across geographical locations. A significant number of public health–promoting organizations, such as the World Health Organization (WHO), the United States Centers for

A. Ansehl (✉)
New York Medical College School of Health Sciences and Practice, Valhalla, NY, USA

Visiting Nurse Services, Westchester Foundation, White Plains, NY, USA
e-mail: amy_ansehl@nymc.edu

J. Ansehl
Westchester VNS, White Plains, NY, USA

© Springer Nature Switzerland AG 2020
P. Murthy, A. Ansehl (eds.), *Technology and Global Public Health*,
https://doi.org/10.1007/978-3-030-46355-7_7

Disease Control and Prevention (CDC), the United Nations (UN), the American Public Health Association (APHA), the United States Food and Drug Administration (FDA), and a plethora of others, have added social media to their overall strategy of population engagement [2].

Based on the public health literature, social media has been found to be a viable tool to promote engagement when integrated with traditional public health channels to support communication goals and objectives. This is because it enables a health-care practitioner or public health organization to reach targeted and diverse individuals and groups. Wen-Ying et al. found that social media use is widespread in the United States, independent of education, race/ethnicity, or healthcare access [3]. Their study focused on sociodemographic characteristics associated with social media support groups, blogs, and networking sites in an effort to "better understand who is accessing and being reached through these emerging communication channels" [3]. Understanding these characteristics creates the opportunity to more effectively target specific audiences by selecting highly utilized social media channels with relevant messaging. A practitioner or organization can tailor social media campaigns to specific audiences to augment access and engagement.

Two key terms that are important for social media and public health are *community engagement* and *community building*. Community engagement is a process of working collaboratively to bring together groups of people with a common interest or geography. Community building refers to the ways people who identify with a particular community interact to bring about a particular community change [2]. The WHO describes social media as a great equalizer [4]. Why? Because, regardless of socioeconomic status, race, gender, or geography, social media enables community engagement and community building by promoting access to information. According to research published by the WHO, approximately 80% of its member states reported that their healthcare organizations used social media for health promotion messages [4]. These countries report that individuals and communities use social media as a direct mode of educating themselves or their communities about specific health issues and for developing community-based health campaigns. Rapid communication and innovation is a key characteristic of social media and networks. This is important since social media enables health organizations to share and receive information quickly. Furthermore, social media generates real-time data, which can help practitioners and organizations determine which communication efforts are working.

Significant value is placed on gathering health research data from nontraditional platforms that are enabled by social media. For example, receiving real-time information on a current disease outbreak is extremely beneficial to public health practitioners. One example is the Zika outbreak in 2015. In cases like this, social media generates valuable information to detect disease outbreaks. It also simultaneously helps prevent the spread of disease by sending important health messages to alert people. In doing so, social media enables public health surveillance. Digital data sources provide public health professionals, government, and nongovernment stakeholders with additional information to detect, investigate, and confirm the outbreak of diseases. This creates a host of opportunities for public health professionals and their collaborators to monitor disease spread, estimate disease incidence, forecast, and promote situational and global awareness [5]. It is also critical to acknowledge that there are important health policy implications in terms of protecting the health data of individuals. Policy is imperative to ensure data are shared appropriately with the goal of advancing public health in a secure manner [6].

Health Promotion and Social Media

Twitter is one of the more popular social media technologies for sharing information about public health. Why? According to Pershad et al., this is because anyone with a Twitter account can contribute to a conversation and can also post public messages. Twitter allows multiple people, including healthcare experts, to post information and join a dialogue. This promotes virtual communities that enable professionals to measure reactions as well as community engagement. Earlier in the chapter, we mentioned the concept of community building. Twitter is an excellent digital modality to build consensus and engagement around specific public health topics by utilizing hashtags. Twitter can advance research by connecting medical practitioners with consumers under the same hashtag. Millions of people can be connected via public tweets for the purpose of disseminating health updates, sharing information about diseases, and coordinating relief efforts [7].

Mobile health, or specifically the utilization of cell phones by individuals for health-related communications, has become ubiquitous in daily life. According to Anderson-Lewis et al. [8], mobile cellular subscriptions have reached more than 90% of the world's population and 80% of the population globally that live in remote areas [8]. Interestingly, minority populations use mobile phones to access health information via the Internet more frequently than populations not so characterized. This creates strategic opportunities for public health practitioners to reach underserved populations for health promotion purposes. Some of the ways public health practitioners can promote health include text messaging, mobile apps, the Internet, streaming, social media, and instant messaging. For example, streaming soap operas has been an effective strategy to reduce the risk of HIV infection. The Text4baby program is another example. This campaign has provided a means to successfully reach underserved pregnant and postpartum women. In another public health campaign, improved outcomes for promoting physical activity among African American women in the United States were demonstrated via Facebook versus leveraging traditional print media. Group text messaging has also been found to increase rates of cervical cancer screening [8].

The continuous identification of new strategies to prevent cancer and diabetes disparities is a high priority for public health practitioners and their respective organizations. Social media is a powerful tool to shape conversations about cancer and cancer prevention. It can also help mobilize people to advocate for social justice and health equity. This helps reduce the social and environmental forces that contribute to cancer and other chronic disease disparities. Examples of successful health advocacy campaigns include targeting obesity and tobacco use as risk factors for cancer and diabetes. The Bigger Picture (TBP) campaign is very active in the state of California [9]. The campaign effectively has used social media to launch a series of partnered health messages to empower youth to protect their own health. TBP has used Facebook, YouTube, and messaging to create meaningful social change. This translates into real health impacts by targeting areas such as diabetes and obesity-related cancers at the individual and community levels. Furthermore, data from Fernandez-Luque et al. [10] showed that consumer electronics, combined with social media, have facilitated the Quantified Self (QS) movement. The QS movement refers to millions of users worldwide who track their daily living activities. Examples of these activities include tracking the number of steps someone takes or the number of calories consumed daily. There is a direct connection between consumer electronics and social media with regard to promoting healthy behavior in individuals. This is evident through an obesity prevention initiative called 360 Quantified Self, which was implemented in Qatar. This initiative demonstrated that combining Instagram and WhatsApp with wearable sensors has the potential to change behavior and reduce obesity in children [10].

Social Media and Chronic Disease

Does social media use have an impact on patients with chronic diseases? According to Abedin et al. [11], Facebook groups can be effective in promoting patient education about diabetes. Specifically, Facebook was found to be an important platform for disseminating education that can help to prevent common complications from diabetes such as foot-related conditions, hospitalizations, and amputations. In the study, Facebook users posted, shared, and "liked" an 11-point checklist. The checklist prompted group members to (1) check feet daily, (2) wash feet daily, (3) dry feet post washing, (4) moisturize, (5) cut nails, (6) wear appropriate foot attire, (7) protect feet from extreme temperature, (8) develop awareness of mitigation strategies for corns and calluses, (9) get annual check-ups, (10) develop awareness of the toxic effects of smoking, and (11) monitor glucose levels. The researchers found that social media directly supported health education by creating online spaces where people could easily learn, meet, support, and share information with others who have the same chronic disease.

A retrospective analysis by AlQarni et al. [12] demonstrated that many people in the Arabic-speaking world use Facebook to share information and manage clinical diseases like diabetes mellitus and others including cancer and chronic obstructive pulmonary disease (COPD). The authors' purpose was to see how people from Arabic-speaking countries use the Internet specifically to manage and make healthcare decisions about chronic diseases. The authors assessed Internet usage to understand whether people sought to share information about their medical journey. Are people trying to better understand their disease and learn from others? The study included 20 Arabic-speaking countries (Kuwait, Lebanon, Qatar, Saudi Arabia,

Bahrain, UAE, Egypt, Libya, Jordan, Oman, Syria, Yemen, Tunisia, Iraq, Sudan, Algeria, Morocco, Djibouti, Mauritania, and Somalia). The most posts were from Egypt and Lebanon. There were no posts from Somalia, Yemen, and Djibouti. The main themes identified from reviewing the posts included raising awareness about diabetes, support for caregivers, and patients, experience sharing, discussing products and services, sharing the latest research, sharing educational practices, and providing spiritual support. Overall, the authors found that using the Internet to share information about chronic disease management is increasing in the Arabic-speaking world.

Al Qarni et al. also had additional findings from their study leveraging social media. First, they found a large increase in obesity in the countries included in their study. They surmised that this was due to changing lifestyles, including westernization, and the rising popularity of fast food. Second, they highlighted the role social media plays in the context of the female gender. Most Facebook posts were from women between the ages of 40 and 60 years old. Why is this information valuable? It is important for healthcare providers and public health professionals to understand both the information people share and specific demographic concerns. This can enable healthcare professionals to better develop and communicate culturally and demographically targeted educational materials to help people manage chronic diseases.

COPD is a chronic disease with significant global impact. It is characterized by a pathology in the lungs that restricts airflow, making it difficult to breathe. By 2030, it is projected that COPD will be the third leading cause of death and seventh leading cause of morbidity worldwide [13]. According to Sobnath et al. [13], mobile health (mHealth), which includes supporting devices such as tablets, mobile phone applications, and personal digital assistants, plays a significant role in managing chronic diseases, including COPD. Since mobile devices are used ubiquitously and have proven effective, the United Kingdom Department of Health has recommended that mobile apps be prescribed as part of the management of chronic conditions. Studies demonstrate that when mHealth is integrated with a multidisciplinary team approach, it can prevent hospitalizations, reduce exacerbations, and reduce mortality from COPD. However, the authors also found that more personalized feedback from people suffering from COPD is necessary [13].

In Australia, a mobile COPD (M-COPD) system was developed to enhance the connection and personalization between patients and their healthcare providers [13]. The components of the system included a web portal and mobile app for patients to assess their symptoms. The authors identified limitations in that patients were not comfortable with many of the routine self-assessment requirements. This included recording vital signs and uploading them to an mHealth device. When considering mHealth, a key finding is the importance of compliance. For example, integrating mHealth with remote or telehealth monitoring can open up a communication channel between patient and healthcare provider to ensure compliance. One opportunity to improve compliance includes combining mHealth with telehealth monitoring. This can help patients share and manage early exacerbations of COPD. Doing so has the potential to improve the quality of daily life for patients and their families by reducing symptoms such as wheezing and difficulty breathing.

Does social media utilization have an impact on patients with chronic disease?

Patel et al. [14] describe social media as providing easy, fast, and low-cost access to information about healthcare management. It is particularly useful to increase awareness. The use of social media to offer social, emotional, or experience-based support in chronic disease management through Facebook and blogs appears likely to improve patient care. The data compiled from a literature review by Merolli et al. [15] related to chronic diseases, including chronic pain, arthritis, diabetes, cancer, and depression. Among their findings, the researchers noted that social media was effective in information sharing, providing support, and improving knowledge. That said, quantifiable, objective data to guide clinicians on using social media are limited, and further analysis is needed. More specific outcome-based research is needed to determine whether components beyond the psychosocial are affected and that physical outcomes have, in fact, been improved. Tailoring social media–driven programs to the person impacted by a particular disease is also critical. While the use of social media platforms holds promise, additional evidence-based research is needed to fully understand their impact for people suffering from chronic diseases.

Social Media and Surveillance

Based on the research of Bragazzi et al. [16], social media plays an important role in recent outbreaks of infectious diseases like Zika virus. Zika is an emerging global public health threat. As such, it generates social media interest worldwide. Social media is highly effective in rapidly alerting populations to emerging threats, capturing information about how many people are impacted, and identifying data streams through Google Trends, Twitter, YouTube, and Wikitrends, for example. The researchers recommend that public health practitioners, including global and local agencies, leverage web searches and interactions to investigate the disease information needs of populations, analyze general community sentiment, and assess risk. Social media is vital in the rapid dissemination of information to enhance surveillance efforts as an inexpensive and effective delivery system.

In another study, researchers implemented and analyzed the dissemination and surveillance of information from Mo-Buzz, a mobile pandemic surveillance system for Dengue fever [17]. Mo-Buzz is an app that was created to digitize the procurement of information from Dengue-affected sites. The app provided educational information, management recommendations, and updates about outbreak mapping for the public. Initial public acceptance and utilization were slow. However, once people understood how to use the app and became comfortable with it, Mo-Buzz ultimately became a viable option for the disease's surveillance. The researchers recommend that mobile and social media interventions like Mo-Buzz play a more significant role in identifying risk and managing disease outbreaks.

Benefits, Challenges, and Opportunities

The amount of people who have been actively participating in social media has been steadily increasing worldwide. Estimates indicate that about 79% of the U.S. population have a social media profile [18]. Facebook has more than 2.3 billion users [19]. There are many benefits to using social media to advocate for health on a personal level or the health of a population affected by a particular disease. Healthcare providers can use social media to reach out to their patients, develop a professional network, and inform the community where their practice is located. Apps, avatars, blogs, direct messaging, hashtags, tweets, tags, and wikis are among the tools that healthcare providers can use as part of a social media strategy to educate their patients about disease management [20]. Clearly, social media is a powerful resource to educate, promote, and inform patients. It is a potent connector on the worldwide stage of healthcare.

In a recent systematic review of the literature performed by Anderson-Lewis et al. [21], mobile health applications were shown to be a cost-effective platform that enables many people to access the Internet, text, or tweet to share health information. SMS text messaging is an easy, fast, and accessible strategy for healthcare providers to reach and communicate with patients to facilitate health promotion and management. Literature reviews also demonstrate that mobile platforms or mHealth, some examples of which have been discussed in this chapter, hold great potential for public health management. Since mHealth use is high in low-socioeconomic-status countries worldwide, the authors highlight the opportunity to decrease health disparities and promote health equity.

As discussed, social media is beneficial for promoting the spread of global health information, education, and data collection. It can also facilitate global awareness and the distribution of health products. Personal care products, which promote public health goals, are widely distributed through a plethora of social marketing channels. For example, in 2017, CVS Health, in partnership with the American Cancer Society, launched the Long Live Skin campaign. Skin cancer is "by far the most common type of cancer" [22]. Prevention and early detection are imperative. The Long Live Skin campaign leveraged a "multiplatform" approach to educating and informing people about skin health, care, safety, and related products [23]. The campaign included a dedicated social media program that encouraged engagement by asking people to share their skin care advice via Instagram and Twitter. Women were invited to participate in sharing their perspective with @CVSPharmacy, #AdviceToMyYoungerSelf. In conjunction with Johnson & Johnson as well, they also created additional content for their stores, circulars, and website to promote skin care and health. Combining social media with digital commerce platforms for chronic disease prevention and management represents a significant partnership opportunity for patients, public health and personal care companies and organizations, consumers, and pharmaceutical companies.

What are the perils of social media? The perils include poor information quality, damage to professional image, breaches of patient privacy, violation of the boundaries between patients and providers, licensing issues, and other legal issues. A strategy to mitigate these perils includes having organizations develop and implement guidelines that are adopted by healthcare providers. Social media creates many opportunities to communicate to a wide range of audiences, but policies for the effective utilization of social media practices are essential and a key component of good healthcare provider practice [20]. According to Antheunis et al. [24], the barriers to social media use differ for patients versus providers. For patients, the primary barriers are privacy and reliability of information presented on a social media platform. For providers, the primary barriers include inefficiency and skill gaps with using social media. The authors emphasize the importance of better understanding of respective users' motives, concerns, and goals.

Conclusion

Utilizing a variety of social media platforms is becoming the norm worldwide. They are used to share health information to rapidly promote awareness, educate patients, prevent exacerbations of chronic disease, inform the public of disease outbreaks, and create access to health/wellness products and services. Social media provides a relatively easy and low-cost way to reach many people and track information as data are collected. Additional research is needed to gain more specific knowledge about the outcomes and efficacy of specific social media platforms and modalities. For example, are certain platforms better able to reach and educate target populations? Are there other platforms that more reliably track data from disease outbreaks?

Social media is a complementary tool and not a replacement for seeking medical care from a healthcare professional [25]. According to Fung et al. [26], social media has a significant and notable role in public health surveillance. Important applications for social media in the intervention of public health emergencies include detection, awareness, monitoring, and communication. We are living in times of disease outbreaks and chronic disease management. Social media technologies are well equipped to quickly spread information globally, communicate strategies to prevent the spread of disease, and provide management tools.

Discussion

You are the new Executive Director of Prevent Colon Cancer, a community-based organization whose mission is to promote awareness and conduct screenings to reduce the prevalence of colon cancer in high-risk populations. Recently, you received credible data regarding the high prevalence of colon cancer in the communities your organization serves. You know you need to plan. Begin your plan by addressing the following questions:

1. Problem Statement: Identify a problem statement reflecting the public health issue. Identify the social media strategies you will employ.
2. Decision Criteria: Develop appropriate decision criteria that you will use in addressing the problem.
3. Planning and Priority Setting: Describe your short-term and long-term goals based on the information in the case study, chapter, and your professional experience.
4. Operational Issues: Identify at least one operational issue you may need to address along with a minimum of one potential strategy you might employ to mitigate it.
5. Evaluation: Identify a minimum of one organizational outcome that you will utilize to evaluate your success. Include in your rationale a consideration of how and how frequently you will measure the outcome.

References

1. U.S. Department of Health and Human Services Centers for Disease Control and Prevention. CDC Enterprise Social Media Policy updated Jan 8, 2015. https://www.cdc.gov/socialmedia/tools/guidelines/pdf/social-media-policy.pdf. Accessed 17 Aug 2018.
2. Heldman AB, Schindelar J, Weaver JB III. Social media engagement and public health communication implications for public health organizations being truly social. Public Health Rev. 2013;35:13.
3. Chou WY, Hunt YM, Beckjord EB, Moser RP, Hesse BW. Social media use in the United States: implications for health communication. J Med Internet Res. 2009;11(4):e48. https://doi.org/10.2196/jmir.1249.
4. World Health Organization. Global diffusion of eHealth: making universal health coverage achievable. 2016. https://www.who.int/goe/publications/global_diffusion/en/. Accessed 17 Aug 2018.
5. Chung-Hai Fung I, Zion THO, King-Wa F. The use of social media in public health surveillance. WPSAR. 2015;6(2):3–6. https://doi.org/10.5365/wpsar.2015.6.1.019.
6. Vayena E, Dzenowagis J, Brownstein JS, Sheikh A. Policy implications of big data in the health center. Bull World Health Organ. 2018;96:66–8. http://www.who.int/bulletin/volumes/96/1/17-197426.pdf. Accessed 17 Aug 2018.
7. Pershad Y, Hangge PT, Albadawi H, Okulu R. Social medicine: twitter in healthcare. J Clin Med. 2018;7(121):1–9. https://doi.org/10.3390/jcm7060121.
8. Anderson-Lewis C, Darville G, Mercado RE, Howell S, DiMaggio S. mHealth technology use and implications in historically underserved and minority populations in the United States: Systemic literature review. JMIR Mhealth Uhealth. 2018;6(6):1–17. https://doi.org/10.2196/mhealth.8383.
9. Schillinger D, Ling PM, Fine S. Reducing cancer and cancer disparities: Lessons from a youth –generated diabetes prevention campaign. Am J Prev Med. 2017;53(3S1):S103–13. https://doi.org/10.1016/j.amepre.2017.05.024.
10. Fernandez-Luques L, Singh M, Ofli F. Implementing 360 quantified self for childhood obesity; feasibility study and experiences from a weight loss camp in Qatar. BMC Med Inform Decis Mak. 2017;17(37). https://doi.org/10.1186/s12911-017-0432-6.
11. Abedin T, Al Mamun M, Lasker MAA, et al. Social media as a platform for information about diabetes foot care: a study of Facebook groups. Can J Diabetes. 2017;41:97–101. https://doi.org/10.1016/j.jcjd.2016.08.217.

12. AlQarni ZA, Yunas F, Househ MS. Health information sharing on Facebook: an exploratory study on diabetes mellitus. J Infect Public Health. 2016;9(6):708–12. https://doi.org/10.1016/j.jiph.2016.08.015.

13. Sobnath DD, Philip N, Kayyali R, et al. Features of a mobile support app for patients with chronic obstructive pulmonary disease: literature review and current applications. JMIR Mhealth Uhealth. 2017;5(2):e17. https://doi.org/10.2196/mhealth.4951.

14. Patel R, Chang T, Greysen SR, Chopra V. Social media use in chronic disease: a systematic review and novel taxonomy. Am J Med. 2015;128(12):1335–50. https://doi.org/10.1016/j.amjmed.2015.06.015.

15. Merolli M, Gray K, Martin-Sanchez F. Health outcomes and related effects of using social media in chronic disease management: a literature review and analysis of affordances. J Biomed Inform. 2013;46(6):957–69. https://doi.org/10.1016/j.jbi.2013.04.010.

16. Bragazzi NL, Alcino C, Trucchi C, et al. Global reaction to the recent outbreaks of Zika virus: insights from a big data analysis. PLoS One. 2017;12(9):e0185263. https://doi.org/10.1371/journal.pone.0185263.

17. Lwin OM, Jayasundar K, Sheldenkar A, et al. Lessons from the implementation of Mo-Buzz, a mobile pandemic surveillance system for Dengue. JMIR Public Health Surveill. 2017;3(4):e65. https://doi.org/10.2196/publichealth.7376.

18. Percentage of US population with a social media profile from 2008 to 2019. https://www.statista.com/statistics/273476/percentage-of-us-population-with-a-social-network-profile/

19. Number of monthly active Facebook users worldwide as of 1st quarter 2019 (in millions). https://www.statista.com/statistics/264810/number-of-monthly-active-facebook-users-worldwide/

20. Ventola CL. Social media and health care professionals: benefits, risks, and best practices. P T. 2014;39(7):491–520.

21. Anderson-Lewis C, Garville D. mHealth technology use and implications in historically underserved and minority populations in the United States: systematic literature review. JMIR Mhealth Uhealth. 2018;6(6):1–17. https://doi.org/10.2196/mhealth.8383:10.2196/mhealth.8383.

22. American Cancer Society. Skin cancer. https://www.cancer.org/cancer/skin-cancer.html

23. Pensa E. CVS Pharmacy launches long live skin campaign to increase awareness around sun safety and skin health. Published May 15, 2017. https://cvshealth.com/newsroom/press-releases/cvs-pharmacy-launches-long-live-skin-campaign-increase-awareness-around-sun

24. Antheunis ML, Tates K, Nieboer TE. Patients and health professionals use of social media in healthcare: motives, barriers, and expectations. Patient Educ Couns. 2013;92:426–31.

25. Hout TA, Alhinnawi H. Social media in public health. Br Med Bull. 2013;108:5–24. https://doi.org/10.1093/bmb/ldt028.

26. Fung I, Tse TZ. The use of social media in public health surveillance. WPSAR. 2015;6(2):3–6. https://doi.org/10.5365/wpsar.2015.6.1.019.

Chapter 3: The Role of Technology in Women's Empowerment and Well-Being and Addressing Gender-Based Violence

Padmini Murthy and Jonathan Ogulnick

Introduction

As the world gets ready to celebrate the 25th anniversary of the Beijing Declaration and Platform of Action in 2020, women and girls globally face discrimination and are being denied their human rights; this has a major impact on their health status. As a result, almost half of the world's population, i.e., women and girls, cannot enjoy a complete state of health as defined by the World Health Organization, which defines health as "a state of complete physical, mental and social well-being and not merely the absence of disease or infirmity" [1]. This asserts and reiterates the link between physical and mental well-being and human rights, which are essential to enable a life without limitations or restrictions.

History

The efforts and drive to engender information and communications technology (ICT) strategies to advance empowerment of women can be traced back to the Beijing Declaration and Platform for Action (BPfA), adopted by the Fourth World Conference on Women in 1995. The PfA identified gender mainstreaming

P. Murthy (✉)
New York Medical College School of Health Sciences and Practice, Valhalla, NY, USA

Medical Women's International Association and NGO Representative to United Nations, New York, NY, USA

American Medical Women's Association, Schaumburg, IL, USA
e-mail: padmini_murthy@nymc.edu

J. Ogulnick
New York Medical College School of Medicine, Valhalla, NY, USA

© Springer Nature Switzerland AG 2020
P. Murthy, A. Ansehl (eds.), *Technology and Global Public Health*,
https://doi.org/10.1007/978-3-030-46355-7_8

as a critical strategy for the advancement of women and girls and the improvement of their quality of life globally. In addition, the PfA, which is considered to be a landmark in promoting gender equity and empowerment, drew attention to the emerging global communications network and its impact on public policies, service delivery, and the private attitudes and behavior of stakeholders. The PfA called for the empowerment of women through enhancing their skills, knowledge, and access to and use of information technologies as a critical tool in promoting gender balance and harmony [2].

Best Practices of ICT

A good illustration of the empowerment of women is the rehabilitation of young sex workers in Nigeria, which is greatly enhanced by their acquisition of ICT skills. These skills, especially lessons in using computers, helped the affected young women to gain meaningful employment and facilitate their reintegration into mainstream society [2]. Despite the numerous barriers and challenges to gender equity in the ICT arena, various stakeholders have harnessed ICT as tools for social transformation and gender equality. Another example is how women artisans in India over the past few years have been directly accessing global markets through e-commerce initiatives and are using the Internet to support their business growth with market and production information. This results in greater income for these women, and the financial independence they gain enables them to improve their health status and that of their families as well [3].

Women of all ages will benefit on many levels from the inroads made by ICT in the domain of knowledge networking. The question we need to be asking ourselves is what are the mechanisms in place in ICT to ensure that the benefits that women accrue in the global community do not remain restricted to mere trickle-down effects but are made available to all and on par with those enjoyed by males? According to an interesting hypothesis put forth by Chandrashekar, at the conceptual level, ICT has the potential to digitally link all women in the world in a star topology network, which can open many windows for information exchange. He further states that this linkage could be used by women in creative ways, both to communicate with other people who are online and to disseminate information to the global community and to "disseminate information to people who are not on-line through the use of convergence and hybrid technologies such as community e-mails, community radio broadcast, tele-centres, newsletters, videos etc." [4]. This mechanism has the potential to change the lives of women in various communities to overcome the constraints of seclusion, mobilize resources, and gather support. This in turn can help them to explore markets to set up small businesses and open various avenues for imparting knowledge and life-long learning. Chandrashekar further suggests that the two spaces that women stand to gain a share in fall into the spheres of empowerment and governance [4].

Impact on Women's Work and Health

ICT is both empowering for women and an important contributing factor in globalization. A thorough analysis of the impact of information technology "on women's work in the context of globalization highlights the differences in the issues of information technology and women's work between developed and developing countries" [4].

The Self Employed Women's Association (SEWA) is a groundbreaking initiative established by Ila Bhatt in 1972 in the Indian state of Gujarat to protect and address the needs of poor textile workers, most of whom were women living below the poverty line. The founder and the board members of SEWA incorporated the principles of ensuring the health and well-being of their members while promoting work and income security to foster growth and gainful employment. These principles are crucial in steering the organization in the direction of their two important goals of full employment and self-reliance. In their inbuilt evaluation and monitoring process, the following 11 questions were incorporated [5].

The Eleven Questions of SEWA [5]:

1. Have more members obtained more employment?
2. Has their income increased?
3. Have they obtained food and nutrition?
4. Has their health been safeguarded?
5. Have they obtained childcare?
6. Have they obtained or improved their housing?
7. Have their assets increased (e.g., their own savings, land, house, workspace, tools or work, licenses, identity cards, cattle, and share in cooperatives, and all in their own name)?
8. Has the workers' organizational strength increased?
9. Have workers' leadership skills increased?
10. Have they become self-reliant both collectively and individually?
11. Have they become literate?

The first seven questions highlight the criteria for evaluating the first goal of full employment, and the remaining four are the criteria for the second goal of self-reliance: to educate women and improve their health status and that of their families. SEWA is unique in that the members themselves have produced short videos on how to address diarrhea through oral rehydration therapy, and these are distributed through their own networks [3]. This is an example of meeting targets of the UN's Sustainable Development Goal (SDG) 3, health for all at all ages, and SDG 5, which addresses women's empowerment using technology.

e-Education

Since the late 1990s and early 2000s, the use of technology, such as television, apps for smartphones and tablets, and radio, has opened up new avenues for informal and continued education for adult learners. These technological innovations have been effective in delivering educational contact to women and girls who may be constrained by lack of access to education due to geographic and cultural barriers. The use of massive open online courses (MOOCS) offers an affordable and flexible way for women to learn new skills, advance their knowledge, and help to reduce the gender gap in education. Nongovernmental organizations and foundations have in recent years become very proactive in working with governments to strengthen the public education system. The Azim Premji Foundation in India has been a leader in using technology to benefit girls and women. The foundation has produced CD ROMs incorporating content based on primary schools' curriculum which is gender sensitive, uses local dialects to promote inclusiveness, and increases rates of education for girls. In addition, the foundation has launched a new initiative that focuses on educational leadership for girls and women [3, 6].

Role of United Nations and Private Sector in Promoting Use of Technology among Women

At the World Summit on the Information Society held in Geneva in 2003, with a follow-up in 2005 in Tunis in 2005, the member states of the United Nations came together to partner and work to promote the use of technology to meet the targets of the Millennium Development Goals. The Tunis commitment recognized the existence of a gender divide in the society, and member states reaffirmed their commitment to encourage and work with stakeholders across disciplines to encourage and increase the full participation of women as contributors in the world of technology in local, national, and international arenas. The crucial role played by technology in promoting the human rights of children and protecting them from abuse was another important commitment made at this conference [7]. The World Health Organization, Pan-American Health Organization, United Nations Population Fund, UNICEF, and World Bank have been incorporating the use of technology to empower and educate women, and these initiatives have resulted in increasing the health status of women and their families. According to a report released by UNICEF, of the 600 million adolescent girls in the world, most live in low- and middle-income countries. Unfortunately, many of these young girls are not able to reach their full potential owing to the various barriers they encounter and challenges they face. For example, almost 1000 young women are newly infected by HIV daily, and more than 13 million young girls become child brides every year. A partnership between UNICEF and Gucci was launched in 2017 known as the Girls' Empowerment Initiative, which utilized partnerships, communication tools, and advocacy efforts by stakeholders. This led to the utilization of U Report, which is a social messaging tool with over 1.3 million young girls, known as U reporters, from 35 countries. This is an empowering platform for girls to discuss their challenges, communicate with each other, and share best practices. In May 2017, a global poll was conducted on menstrual hygiene in which 45,000 girl U reporters participated. There was a discussion on the challenges young girls faced during their menstrual cycle and how they could not attend school because of the lack of bathrooms and other sanitary products for girls. This is a great example of best practice where technology was used to empower girls to have discuss menstruation and how they could address the challenges they face globally. It is also an illustration of addressing SDGs 3 and 5. UNICEF, based on the data collected from platforms such as U Report, has launched initiatives and solutions in partnership with governments, foundations, and the private sector to help girls manage their periods by providing access to feminine hygiene products. UNICEF also supports water sanitation and hygeine (WASH) to ensure separate toilets for girls in schools [8]. Thus, technology is a powerful tool in promoting the health and well-being of women and girls and addressing the global pandemic of gender-based violence.

Role of Technology in Violence Against Women

It would be naive to take a black-and-white stance regarding the role technology plays in either enhancing or harming people's lives in our contemporary, global community. Rather, the proper approach would be to view technology's role in the same way we would view one of our friends – it has flaws and imperfections, sometimes detrimental, that we accept in light of its net positive contributions to our lives. With regard to women around the globe today, this dichotomy is especially unforgiving and needs to be addressed by officials at all levels of government, medicine, and industrial technology in order to resolve problems amenable to solution that have the potential to ruin, or even end, women's lives. This chapter will explore the length of the spectrum of ways in which technology affects women's lives, from enhanced empowerment and safety, cyberbullying, and the deleterious effects of social media on mental health to scams targeted at older women.

Technology and Women's Safety

One of the unfortunate truths of human existence that has been universally true in all of recorded history is the vulnerability of women to abuse of virtually every imaginable category. But fortunately, while this truth holds true in contemporary society, it is progressively being mitigated with the help of convenient and increasingly ubiquitous technological advances. The technological advancement that will be closely looked at in this chapter, due to both its practicality and global pervasiveness, is the use of smartphone apps to promote women's safety and their ability to help women escape from either potentially or imminently dangerous situations. Varsha et al. compiled a survey of Android apps that can be used to protect women from violence and harassment [9]. Many of these apps operate by sending either trusted contacts or emergency responders the victims' GPS location. Certain apps that are already commercially available for both Android and iOS systems [10] will be summarized in this chapter.

1. *Circleof6*: This app, originally marketed to college students, won the Obama Administration's Apps Against Abuse challenge back in 2011. Users choose up to six trusted contacts and have the option to use any of the following features: Come Get Me, which sends a text with the user's GPS coordinates to contacts, and Call Me, which sends a text to contacts that reads "Call and pretend you need me. I need an interruption" [10].

2. *uSafeUS*: This app is free to download. However, the purpose of the app is for institutions, such as universities, to license the app and customize the content based on the population for whom its licensing was intended. It connects users to local resources such as law enforcement and counseling. The app also has a list of steps to take following a sexual assault. Its target audience is all members of a university community, such as students, faculty, staff, alumni, and others. The app has several features such as "Time to Leave," which sends an automated call sounding like an urgent request from a roommate; "Expect Me," which will alert a friend if you do not show up to an expected destination; and "Angel Drink," which can communicate to a bartender that the user feels as if they are in an unsafe situation [10].

3. *bSafe*: This app champions the slogan "Never Walk Alone." It has voice features, such as voice alarm activation, video and audio recording, and live streaming, that allow trusted contacts to actively monitor the user's activities. Like several other personal safety apps, it has a fake call feature, allowing the user to escape a potentially dangerous situation. Its most salient feature is an SOS signal that can be sent with a voice command, even when the user is not physically holding her phone. This enables trusted contacts to be quickly alerted of any distress being felt by the user [9].

4. *VithU*: A very simple app in terms of design and concept but with an element of surreptitiousness that other apps do not. It simply has a panic button that, when pressed twice, sends an alert to trusted contacts that reads "I am in danger. I need help. Please follow my location." This message gets sent repeatedly every two minutes, each time with the user's real-time location. As with the other apps, the user inputs a list of trusted contacts beforehand. Additionally, VithU has a function that sends the user tips during an active emergency [9].

Of course, while potentially quite useful, these apps have limitations. For example, one cannot assume that an inebriated person will necessarily have the wherewithal to launch and successfully operate a safety app. In addition, while their use is becoming increasingly widespread, these apps are not necessarily accessible to women who either cannot afford or choose not to have a smartphone. The apps that rely on the use of GPS coordinates pose another problem: keeping GPS tracking enabled on one's smartphone raises potential privacy issues in that an abuser may be able to determine a woman's location, which clearly poses a problem. Because of these apps' novelty, more studies are needed, at least at the time of this chapter's writing, to analyze the efficacy of women's safety apps, though some investigations have shown promising results. Glass et al. demonstrated in their 2015 paper that a decision-making app they developed was effective at preventing dating violence among homosexual women college students [11]. Despite the potential quibbles, when all is said and done, anything that helps to reduce violence against women on any scale is very welcome.

Cyberbullying and Cyberstalking

While social media does present the opportunity for people to stay connected in a truly globalized world, this increased connectedness does have potential drawbacks, namely, regarding cyberbullying and cyberstalking. This chapter will specifically address ways in which cyberbullying and cyberstalking commonly manifest, how women are disproportionately affected, how prevention should be front and center in the discussion on these crimes and approaches to dealing with the consequences of cybercrime. Given the fact that cyberstalking and cyberbullying are relatively new phenomena, the data collected in recent years is somewhat limited. However, some trends have been identified. Victims of cyberstalking are overwhelmingly women and girls. Two factors in addition to being a woman that predispose a person to being a victim of cyberstalking are being young and being gender nonconforming. While Internet stalking by strangers is, of course, a significant problem, it cannot be forgotten that some of the most common perpetrators of Internet stalking are intimate partners. A survey of 152 domestic violence advocates and 46 domestic violence victims shows that Internet-accessible technology, such as phones, tablets, and computers, as well as social networking sites, is commonly abused to facilitate the stalking of intimate partners [11]. According to Woodcock's survey, the most common ways in which these media are used to harass domestic violence victims include threatening to share sexual content of the victims online to humiliate them and creating a sense that the perpetrator is omnipresent and the victim is isolated. In the realm of cyberbullying, the most alarming statistic is its sheer prevalence and the fact that it is so pervasive in intimate relationships. Durán et al. showed in a retrospective study of 219 college students that 48.4% of participants reported having bullied their partners during the last year via mobile phone and 37.5% via Internet [12]. These data clearly demonstrate that cyberbullying and cyberstalking are sufficiently widespread and destructive that governmental and nongovernmental organizations owe it to women everywhere to reform society's current approach to Internet crime.

First and foremost, no matter what laws are in place to prevent Internet violence and penalize their perpetrators, they will be of absolutely no use if women do not feel sufficiently safe, comfortable, protected, and private when responding to the crime of which they were a victim. In addition, would preventing cyberbullying and cyberstalking in the first place not be preferable to victims having to face the psychological consequences of dealing with their perpetrators' actions? In a poll of 1004 university students on the ways in which respondents felt cyberbullying and cyberstalking should best be addressed in a university setting [13], the most common recommendations were for the university to post advertisements with famous people condemning Internet violence, enabling anonymous reporting, and terminating Internet privileges of perpetrators. The proposals that were least appealing to students were those that involved police interventions, mandatory reporting, or suspension, communicating that students are indeed in favor of primary prevention as opposed to necessarily promoting punitive measures. Despite the fact that this study only included university students, it makes a salient point – that a comprehensive preventive approach that incorporates real feedback is the best way to prevent crimes whose consequences to the women victimized are so numerous and severe that they cannot be addressed in the context of this chapter.

Just as important to women who have already been victims of cybercrime is how they deal with the consequences. While research on the help-seeking behavior of cybercrime victims is limited, a survey of 477 cyberstalking victims showed that "cyberstalking victims who experienced more serious offenses had increased odds of engaging in reporting and both types of help-seeking behaviors. Furthermore, victims who were cyberstalked by their current intimate partner had greater odds of engaging in reporting and professional help-seeking behaviors" [14]. This survey shows that the willingness of victims to engage in self-help behavior is directly related to how severe the crime was and how intimate they were with the perpetrator. However, a limited numbers of studies demonstrate specific help-seeking behaviors women engage in and how the residua of the crimes are dealt with. It is essential to note that these limitations in and of themselves express society's need to engage victims of cybercrimes more empathetically and with greater alacrity.

Social Media and Self-Image

In addition to facilitating cyberbullying and cyberstalking, as addressed earlier in this chapter, social media also represents a medium that can be used to promote deleterious notions of women's self-image and perceptions of what an ideal image is. This is, once again, an unfortunate side effect of something that allows for non-physical, potentially meaningful relationships as well as facilitated communication in already existing relationships. This section will focus on how social media can negatively affect a woman's self-image outside the context of cyberbullying, focusing more on the propagation of societal standards. The most salient problem with social media–related self-image issues is the exposure of women to an idealized version of what a twenty-first-century woman should look like. On a more immediately tangible level, part of this stems simply from one's ability to manipulate images one posts on social media. A variety of filters are available on most mainstream social media sites (e.g., Instagram, Facebook) that can ostensibly enhance one's appearance by covering up blemishes and giving the photo more aesthetically pleasing lighting. This is obviously not a realistic portrayal of one's true appearance, and while it is not inherently harmful to try to make a photo of oneself more flattering, it certainly encourages one to compare oneself with others, which can be detrimental to one's self-image. Besides exposure to enhanced photos of one's peers, the response to one's own photos has the potential for negative consequences. This could manifest itself either as a perceived lack of positive feedback (e.g., not enough "likes" on one's photo or not enough positive commentary) or critical feedback, which has also been shown to be one of the factors, even outside the context of cyberbullying, that have a negative impact on women's and girls' self-esteem.

The third issue that promotes a negative self-image via social media is exposure to celebrities, whom we are led to believe represent the ideal standard of beauty. Thankfully, research has shown that these issues can be mitigated, the most effective method to do so in women being increased exposure to social media literacy [15]. Even more promising is that the same study by Gooding et al. demonstrated that these exposure mitigation effects were independent of internalization or body comparison [16]. Another promising feature of these results is that social media literacy education is inexpensive and easily disseminated. Since adolescent girls are often just beginning to incorporate social media into their lives and are also the most susceptible to having labile body images, it only makes sense that social media literacy should be introduced by schools as a means of primary prevention. Numerous companies and organizations already provide this type of education, removing another barrier for schools. One such organization is Future Classroom Lab by European Schoolnet, which has a multitude of online classes, webinars, interactive classrooms, learning labs, and projects for students to do [17]. It is clear not only that this is a problem worth addressing but that there is a means to do so; and given its feasibility, the onus is on schools to incorporate social media literacy into their curricula. Is being happy and content not worth it for its own sake? If there are feasible and readily accessible methods to reduce the discontentment associated with body-image issues, are those not worth incorporating into schools for no other reason than to help women and girls live happy lives? With all the issues women face whose solutions are not so clear cut, and even though social media–induced negative self-image is too complex an issue to be cured with a magic bullet, it only makes sense to do what we can when we can do it.

Online Scams Targeting Middle-Aged and Older Women

While the issues previously discussed in this chapter do, by and large, primarily affect younger women and girls, older women are not immune to being victimized, with technology as the weapon. A study by Monica Whitty demonstrated that "Romance scam victims tend to be middle-aged, well-educated women. Moreover, they tend to be more impulsive (scoring high on urgency and sensation seeking), less kind, more trustworthy, and have an addictive disposition" [18]. These scams are perpetrated most commonly on social media and dating sites and by e-mail, although sometimes even telephone calls are used. This type of scam is commonly referred to as "catfishing." Scammers will typically lure in their victims with false and often alluring profiles, incorporating fake names or fraudulently used names of real people such as military officers or foreign doctors and pictures of attractive people other than themselves, and will generally express loving and passionate emotions very early on. Most commonly, they pretend to be from foreign, Western countries but work overseas. They will do whatever it takes to build the victim's trust, such as by sending gifts, using loving words, and even falsely making plans to visit. Once they gain the victim's trust, they will often then pretend to need the victim's money for some sort of emergency, such as urgent medical or travel costs. Once the victim has been successfully bamboozled, the monetary losses and emotional betrayal are often difficult, and even impossible, to recover from [19]. Primary prevention of this type of crime mostly relies on potential targets being aware of the warning signs: poorly written messages, proposals to move away from the dating site to a more private method of communication, expressions of strong emotions after only a few contacts, requests for money after gaining the victim's trust, and failures to keep promises to meet the victim in person. Being aware of this is, of course, easier said than done. Dating websites can take the initiative by providing mandatory materials to new members that promote awareness of potential risk factors for romance scams. Social media sites can play their part by advancing screening for new members such as with automatic cross-referencing of profile pictures and names with those found on search engines. Despite the reality that most victims of cybercrimes are young women and girls, middle-aged and elderly women are not immune to such crimes. Romance scams disproportionately affect women, especially middle-aged widowers, and result in tremendous emotional and financial consequences. If increased action on the part of online dating sites and social media platforms can help to reduce the incidence of these crimes, then it is their responsibility to society to do so.

Conclusion

Throughout human history, women have always faced a set of societal issues targeted directly at them, and unfortunately, as we move into a globalized, technological era, the issues that face women evolve concurrently with technology. But when all is said and done, technology-facilitated violence against women (TFVW) can be conquered if bright and enthusiastic minds direct their focus toward it. It has been done before – as recently as 2018, when women in Saudi Arabia were finally granted the right to drive automobiles [20]. In time, with sufficient effort, TFVW will be eliminated much like bans on women driving. As discussed in this chapter, technology can also be pivotal in empowering women and ensuring that they enjoy health in the complete sense as defined by the constitution of the World Health Organization.

References

1. World Health Organization. Constitution. 2019. Retrieved from https://www.who.int/about/who-we-are/constitution. Accessed 10 July 2019.
2. United Nations. Division for the Advancement of Women (DAW) International Telecommunication Union (ITU) United Nations ICT Task Force Secretariat. In: Marcelle MG, editor. Information and communication technologies (ICT) and their impact on and use as an instrument for the advancement and empowerment of women. 2003. Retrieved from https://www.un.org/womenwatch/daw/egm/ict2002/reports/Report-online.PDF. Accessed 10 July 2019.
3. Lal SB. Impact of information and communication technologies on women empowerment in India. Syst Cybern Inform. 2011;9(4). Retrieved from http://www.iiisci.org/Journal/CV$/sci/pdfs/QN001HZ.pdf. Accessed 10 July 2019. ISSN: 1690-4524.
4. Chandrasekhar CP. Promoting ICT for human development in Asia: realizing the millennium development goals, India Country Paper, for Regional Bureau for Asia and the Pacific. United Nations Development Programme (UNDP). 2003.
5. Self Employment Women's Association – SEWA. 2009. Retrieved from http://www.sewa.org/About_Us_Goals.asp. Accessed 10 July 2019
6. Azim Premji Foundation. Who we are. 2017. Retrieved from https://azimpremjifoundation.org/about/who-we-are. Accessed 10 July 2019.
7. United Nations. World Summit on the information society Geneva-2003 Tunis – 2005. WSIS-05/TUNIS/DOC/7-E. 2005. Retrieved from http://www.itu.int/net/wsis/docs2/tunis/off/7.html. Accessed 10 July 2019.
8. Malhota A, Alleman P. Empowering adolescent girls is investing in a bright future. UNICEF. 2017. Retrieved from https://blogs.unicef.org/blog/empowering-adolescent-girls/. Accessed 10 July 2019.
9. Varsha SK, Seetha G, Sasikala S, Srikanth GU. A survey on android applications for personal security. Int J Mod Trend Eng Res. 2017;4(2):1–7. https://doi.org/10.21884/ijmter.2017.4043.sgbkp.
10. Aubrey A. Feel in danger on a date? These apps could help you stay safe. NPR. https://www.npr.org/sections/health-shots/2017/12/18/571086219/on-a-bad-date-these-apps-could-help-you-stay-safe. Published 18 December 2017. Accessed 30 June 2019.
11. Bloom T, Gielen A, Glass N. Developing an app for college women in abusive same-sex relationships and their friends. J Homosex. 2015;63(6):855–74. https://doi.org/10.1080/00918369.2015.1112597.
12. Woodlock D. The abuse of technology in domestic violence and stalking. Violence Against Women. 2016;23(5):584–602. https://doi.org/10.1177/1077801216646277.
13. Martinez-Pecino R, Durán M. I love you but I cyberbully you: the role of hostile sexism. J Interpers Violence. 2016;34(4):812–25. https://doi.org/10.1177/0886260516645817.
14. Cunningham CE, Chen Y, Vaillancourt T, et al. Modeling the anti-cyberbullying preferences of university students: adaptive choice-based conjoint analysis. Aggress Behav. 2014;41(4):369–85. https://doi.org/10.1002/ab.21560.
15. Fissel ER. The reporting and help-seeking behaviors of cyberstalking victims. J Interper Violence. 2018:088626051880194. https://doi.org/10.1177/08862605188019428. Tamplin NC, Mclean SA, Paxton SJ. Social media literacy protects against the negative impact of

exposure to appearance ideal social media images in young adult women but not men. Body Image 2018;26:29–37. https://doi.org/10.1016/j.bodyim.2018.05.003.

16. Hausmann JS, Touloumtzis C, White MT, Colbert JA, Gooding HC. Adolescent and young adult use of social media for health and its implications. J Adoles Health. 2017;60(6):714–9. https://doi.org/10.1016/j.jadohealth.2016.12.025.

17. About – FCL. Go to FCL. http://fcl.eun.org/about;jsessionid=7634765D169ECE32217BA380 EA8AAB47. Accessed 3 July 2019.

18. Whitty MT. Do you love me? Psychological characteristics of romance scam victims. Cyberpsychol Behav Soc Netw. 2018;21(2):105–9. https://doi.org/10.1089/cyber.2016.0729.

19. Australian Competition and Consumer Commission. Dating & romance. Australian Competition and Consumer Commission. https://www.scamwatch.gov.au/types-of-scams/dating-romance. Published 4 January 2018. Accessed 3 July 2019.

20. Sant SV. Saudi Arabia lifts ban on female drivers. NPR. https://www.npr.org/2018/06/24/622990978/saudi-arabia-lifts-ban-on-women-drivers. Published 24 June 2018. Accessed 3 July 2019.

Chapter 4: Telehealth and Homecare Agencies

Amy Ansehl and Timothy Leddy

Introduction

The world is facing a marked increase in the population older than 60 years of age. The world's population over 60 years will nearly double from 12% to 22%. By 2020, the number of people over 60 will be much greater than the number of children aged 5 years and younger. Furthermore, there will be unprecedented challenges based on these demographics. The pace of population aging is moving much faster than in past decades. Global life expectancy will increase from 68.6 years in 2015 to 76.2 years in 2050. The global population of people over the age of 80 years is expected to triple between 2015 and 2050. In Asia and Latin America, the oldest population is expected to quadruple. Worldwide noncommunicable diseases, as well as communicable diseases, will continue to be a huge burden. Noncommunicable diseases are also known as chronic diseases and include heart failure (HF), diabetes, hypertension, and chronic obstructive pulmonary disease (COPD). Chronic diseases pose a significant risk to global population health, much like communicable or infectious diseases do. In the United States, in the period 2012–2050, there will be formidable growth in the older population. For example, by 2050, the over-65 population will nearly double in size based on current estimates and be at approximately 84 million people. The population referred to as the baby boomers that were born post-World War II will be over the age of 85. The percentage of females in the age bracket over 85 is expected to represent 66.6% of the population. An interesting concept is the dependency ratio. Dependency ratios are an indicator of the potential

A. Ansehl (✉)
New York Medical College School of Health Sciences and Practice, Valhalla, NY, USA

Visiting Nurse Services, Westchester Foundation, White Plains, NY, USA
e-mail: amy_ansehl@nymc.edu

T. Leddy
Westchester VNS, White Plains, NY, USA

© Springer Nature Switzerland AG 2020
P. Murthy, A. Ansehl (eds.), *Technology and Global Public Health*,
https://doi.org/10.1007/978-3-030-46355-7_9

burden of a particular population. By 2030, there will be an equalization of the youth and old-age population, specifically meaning they will each be half of the population. Another important trend is that as people age in the United States, the older population is becoming more diverse, with minorities representing 39.1%, an increase of 19% over 2012.

The United States is not alone in this aging-of-the-population trend. Drivers of mortality or survivorship in developed nations have increased. In Sweden, life expectancy at age 65 increased from 15.7 years in 1972 to 19.8 years in 2010. Life expectancy at age 85 in Sweden increased from 4.9 years in 1972 to 6.2 years in 2015. Interestingly, the United States population is still not as old as that of many other developed countries. For example, Germany, Italy, and Japan have seen increased numbers of older people over the age of 65. By 2013, Japan will be the oldest country with close to one-third of its population over age 65. Germany follows at 27.9% and Italy at 25.5%. In contrast, the United States is projected to be at 20.3% by 2030. Youth dependency ratios in Japan, Italy, Spain, and Poland are projected to decrease between 2012 and 2030. Canada, France, and the United Kingdom show slight dependency ratio increases. China, which has the world's largest population, will also have the oldest population, and India will have the second oldest population. The size of the older population in China will be greater than the total United States population [1–5].

This chapter will identify, explore, and discuss those challenges in the contextual framework of an aging population worldwide that will place even greater stress on the healthcare system and require the utilization of information and communications technology (ICT) [6]. We will explore together on a global scale the evidence-based research that looks at home care agencies and the continuum of the provision of healthcare services and in particular telehealth. Why? Home care agencies are an integral part of promoting health and keeping people with chronic diseases from utilizing emergency rooms and being rehospitalized. Most people prefer to recuperate in their own homes rather than recover in a hospital. There is also promising evidence that home care services are less costly in many cases where appropriate than care delivered in the hospital. Technology plays a pivotal role in enabling people to access supportive services in their homes.

The Role of Home Care Agencies in the Aging Worldwide Landscape

As people worldwide live longer, they have more chronic healthcare conditions. Home health agencies are defined as organizations that are engaged in providing skilled nursing services and other rehabilitation services in people's homes. Home health services play a critical role in achieving healthcare policy goals to enhance care coordination among providers to extend care beyond the four walls of the physician's office to prevent initial hospitalizations. Home health agencies also have a meaningful role in care transitions. Care transitions refer to providing care to a patient after an acute episode or return from the hospital. The home health agency team provides medication reconciliation in a patient's home, and this intervention is led by a registered nurse who coordinates the care instructions from multiple physicians and the hospital. Home health services are one of the fastest growing businesses in the healthcare sector. At the same time, there are major challenges. For example, there is an urgent need for technological innovation so that the care provided is both efficient and effective [7]. Telehealth is a remote monitoring technology that is emerging as a potential solution in the management of people with chronic diseases in their homes [8]. A wide spectrum of services can be provided in home-based care to support patients, which includes personal care, skilled nursing, and rehabilitative services. Rehabilitative services include physical therapy, speech and language therapy, and occupational therapy. It is paramount that care be delivered in the most efficient and effective way. According to the U.S. Medicare Payment Advisory Commission, 9.5% of fee-for-service beneficiaries used home healthcare services. In addition, 86% of home healthcare users are 65 years of age or older, 63% are 75 or older, nearly 30% are 85 or older, and 83.2% of patients receiving home healthcare services are over 85 years of age. As more senior citizens live longer, home healthcare has an important role in keeping people healthy, improving healthcare quality, and outcomes [7]. The concept of the Triple Aim developed by the U.S. Health and Human Services Administration in 2009 is extremely relevant at present and will be in the future as it applies to the delivery of healthcare services. It has three goals: improving the patient experience of care, improving the health of the population, and reducing costs. Patient satisfaction and quality of services are inherent in the Triple Aim [7]. The vision and framework for the future of home-based care include expanding and offering more people worldwide the option to receive care in their home. This can include primary care services for acute care services. New and alternative healthcare delivery models can play a vital role in providing high-quality and efficient services. Four pillars for the home care agency of the future are postacute care, acute care, primary care, and long-term care. Home care agencies of the future need to be considered key partners with other healthcare organizations, and they must have interoperability with their respective partner's health information technology platforms to receive and communicate important healthcare data in a secure manner [7].

What Is Telehealth and How Is It a Component of E-Health?

"E-health is defined as the use of information and communication technologies in support of health to improve the efficiency and effectiveness of healthcare management and delivery" [6]. E-health has many benefits in supporting system management, thereby improving the effectiveness of the delivery of healthcare services to the population. There are many benefits of e-health. These include access to healthcare services, reducing shortages of healthcare professionals, reducing healthcare professional isolation, improving healthcare worker retention, and presenting opportunities for both patient and provider communication and education. E-health facilitates the expansion of healthcare delivery and can optimize patient outcomes in developed and underdeveloped countries. A recent study in Uganda demonstrated that improving healthcare providers' ICT skills has the potential to improve individual and population-based health [6]. This is a very important consideration because a systematic review of the literature developed by Radhakrishnan et al. [9] also confirmed the importance of training home care providers in telehealth in order to achieve sustainability of telehealth and e-health initiatives in home care agencies.

The terms telehealth and telemedicine have different meanings, though in many articles and other media sources they are used interchangeably. Telehealth refers to a broader range of healthcare services, whereas telemedicine is narrower in focus. Telemedicine refers to remote clinical services. Telehealth also incorporates surveillance, health promotion, and public health functions. E-health is a bigger umbrella term that includes both telemedicine and telehealth. E-health includes the delivery of health information to a wider audience. This wider audience captures consumers, healthcare professionals, health workers and their education and training, and health systems management through the World Wide Web.

Key Terms and Definitions

We have already discussed the concepts of e-health, telehealth, and telemedicine. In this new frontier of technology in the home, other important technological strategies are also used to advance the care of patients. Telehomecare is a type of telehealth that is used in the patient's home. The advantage of telehomecare is that clinical information is communicated using telephone lines. Various information can be communicated using telephone lines that includes but is not limited to the patient's vital sign statistics such as body weight, blood pressure, pulse or heart rate, and body fluid input and output. The interaction of voice and video enables home care providers to recognize the early warning signs of an acute exacerbation of a patient's chronic or episodic health condition. The reason this is important is twofold in preventing the patient from having to be seen in an emergency department or being readmitted to a hospital [7].

Teleeducation refers to using the live interaction of educational information remotely for the purpose of teaching or training patients in strategies to self-manage their chronic conditions. For example, in diabetes this means education on how to inject insulin [8]. Telemonitoring is a process whereby the health status of patients with chronic conditions is monitored remotely. In home care, many agencies were early adopters of teleheart programs to monitor the vital signs of patients who were discharged from the hospital with HF. Telerehabilitation is an application of telehealth that uses telecommunication approaches to provide interventions that necessitate rehabilitation. The benefit of this approach is that it enables patients to receive a physical or occupational therapy session without having to leave their home. For many elderly or disabled patients, this increases access to health-promoting treatment. Telerehabilitation is an approach supervised by a therapist that encompasses checkup, monitoring, education, and training. It can also be an adjunctive therapy that is part of a patient care plan that also includes office-based physical or occupational therapies [8].

Telehealth, Chronic Diseases, and Home Care Agencies

Tele-homecare is defined as a communication and clinical information system that enabled the interaction of voice, video, and health-related data using ordinary telephone lines from the patient's homes to home health agencies in conjunction with skilled nurses' home visits [8].

The Alliance for Home Health Quality and Innovation reports that the delivery of services in a patient's home is the least costly postacute setting for delivering services. Home healthcare represents only 38.7% of all Medicare episodes using postacute care but accounts for only 27.8% of payments [9]. Numerous home healthcare studies illustrate the value of home healthcare agencies as a provider of subacute care, skilled nursing, and rehabilitative services. A recent case study compendium from the Visiting Nurse Associations of America (VNAA) demonstrates the importance of using technology in changing and adapting new programs to build partnerships between organizations to improve the delivery of home health services [10]. Typically, home care patients have multiple chronic conditions, and agencies have become "engines of innovation." Examples of this include reconciling medications and coordinating care through electronic communications. A nurse call button is linked to a call center, and the staff at the call center respond to the client and review the discharge instructions, arrange for food delivery, doctor appointments, and medication reminders. In essence, the call button provides "discharge security." As a result of this call button strategy, patients report increased satisfaction rates and decreased hospitalizations. Also reported was a decrease in high-risk patients going to the emergency department at their local hospital. In sum, acute hospitalization rates were reduced by four percentage points. Issues included some technical problems and language barriers because the teleremote company did not have a language interpreter in several cases.

Telehealth is being used by home care agencies in the management of HF or COPD. It is a widely used tool to provide daily monitoring to prevent symptom severity and rehospitalization. It also reinforces self-care among patient participants. Approximately half of patients in a teleheart program or telelung program demonstrated improvements in self-care. Patient satisfaction scores were high. Cost savings were estimated at more than $100,000 during the pilot year as a result of preventing avoidable hospitalizations. Integrated care models (ICMs) are designed to facilitate a more patient-centered care approach that embraces the concept of the Triple Aim, as discussed earlier in the chapter. Specifically, an ICM goal includes improving the quality of care and patient satisfaction while lowering associated costs. Many home care agencies use this integrated approach and send out to patient homes multidisciplinary teams composed of nurses and professionals from other fields like social work, physical therapy, speech and language therapy, and occupational therapy. This enables a whole-patient perspective. A whole-patient perspective is vital. The clinician must look at the patient in the context of the social determinants of health. This specifically relates to the patient and his or her environment. We look at the patient as more than just the sum of her diseases. How does the social context determine whether the patient is able to take her medications or take responsibility for her own care? Does the patient have a support system in place? How does where the patient lives and who if any are the patient's support system fit into the context of preventing illness or further exacerbation of an existing illness? This is what we mean when we discuss the social determinants of health as it relates to a patient in home care. The thought process behind it is that this approach will be more in line with meeting the goals of the triple aim.

The old model of delivering home health services was a traditional fee-for-service model, and healthcare providers were in silos. Many home care agencies are moving away from automatically having a nurse manage the team. Since the team providing the care is composed of professionals from different disciplines, there is no reason why a rehabilitation specialist cannot manage the team. ICMs focus on competency-based self-care management skills to enable patients to develop experience and confidence in managing their care. On a broader scale, it is not sustainable to develop patient dependence on a nurse or other healthcare provider if patients can be empowered to take on a meaningful role in their own care and learn prevention strategies from healthcare professionals to prevent further exacerbations. Embedded in an ICM paradigm is hardwiring the model so that consistent and high quality of care is front and center in healthcare service delivery. This requires the electronic medical record (EMR) to be fully functional and interoperable with other platforms. Why is this essential? Real-time data must be critiqued and evaluated for the purpose of identifying barriers to patient adherence early on as well as establishing metrics to demonstrate progress and assist the healthcare team in achieving the quality of care and patient satisfaction goals.

An EMR is an integral tool as part of any continuous quality program of a home care agency or any other organization that provides the delivery of healthcare services. In addition, in another VNAA compendium study, EMRs that were used to disseminate an ICM demonstrated a reduction in acute hospitalizations from 29% to 14%. The turnover of registered nurses was reduced from 20% to 6%, and there was also evidence of an increase in patient satisfaction [10]. To drive meaningful and sustainable change, technology must be partnered with benchmarks that capture what other home care agencies are doing in a given area as well as at the state and national levels. Critical thinking about the way an organization and its healthcare professionals deliver care to their patients is the most effective and efficient way to drive the right type of organizational change. An interesting pilot study focusing on bringing primary care services to the homes of seniors over 80 years old who are afflicted with mobility limitations found that technology had an important role to play. Technology, whether through telehealth or another modality, has been found to increase access to primary care and decrease acute exacerbations of chronic illnesses, which often lead to unwanted emergency department visits. Other specific benefits of this pilot study include disease management education, peace of mind for patients and their families, and cost savings. The Agency for Healthcare Research and Quality reported that telemedicine was beneficial for patients with chronic health conditions [10].

Chronic Disease Telehealth and Nutrition

"Telehealth interventions allow healthcare providers and patients to communicate by phone, email, web-based programs, or other electronic digital media. Healthcare providers and patients may also interact in person, though in comprehensive telehealth interventions, most of the interactions are distance-based" [11]. A systematic review of the literature confirmed that long-term management of chronic disease is beneficially impacted by the adoption of dietary recommendations that can be very complicated. Anyone who has a chronic disease or is a caregiver for another person with a chronic disease understands how overwhelming it can be to follow or be in compliance with multiple medication regimens and manage a restrictive dietary regimen. Good nutrition is a hallmark activity for patients with chronic disease. It has an impact on helping them get well. Telehealth interventions can have a significant and positive impact on facilitating the changes in behavior that are necessary to improve symptoms in patients suffering from chronic diseases [12]. Healthy nutritional practices have a major role in the management of chronic diseases. Self-management and practicing a healthy lifestyle, which includes increasing physical activity, eating a healthy diet, and not smoking, are some important behaviors that are essential management strategies for dealing with chronic diseases. Many patients, and especially homebound patients that qualify for home healthcare services, are limited in their capacity to assess health-promoting education from clinicians because they are unable to access the clinician face to face at the site where the clinician works. Telehealthcare enables such access. Telehealth-delivered dietary interventions have tremendous potential to be part of the care plan for people with chronic diseases [13]. An interesting fact is that patients with cerebrovascular disease (CVD) and other chronic diseases have been identified as having higher levels of nonattendance in face-to-face consultations with their health-related consultations. Telehealth interventions have a significant impact on the reduction of sodium from the diet, which has a significant impact on blood pressure and the secondary prevention of CVD. There is also a significant impact on the improvement of diet quality, specifically fruit and vegetable intake [14]. In 2017, for the first time, the Community Preventive Services Task Force (CPSTF) recommended "comprehensive telehealth interventions to supplement the care of adults who have chronic diseases affected by diet, such as cardiovascular disease and diabetes. This finding is based on the evidence that shows comprehensive telehealth interventions improve patients' diets" [15].

Telehealth and Postacute Care

Telehealth also provides important links to patients following an acute care event. For example, a hospitalization is considered an acute care event. As a direct result of achieving cost-effectiveness in the delivery of healthcare services, same-day joint replacements have used telehealth to provide postacute services to their patients. Through the use of web-based technology, an avatar is embedded in a tablet and provided to patients. The role of the avatar is to teach patients important self-care strategies to promote their recovery after the surgical procedure. The patient is instructed on how to handle pain, change dressings, and what to expect regarding their recovery. The results of the study demonstrated strong clinical results, including no hospital readmissions and cost savings [16]. Surgical infections are another high-risk, painful, and costly unwanted event. Surgical wounds require attention by a skilled nurse, and telehealth is an important modality in ensuring that wounds are photographed and monitored. Technology is significant in preventing infection [17]. The Alliance of Home Health Care Quality and Innovation reports that home healthcare is the least costly postacute setting representing almost 40% of all Medicare episodes but accounting for less than 29% of all payments [18]. This means that as a postacute care setting, home healthcare is underutilized. A key question that healthcare professionals and policymakers globally need to consider is how to manage the growing number of people affected by chronic diseases and the associated increasing healthcare costs while facilitating patient satisfaction as reflected in their quality of life.

Benefits, Challenges, and Opportunities

The adoption of technology and the acceleration in technological change pose a major challenge for providers and a significant opportunity. The American Medical Association (AMA) has recognized the importance of the adoption by physicians nationally of digital health applications in order to improve the integration and delivery of healthcare services to their patients [19]. Furthermore, the AMA convened a summit for the purpose of focusing on how to use digital applications and innovations to advance the quadruple aim of better healthcare outcomes, improved patient experience, improved clinical experience, and lower cost of care. Many novel innovations fail because they are not scalable, sustainable, or cost-effective. The healthcare system is plagued by widespread burnout partly because of widespread inefficiencies. This is due to the overwhelming volume of patients affected by chronic disease, which contributes to worse health outcomes and exacerbates the cost of healthcare.

New digital technologies need to be interoperable between multiple health systems. They need to be designed in such a way that the technology enables easy and quick utilization by the healthcare provider. Training is a vital component, as is security. The ability to safeguard patient information is a hallmark of any technology that communicates with stakeholders [20]. Monitoring people with chronic conditions, known as telemonitoring, is becoming more widespread and presents opportunities for the management of people living with chronic conditions. This is especially relevant for people living in rural or other areas where access to specialists is very limited. For the homebound elderly, this can be essential. According to Cellar et al. (2017) [21], approximately 70% to 80% of the healthcare budgets of industrialized nations are spent on managing people with multiple chronic diseases. In an effort to understand whether telemonitoring would have an impact on chronic diseases, a before-and-after control intervention analysis model was adopted in Australia and New Zealand. Data were analyzed over a 3-year period. The results showed a particularly robust positive impact on reducing healthcare expenditures, admissions to the hospital, and reduction in mortality. A marginal benefit was achieved in reducing pharmaceutical costs. Additional research demonstrated that in a randomized control trial that included patients in 26 different municipalities, with a focus on patients with COPD in Denmark, telehealthcare had the advantage of promoting clinician communication and follow-up with patients on a more timely basis because data can be transmitted more frequently and over greater distances. Although communication was positively impacted, there was no reported benefit to quality of life. More research is needed to identify and understand how to improve quality of life. Smartphones and health apps are extremely beneficial in the spheres of health promotion and the management of chronic diseases. There is a plethora of apps for weight management, nutrition, and diabetes and other chronic diseases. Apps support patients in their homes. A recent study in Germany using smartphones and health apps found a significant relationship between health app use and behavior in the management of chronic conditions. These conditions included smoking, physical activity, diet, weight loss, medication adherence, improvement in blood pressure control, and improvement in blood sugar control [22]. It is fundamental that technology needs to be able to communicate across many systems. Yet this remains a formidable challenge such that even with the advances that have been made, there remains an integration and communication problem between organizations and patients. There is a significant need to establish and maintain priorities for telehealth research. Telehealth technologies are becoming an important part of healthcare systems worldwide. In the United States, the Department of Health and Human Services estimates that more than 60% of healthcare organizations and up to 50% of hospitals use some type of telehealth. Private insurers are increasingly considering reimbursement for telehealth. Recommended areas for research include physician leadership, reimbursement, licensure, liability, human factors, device interoperability and data integration, privacy and security, performance measurement, patient engagement, patient-physician relations, and research design and methods [23].

In a recent report to Congress in the USA, it was reported that as alternative payment methodologies like value-based purchasing and bundled payments become more important, the role of telehealth will only increase. Telehealth will expand access to healthcare and promote greater levels of accountability for healthcare delivery, access, and outcomes. Telehealth has an important role to play in serving the more than 50% of the population in the USA that lives with chronic diseases [24].

Conclusion

Important lessons can be taken from systems thinking or taking a systems-based approach. Systems theory is "an enterprise aimed at seeing how things are connected to each other within some notion of a whole entity" [25]. Systems thinking is very applicable to home care in that the home is the system and multiple components need to work together to improve patient health. For example, there must be supports in the home environment that facilitate the patient's recuperation. Simply stated, can the patient take her medicine? Does the patient have safety systems and reminders in place? Technology has an important role to play in optimizing wellness. To give people worldwide the right and choice to manage their health in their own homes and with the support of family and nonfamily caregivers, the use of technology and telehealth represents a significant approach that has the ability to transform the lives of patients and their families by providing synchronous and real-time access to healthcare providers. It makes it easier for patients and their caregivers to incorporate health-promoting care plans into their lives. The home health industry, with the support of multiple stakeholders and advances in technology, must commit to transforming the way healthcare services are delivered. Collaborations on a global scale are needed.

echnology has no boundaries. We must commit to learning from each other and promoting best practices. Clearly, as the aging population grows, along with the economic burden in both developed and underdeveloped countries, there is an economic imperative to control unnecessary costs. We have the ability through the adoption of cutting-edge technologies to improve the way health is delivered globally. In sum, the World Health Organization (WHO) describes the rapid increase in the number of elderly people as a global phenomenon. By the year 2030 more people than ever will be considered elderly and be at risk for multiple chronic diseases and have significantly greater needs, including the need for medical services. The WHO embraces the concept of home healthcare, which will make it easier and possible for people to remain at home rather than receive institutional care. Technology-enabled homes have tremendous potential to facilitate the human right to age in one's own home [26].

Discussion

Blue Horizons Homecare Company is a 50-year-old agency that provides skilled nursing and rehabilitation services for a population composed predominantly of older adults. The mean age of a patient requiring service is 79 years. You are the director of the agency and are confronted with new payment modalities that are putting pressure on your agency. You can no longer bill as needed on a fee-for-service basis. You embrace the concept of the triple aim, which means better healthcare quality of services that are cost effective. You know you need to make a plan. Begin your plan by addressing the following issues:

1. Problem statement: Identify a problem statement reflecting the situation in which you find yourself.
2. Decision criteria: Develop appropriate decision criteria that you will use in resolving the problem.
3. Planning and priority setting: Describe your short-term and long-term goals based on the information in the case study, chapter, and your professional experience.
4. Operational issues: Identify at least one operational issue you may need to address along with a minimum of a potential strategy you might employ.
5. Evaluation: Identify at least one organizational outcome that you will utilize to evaluate your success. Include in your rationale how and how frequently you will measure the outcome.

References

1. Beard J, Officer A, Cassels A. World report on ageing and health. Geneva: World Health Organization, 2015. http://www.who.int/ageing/publications/world-report-2015/en/. Accessed 27 July 2018
2. United Nations, Department of Economic and Social Affairs, Population Division. World Population Ageing 2017- Highlights (ST/ESA/SER.A/397). 2017. http://www.who.int/news-room/fact-sheets/detail/ageing-and-health
3. World Health Organization. Ageing and Health Feb 5, 2018. http://www.who.int/en/news-room/fact-sheets/detail/ageing-and-health. Accessed 27 July 2018.
4. Ortman JM, Velkoff VA, Hogan H. An aging nation: the older population in the United States, current population reports, P25-1140. Washington, DC: U.S. Census Bureau. https://www.census.gov/prod/2014pubs/p25-1140.pdf. Published May 2014. Accessed 26 Oct 2017.
5. Cire B. World's older population grows dramatically. NIH-funded Census Bureau report offers details of global aging phenomenon. National Institutes of Health Website. https://www.nih.gov/news-events/news-releases/worlds-older-population-grows-dramatically. Published March 28, 2016. Accessed 26 Oct 2017.
6. Olok GT, Yagos WO, Ovuga E. Knowledge and attitudes of doctors towards e-health use in healthcare delivery in government and private hospitals in Northern Uganda: a cross-sectional study. BMC Med Inform Decis Mak. 2015;15:87. https://doi.org/10.1186/s12911-015-0209-8.
7. Landers S, Madigan E, Leff B, et al. The future of home health care: a strategic framework for optimizing value. Home Health Care Manag Pract. 2016;28(4):262–78. https://doi.org/10.1177/1084822316666368.
8. Smith, A. Telemedicine vs. telehealth: what's the difference? Chiron Health Website. https://chironhealth.com/blog/telemedicine-vs-telehealth-whats-the-difference/. Published December 4, 2015. Accessed 26 Oct 2017.
9. Radhakrishnan K, Xie B, Berkley A, Kim M. Barriers and facilitators for sustainability of tele-homecare programs: a systematic review. Health Serv Res. 2016;51(1):48–75. https://doi.org/10.1111/1475-6773.12327.

10. Visiting Nurse Associations of America. VNAA case study compendium: innovative models for the evolving home health and hospice industry. http://www.vnaa.org/files/Education-Quality/VNAA%20CSfinal.pdf. Published October 2013. Accessed 26 Oct 2017.
11. Visiting Nurse Association of America Case Study Compendium. https://urldefense.com/v3/__ https://members.elevatinghome.org/Files/Education-Quality/Case-Study-Compendium/2015/VNAA-Case-Study-Compendium-2015.pdf__;!!HoV-yHU!6Zo_v4hgNKElWrd1iU-pw1ONyQ0qSKdrk4wWqhD0Q6go-aqIf6IO4-iTVwqJoIEboD0$. 2015.
12. Summerfelt WT, Sulo S, Robinson A, Chess D, Catanzano K. Scalable hospital at home with virtual physician visits: pilot study. Am J Manag Care 2015;21(10):675–684. http://www.ajmc.com/journals/issue/2015/2015-vol21-n10/scalable-hospital-at-home-with-virtual-physician-visits-pilot-study. Accessed 26 Oct 2017.
13. van den Berg M, Crotty M, Liu E, Killington M, Kwakkel G, van Wegen E. Early supported discharge by caregiver-mediated exercises and e-health support after stroke. Stroke. 2016;47(7):1885–92. https://doi.org/10.1161/STROKEAHA.116.013431.
14. Oksman E, Linna M, Hörhammer I, Lammintakanen J, Talja M. Cost-effectiveness analysis for a tele-based health coaching program for chronic disease in primary care. BMC Health Serv Res. 2017;17(1):138. https://doi.org/10.1186/s12913-017-2088-4.
15. Rubinstein AL, Irazola VE, Poggio R, Gulayin P, Nejamis A, Beratarrechea A. Challenges and opportunities for implementation of interventions to prevent and control CVD in low-resource settings: a report from CESCAS in Argentina. Glob Heart. 2015;10(1):21–9. https://doi.org/10.1016/j.gheart.2014.12.011.
16. Ernsting C, Dombrowski SU, Oedekoven M, et al. Using smartphones and health apps to change and manage health behaviors: a population-based survey. J Med Internet Res. 2017;19(4):e101. https://doi.org/10.2196/jmir.6838.
17. Lilholt PH, Witt Udsen F, Ehlers L, Hejlesen OK. Telehealthcare for patients suffering from chronic obstructive pulmonary disease: effects on health-related quality of life: results from the Danish 'TeleCare North' cluster-randomized trial. BMJ Open. 2017;7(5):e014587. https://doi.org/10.1136/bmjopen-2016-0145874.
18. Totten AM, Womack DM, Eden KB, et al. Telehealth: mapping the evidence for patient outcomes from systematic reviews. Technical brief no. 26. (Prepared by the Pacific Northwest Evidence-based Practice Center under Contract No. 290-2015-00009-I.) AHRQ Publication No.16-EHC034-EF. Rockville: Agency for Healthcare Research and Quality; June 2016.
19. Kelly JT, Reidlinger DP, Hoffmann TC, Campbell KL. Telehealth methods to deliver dietary interventions in adults with chronic disease: a systematic review and meta-analysis. Am J Clin Nutr. 2016;104(6):1693–702.
20. Health Affairs Blog Diffusion of Innovation. Health Care industry requires a roadmap to accelerate the impact of digital innovations. June 8, 2018. http://www.healthaffairs.org/do/10.1377/hblog20180606.523635/full/. Accessed 27 June 2018.
21. Celler B, Varnfield M, Nepal S, Sparks R, Li J, Jayasena R. Impact of at-home telemonitoring on health services expenditures and hospital admissions in patients with chronic diseases: before and after control analysis. JMIR Med Inform. 2017;5(3):1–19.
22. Tuckson RV, Edmunds M, Hodgkins ML. Telehealth. N Engl J. 2017;377(16):1585–91.
23. Ernsting C, Dombrowski SU, Oedekoven M, et al. Using smartphones and health apps to change and manage health behaviors: a population-based survey. J Med Internet Res. 2017;19(4):1–17.
24. Lilholt PH, Witt Udsen F, Ehlers L, Hejlesen OK. Telehealthcare for patients suffering from chronic obstructive pulmonary disease: effects on health-related quality of life: results from the Danish 'TeleCare North' cluster-randomized trial. BMJ Open. 2017; 7(5):e014587. https://doi.org/10.1136/bmjopen-2016-0145874. U.S. Department of Health and Human Services. Report to Congress E-health and Telemedicine 2016. https://aspe.hhs.gov/system/files/pdf/206751/TelemedicineE-HealthReport.pdf. Accessed 6 Aug 2018.

25. Peters DH. The application of systems thinking in health: why use systems thinking? Health Research Policy and Systems. 2014; http://www.Health-policy-systems.com/contents/12/1/51. Accessed 12 June 2018.
26. World Health Organization. Regional Office for the Eastern Mediterranean. The growing need for home health care for the elderly: home health care for the elderly as an integral part of primary health care services. 2015. http://applications.emro.who.int/dsaf/EMROPUB_2015_ EN_1901.pdf?ua=1 . Accessed 8 Aug 2018.

Chapter 5: Health Transformation in Saudi Arabia via Connected Health Technologies

Hebah ElGibreen

Introduction

The Kingdom of Saudi Arabia (KSA) is the second largest Arab state with a population estimated at more than 33.5 million [1]. Recently, the KSA began an important economic and social journey in its healthcare system. From the Ministry of Health (MoH) annual report [2], it was found that billions of Saudi riyals are spent on services that can be replaced with e-health and connected health technologies. In particular, connected health technologies can be of great benefit to patients who live in rural areas by reducing the travel time, expense, and stress involved in traveling long distances to reach the appropriate health service [3]. The widespread population and vast expanse of the country are other factors that motivate the drive to adopt connected health in the KSA.

Connected health can open new communication channels and overcome geographical barriers between patients and healthcare professionals around the world. It enables health providers to shift to a more proactive model that connects all stakeholders and focuses on patients as the center of the process throughout their lifespan [4]. Users' acceptance of connected health technologies in the KSA has been studied by multiple researchers [5–9], and it has been found that a high percentage of users tried connected health technologies through the use of wearable devices, remote consultation, remote monitoring, applications, websites, and social media.

Consequently, this chapter focuses on connected health technologies and their development in the KSA. Progress in the Saudi healthcare transformation model and the Saudi model of care (MoC) will be outlined. Use cases related to Saudi culture will

---

The original version of this chapter was revised. The correction to this chapter is available at
https://doi.org/10.1007/978-3-030-46355-7_28

H. ElGibreen (✉)
College of Computer and Information Sciences, King Saud University, Riyadh, Saudi Arabia
e-mail: hjibreen@ksu.edu.sa

© Springer Nature Switzerland AG 2020, Corrected Publication 2020
P. Murthy, A. Ansehl (eds.), *Technology and Global Public Health*,
https://doi.org/10.1007/978-3-030-46355-7_10

also be explained. In particular, since the healthcare system is mainly owned by the government, the MoH efforts to improve the connected health infrastructure in the KSA and advocate its use will be highlighted. Both governmental and academic questions and directions for future research will also be proposed at the end of this chapter.

Connected Health

There is no standard definition of connected health in the literature. However, the term encompasses different terminologies and utilizes technologies such as telehealth, telemedicine, mobile, electronic, virtual, digital, and wireless to offer a conceptual model of health management in which data are shared and interventions, services, and devices are designed around patients' needs to provide them with the most efficient and proactive healthcare possible [4].

Through connected health, all traditional health information and services can be accessed from home through smart devices or online platforms. The patient can download an application online and easily register to request a service or gain access to medical information. This increases patient satisfaction rates and saves time and money. As illustrated in Fig. 1, connected health changes the healthcare system and reduces the need for in-person visits while using the Internet to connect healthcare stakeholders.

To operate efficiently, connected health must be complemented with information technology (IT) and information and communications technology (ICT) [8]. IT and ICT are needed to access health information, consult with patients, provide diagnoses, and recommend treatments remotely. These services extend healthcare to a larger population and improve the quality of care by connecting with higher levels of expertise while reducing the costs of travel or face-to-face appointments.

Relevant Technologies

Connected health, also known as technology-based care, converges through the use of various digital technologies. To understand how it works, it is important to be familiar with the most widely known technologies that it offers. As summarized by Taylor [10], electronic health (**e-health**) is a technology that uses services that transmit healthcare and its resources through electronic means. An electronic health record (**EHR**) is one important component of connected health that stores, manages, and transmits a patient's information in any healthcare system online. Another related technology is mobile health (**m-health**), which represents public and medical health that is practiced through mobile devices, such as smart phones or tablets.

Technologies such as virtual care, telemedicine, and telehealth are sometimes confused and used interchangeably. However, it must be emphasized that, although they contribute to connecting health, they are not the same. **Telemedicine** is one of the connected health roots and is a combination of two terms: "tele," which

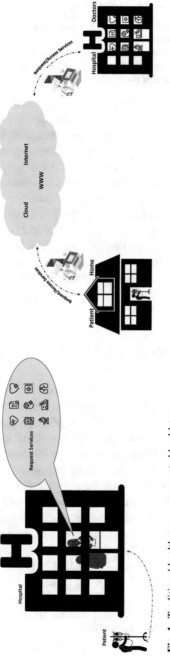

Fig. 1 Traditional healthcare vs. connected healthcare

represents communication from a distance, and "medicine," which represents healing. The two terms together denote "healing from a distance" [11]:

The World Health Organization (WHO) defines telemedicine as:

the delivery of health care services, where distance is a critical factor, by all health care professionals using information and communication technologies for the exchange of valid information for diagnosis, treatment and prevention of disease and injuries, research and evaluation, and for the continuing education of health care providers, all in the interests of advancing health of individuals and their communities [12].

Thus, its common theme is to deliver healthcare services and information from a distance through the use of ICT to improve the cost, quality, and ease of access [13].

Telehealth is a broader term that incorporates remote and automatic monitoring and management of patient health conditions to provide preventive care and avoid hospital admissions. Unlike telemedicine, telehealth can refer to remote, nonclinical services, such as training and education. **Virtual care**, on the other hand, is a component of telehealth. This term combines two terms: "virtual," which represents something that is extended by software or temporally simulated, and "care," which represents treatment and nursing [14]. Virtual care extends telemedicine and supplements its delivery in healthcare. Instead of connecting patients online and in real time with their physicians, virtual care connects anonymous users asynchronously and can even outsource services to people outside of the healthcare profession [14]. It provides users with more healthcare choices for where, when, and how to connect.

Healthcare Transformation in KSA

The healthcare system in the KSA is mainly owned and operated by the government. The MoH is one of the major governmental entities responsible for 60% of the healthcare services in the country [1]. Through Vision 2030, the MoH was given clear directions and a set of reforms that will transform the entire health sector, including the care model, healthcare financing, governance, segregation of health facilities, privatization, manpower, and digital transformation. The MoH 2017 annual report [2] showed that billions of Saudi riyals (SAR) are consumed on services that can be replaced with e-health and connected health technologies.

One important issue that technology can overcome is the lack of expertise and the difficulty of covering vast areas of the country. In the KSA, the government is responsible for many expenses that are clearly caused by shortages of specialists or services rather than facilities. As noted in the MoH 2017 annual report [2], 306,140 medical referrals were recorded in 2017, of which 40.53% were caused by the absence of the required service and 36.24% were due to the lack of a specialist in that institution. Moreover, international referrals in 2017 cost the government SAR2,493,112,874,91 (USD66,483,009,997) for treatment, in addition to SAR422,285,921,34 (USD11,260,957,902) in total costs for living abroad during such treatments.

Connected health services offer cost-effective alternatives that are more efficient long term. Its technologies will allow physicians to perform procedures from a distance, provide teleconsultations, follow up with patients regularly while allowing patients to remain at home, and reduce expenses caused by long-distance travel or medical evacuation. The government recognized such benefits and proposed a novel transformation plan for healthcare in the KSA.

It was estimated that the national transformation initiatives will have significant economic and financial impacts [2]. They will create 31,300 new jobs, achieve additional government revenue equal to SAR30.8 billion, save SAR7 billion in government capital expenses, and increase savings in government operating expenses, projected to save SAR18.8 billion by 2020. Hence, health transformation initiatives must be highlighted, and the relevant connected health services will be discussed in more detail.

National Transformation Program

On April 25, 2016, the KSA announced 12 Vision Realization Programs (VRPs) to achieve the objectives and expectations of Vision 2030. On June 6, 2016, the National Transformation Program (NTP) was launched to build the capabilities and capacities necessary to achieve the Vision 2030 goals. The NTP was launched as one of the VRPs and involved 24 government agencies, including healthcare organizations. The details of the NTP were documented in its 2018–2020 delivery plan report [15]. One of the NTP objectives is to enhance living standards by engaging healthcare stakeholders in identifying challenges, implementing the program's initiatives, and accelerating digital and primary infrastructure implementation. Thus, six main Saudi entities were engaged: the MoH, the Saudi Health Council, the Saudi Food and Drug Authority, the King Faisal Specialist Hospital and Research Centre, the Saudi Red Crescent Authority, and the Ministry of Education.

As illustrated in Fig. 2, the NTP's strategic objectives were mapped into eight achievable themes. The Transform Healthcare theme is concerned with

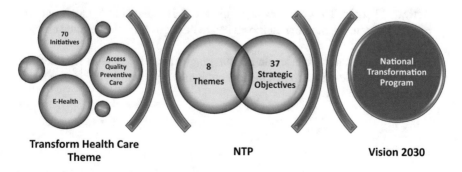

Fig. 2 Health Transformation in Saudi Vision 2030

restructuring the health sector in the KSA into an effective and comprehensive system that can achieve a vibrant society. The Transform Health theme focuses on challenges related to the difficulty in accessing health services, inefficiency and quality limitations, and limitations in preventive healthcare.

To overcome these challenges and promote public health, e-health was proposed as a key element of the Saudi health transformation. Seventy different initiatives were proposed to improve healthcare efficiency under the transform healthcare theme through different state-of-the-art technologies such as ICT, telemedicine, and teleconsultation. These initiatives tacklèd different connected health services such as electronic services, virtual training, online appointment systems, and national health records.

One innovative initiative that is of particular interest and new to the Saudi healthcare system, is the MoC. This initiative introduces a new healthcare approach and goes beyond disease treatment. Its ultimate goal is to improve the quality of peoples' lives. Therefore, the next section will investigate the MoC and its aspects that promote connected health services.

Saudi Model of Care

The MoC integrates the role of health service providers with the role of institutions, society, and individuals to enable best practices in access to healthcare. It has a great impact on national cost savings. It was indicated by the Healthcare Transformation Strategy (HTS) report [16] that the new MoC is estimated to result in a net savings of SAR10.5 billion (USD2.8 billion) by 2021. This financial advantage will result from increasing healthcare productivity and reducing patient demand. The MoC is not only designed to improve the financial status of the healthcare system but also to ensure that healthcare is sustainable and effective in the future and to improve the population's health outcomes [5].

Figure 3 shows that the MoC consists of six intersecting systems that work together to deliver care across different service layers. Accordingly, the MoC is divided into six service layers, and each layer can be described as follows:

- Activated People: The core service of the MoC. Highlights individuals and the role they play in maintaining their own health through awareness, empowerment, and self-care.
- Healthy Community: Focuses on encouraging activated people to lead healthy lifestyles, provide access to healthcare community, wellness facilities, and accurate information.

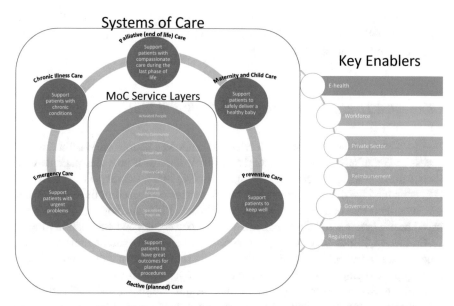

Fig. 3 New Saudi Model of Care [16]. (Source: Adapted from Healthcare Transformation Strategy. Vision 2030. Vol 3, p. 17. Ministry of Health. Kingdom of Saudi Arabia. Retrieved from https://www.moh.gov.sa/en/Ministry/vro/Pages/Health-Transformation-Strategy.aspx)

- Virtual Care[1]: Provide effective and nontraditional sources of health advice to improve people's access to medical information and guide them in using healthcare systems and getting appropriate care.
- Primary care, general hospitals, and specialized hospitals are the traditional layers that currently exist in the healthcare system. They are concerned with primary, secondary, and tertiary care.

The MoC is designed based on systems rather than settings or specialties. Hence, each service layer supports a certain purpose and, accordingly, is delivered by a different system, as described in the HTS report [16]. Each MoC system supports different care stakeholders, including preventive care, palliative care, chronic illness care, maternity and child care, elective care, and emergency care.

To implement the aforementioned systems, key enablers must be supported. These include e-health, the workforce, the private sector, reimbursement mechanisms, political leaders, and regulators. Hence, the MoC shifts the focus of the healthcare system from being service- and resource-oriented to being patient-oriented. The MoC systems will operate more in communities and homes rather

---

[1] From the initiatives discussed in the HTS report, it was clear that the tools proposed encompass more than virtual care, making connected health terminology more appropriate to clarify the spectrum of the new model. Thus, it was decided that the term "connected health" should be used instead of "virtual care" throughout this section.

than in hospitals. Connected health services must be supported in the new MoC. The model will deliver 42 interventions involving virtual self-care tools, virtual education tools, and systematic data collection.

Connected Health Technologies in the Saudi MoC

The MoC uses connected health services to empower people and facilitate their access to health advice from the comfort of their homes. It provides patients with tools, information, and access to care for themselves independently. The HTS report [16] explained the details of connected health services proposed in the new MoC. It was identified that connected health platforms should be developed through web-based health systems to supply patients with empowerment and accessibility tools.

Connected health services will be promoted as empowerment tools by using them to educate people about their health while refining the health system's transparency. It will empower people by offering them accurate information to increase their awareness and knowledge about their health, wellness, and self-care. This empowerment can be enhanced by providing online access to information and guidelines about decision-making tools and patients' rights.

The MoH is working on different programs under the Transform Healthcare theme to convey target outcomes of each of the proposed interventions. One related program is the Health Coach Program, through which people will have access to an online health coach to help them self-manage their health and adopt a healthy lifestyle. Communication can occur via virtual portals, telephone, and user communities. Workplace Wellness Program is another program that aims to improve employees' satisfaction and work productivity by providing health programs in workplaces. Another program, the Health Edutainment Program, uses educational and entertaining programs favored by different age groups to promote healthy lifestyles. It provides fun ways to learn about health through sports challenges, TV shows, quizzes, and game apps and websites.

USE Case: Connect Health in Chronic Illness

To understand how the MoC can be used to promote well-being through its connected health services, a scenario can be proposed based on the HTS report [16]. A Saudi woman named Nora is a 35-year-old working mother who is obese and does not have time to exercise. Due to long working hours, Nora skips lunch, drinks coffee, and eats sweets instead. Additionally, she eats one large meal after she puts her kids to sleep at night. Nora's mother had diabetes, but Nora does not have time to wait for a hospital appointment for routine checks on her blood sugar and blood pressure.

With the MoC it will be possible to resolve Nora's issues through the model new programs. Using the Health Edutainment Program, Nora can play fun games with her kids that teach them about healthy eating habits and explain the implications of unhealthy habits from a young age. Moreover, workplace wellness programs can help Nora to overcome the negative effects of long working hours because the programs will challenge her to engage in fun physical activities while working. Finally, the Health Coach Program will enable a colleague at work, who happens to be a champion in the program, to refer Nora to a coach in the program. Nora can call her coach for advice on losing weight or a recommendation for a discounted, healthy food delivery restaurant.

Connected Health Development in KSA

The Saudi government established an e-health center in 1993 to deliver telemedicine services, such as online consultation and video conferencing [3]. Since then, various national projects have been enacted and contributions made to connected health.

Governmental Contribution

The MoH studied the possibility of implementing telemedicine in the KSA and the challenges and barriers the healthcare system faces. The first telemedicine application was successfully implemented in 1994 by King Faisal Specialized Hospital and Research Centre (KFSH&RC) [17]. KFSH&RC established its own network in 1998 to connect hospitals in various rural areas around the country. In 2010, the MoH cooperated with Canada Health Infoway, a pioneer in telemedicine technologies, to establish a key national project to implement telemedicine that includes all healthcare facilities around the country. In 2011, the MoH launched the first national telemedicine project: the Saudi Telemedicine Network (STN) [18]. The STN made it possible to connect 27 hospitals as health partners to KFSH&RC by 2013.

In 2016, KFSH&RC announced the launch of its new telemedicine center [19]. The center was equipped with the latest technologies to ensure the most efficient and effective healthcare services. Services covered by this center include, but are not limited to, educational and training programs, histological laboratory tests, X-ray equipment, second medical opinions, virtual clinics, and remote intensive care. These services demonstrate that the center offers more than telemedicine. It provides services related to virtual care and e-health and thus contributes to connected health in general. Through the center, it was possible to connect 32 hospitals around the country to monitor patients. More than 1000 patients have been treated by the virtual clinic in 17 specialties, including consultations, diagnoses, and follow-ups. The center includes 27 virtual clinics operating under the MoH, and the number continues to increase.

To complement the MoC and accomplish the proposed health initiatives, the MoH developed and launched various connected health project, as reported in the MoH 2017 annual report [2]. For example, connected health technologies were introduced to manage hospital beds around the country. The system provides accurate information about hospital beds by tracking number of available beds, providing monthly reports about status, usage rates, and other information related to the occupation and condition of beds.

Another system developed by the MoH was proposed to keep track of patients' EHRs. A medical record management system was developed to govern electronic records policies and regulations. The records of 32 hospitals were archived electronically in the first phase, and the process is in progress for another 65 hospitals. The MoH is continuously developing its unified electronic system to connect it to healthcare systems used by patients, such as Ehalaty for medical referrals and Elajee for consultations.

In 2017, a total of 91 ICT projects were completed and launched by the MoH. Another 92 projects are still in progress, including online monitoring for newborn babies and a pilot telehealth system for rural areas. Moreover, 93 projects were under analysis to utilize ICT and improve the country's healthcare system. All these projects are important to create connected systems that can efficiently support all stakeholders of healthcare systems, including patients, physicians, staff, and other healthcare providers.

In 2018, the MoH announced that telemedicine would cover the country in 2 months [20]. Various healthcare applications were launched to promote not only telemedicine but also connected health [21]. For patients and physicians, the MoH officially launched an application called Seha for online consultation. The application allows citizens nationwide to have remote, face-to-face consultations with their physician. Users log in to the application to communicate directly with their specialist at a designated time and date. The MoH also launched the Mawid app, which patients can use to book their appointments online.

Various institutions have also contributed to connected health to enhance the healthcare system and reinforce the MoC in the KSA. An innovative program called Health Outreach Services was initiated by KFSH&RC [22]. The program aims to improve healthcare by developing partnerships between key regional institutions around the country. It provides various services, including virtual clinics to connect patients with their physicians using telemedicine tools and tele-ICU services that use videoconferencing devices to allow critical care nurses and doctors to monitor patients in intensive care units in remote hospitals. The KFSH&RC telehealth portal [23] is another technology that facilitates telemedicine applications and patient outreach for healthcare services.

Various developments were initiated in the healthcare system for the Hajj[2] season. For example, the concept of connected health was introduced to help educate the volunteer healthcare team in Hajj. A learning management system was developed to provide simulations and virtual training online. The system offers 92 courses and trains more than 4500 volunteers from different fields each season.

During Hajj, telemedicine has been employed through the use of different visual communication technologies (Polycom RMX) to connect with physicians. The networking and communication infrastructure in Makkah was also developed and improved to obtain the best possible connections with healthcare experts during the Hajj season. The MoH also activated EHR systems (such as Picture Archiving & Communication System "PACS") to connect radiology devices operating in four major hospitals in Makkah. Medical images and X-rays were stored in the central system and linked to the ministry's data center to be accessed by other hospitals in the country in case online consultation is needed.

The Ministry of Hajj and Umrah has also contributed to Makkah's ICT infrastructure as one of its digital transformation initiatives. In 2018, the ministry announced the signing of a memorandum of understanding (MoU) with SAP, a European multinational software corporation, to develop different cloud-based solutions. It also signed a MoU with Cisco to enhance the digital infrastructure and services. The initiatives will transform the experience for pilgrims to support different aspects of Hajj. It was anticipated that these agreements would increase government IT savings by 25–50% [24].

Literature Development

In addition to MoH initiatives and government contributions, researchers and scientists have also contributed to connected health and exploited its applications and tools. Connected health technologies such as smart beds, EHRs, mobile EHR access, video imaging technologies, smartphones, and virtual desktop infrastructure can help the MoH to serve patients more effectively. Patients in rural areas can connect to their physicians online for consultations using virtual self-care tools. Medical students and physicians can be educated or trained on new healthcare devices through the web. A summary of the latest literature on contributions to connected health in the KSA is given in Table 1.

A comprehensive connected health intervention was also developed and implemented in the KSA by Aldahmash et al. [36]. In 2019, the authors published a paper regarding an innovative intervention called Remotely Accessible Healthcare @ Home (RAHAH). RAHAH is a connected health intervention that utilizes many of the tools and technologies discussed earlier in this chapter. It encompasses services

---

[2]The Hajj pilgrimage is a religious duty that happens yearly in the Holy City of Makkah in the KSA. It is one of the world's largest annual religious events, in which more than two million pilgrims come to Makkah to perform the ritual.

Table 1 Recent literature on connected health in KSA

Literature area	Year	Technology	References
Tools and applications	2014	Telehealth	[13]
Mental health	2017	M-Health	[25]
Chronic diseases	2017	M-Health	[26]
Chronic diseases	2017	M-Health	[27]
Analysis study	2017	EHR	[28]
Analysis study	2018	ICT	[5]
Obesity management	2018	Social robots	[29]
Medical emergency	2018	M-Health	[30]
Obesity management	2018	M-Health	[31]
Telecardiology Mobile	2018	Telehealth	[32]
E-visits	2018	Virtual care	[33]
Social virtual care	2019	Virtual care	[34]
Analysis study	2019	Internet of Things (IoT)	[35]

related to EHRs, mobile devices, wearable devices, telemedicine, and web platforms. RAHAH was implemented in the KSA and Pakistan under the support of the Prince Naif bin Abdul Aziz Health Research Center at King Saud University. It remotely trains, educates, and monitors patients in long-term care. The system was developed in April 2017 and is currently in its initial stage. It is anticipated that a successful implementation of RAHAH will be crucial to efficiently manage the chronic care population, which is continuously increasing in the KSA.

Advocating Connected Health in KSA

Regardless of the progress discussed earlier, several studies have noted that connected health, particularly telemedicine, lacks durability in its success. Although some projects have succeeded thus far, many have failed after a period. Such failures have been mostly attributed to the complex healthcare culture, human factors [3], and providers' lack of understanding of users' acceptance, especially with respect to Saudi culture [9]. This section will present the new directions of government plans to empower and promote connected health. It will also identify research questions that must be explored.

Future Government Directions

In the MoH 2017 annual report [2], various recommendations and solutions were proposed to improve different aspects of health services in the KSA. One is to simplify access to healthcare services, which can be done through appropriate planning with respect to human resources needs in the health sector. It is also important to encourage employment in deficient healthcare-related careers and improve the performance of healthcare facilities. Moreover, virtual dietary clinics should be launched and extended health services such as in-home and chronic illness healthcare should be expanded. Finally, to further simplify access to healthcare services, primary care services must be repaired and restructured according to the innovative services proposed.

Another aspect of the report related to improving the earned value of health services. This can be achieved by regulating and building an effective infrastructure for electronic health services. Sustainable healthcare expenses and human resource education in the healthcare sector are also important. Assessing users' satisfaction and enhancing health services' quality and safety also improve earned value.

Although the MoH is promoting connected health and has allocated a large budget for its technologies, physicians still have serious concerns and see many drawbacks in the quality, efficiency, and implementation barriers of current services [8]. Hence, researchers must work to address these challenges and overcome these drawbacks.

Future Research Directions

The KSA is prepared for connected health thanks to the success of existing projects and the support of Vision 2030. However, connected health projects were bound to fail in many cases. Alaboudi et al. [9] highlighted that 75% of telemedicine projects worldwide either failed or were abandoned, and the rate reached 90% in developing countries. One of the most common challenges that caused such failures is a lack of understanding of users' acceptance when new health technologies are opposed by patients. In general, the HTS report [16] identified eight major challenges for health systems that must be addressed:

1. Variation in the Saudi economy and public expense suppression.
2. Significant gaps in Saudi employment capabilities and capacity.
3. Changes in staff and resources that are patient- or person-centric.
4. Variations in access and investment due to assessment using served populations instead of treated patients.
5. Significant gaps in the quality of services provided to patients due to inconsistent and inadequate policies and treatment pathways.
6. Inconsistent and inadequate primary care services and poorly distributed secondary and tertiary hospitals and their resources around the kingdom.
7. High rates of noncommunicable disease and major risks of communicable disease outbreak due to high visitation seasons such as Hajj.
8. Vast population of residents and overseas long-term visitors concentrated in cities. A 2016 study indicated that 83.3% of the population was urban, and this figure was projected to grow to 85.9% by 2030.

Based on the challenges discussed earlier, it is clear that further research must be conducted to promote connected health further. Moreover, studies have emphasized the importance of decision makers' involvement in connected health implementation to support it with policies and regulations that protect users' rights and increase its acceptance [27].

Case Study: Saudi Arabia Hack 2018

To advocate new digital interventions in the health community and encourage digital health partners to work on innovative technologies that serve healthcare services, public events and conferences should be conducted periodically [5]. Such events demonstrate technological developments and identify clinical problems among the Saudi population. Healthcare hackathons are one form of gathering that can be used as a process and toolset to accelerate team creation and the development of solutions that tackle complex healthcare problems. Connected health solutions can be promoted through such events by creating an ecosystem that combines expertise from different fields to overcome current healthcare obstacles. Participants can hail from various fields such as business, regulatory, industry, academic, engineering, design, and health.

One of the most powerful models in healthcare hackathons is MIT Hacking Medicine. It is "*a scalable and practical approach to integrate interdisciplinary collaboration and training in rapid innovation techniques into the clinical innovation programs of academic medical centers*" [37]. Started in 2010, MIT Hacking Medicine has grown to become a global brand with more than 80 healthcare hackathons per year [38]. In December 2018, the MIT-Ibn Khaldun Fellowship (IBK) Alumni Society organized to bring the MIT Hacking Medicine model to KSA [43]. In colaboration with the MIT Hacking Medicine and the King Abdulaziz City for Science and Technology (KACST), one of the largest healthcare hackathons in the region was held for the first time [39]. It was a 3-day event involving more than 1000 participants to provide a collaborative environment to influence the way healthcare is delivered to millions of people in the KSA.

The main goal of the Saudi hackathon was to advocate innovative digital models in the healthcare field by providing means of collaboration and digital integration between health and IT sectors. One of the tracks proposed was "Connected Health: Virtual Care, Telehealth, and Telemedicine." The main goal of this track was to promote connected health and empower it with innovative ideas around technologies and applications for physical, mental, and social well-being. As announced by the organizers, "*In the connected health section, Harara Tech won first place for a system that accesses and directs treatment to victims after large-scale disasters. Dream Team came second for a project that uses realistic human models to simulate training experiences*" [40].

Although two winners were named in each track (20 teams), this hackathon resulted in many digital solutions to current healthcare challenges that can improve the lifestyles and healthcare quality of Saudi citizens in the realization of Vision 2030. Thus, as encouraged by the MIT Hacking Medicine model, the support did not end with this hackathon. Post-hackathon events were also conducted to mentor the teams and help in shaping their ideas and develop real products. Teams were also linked with incubators and entrepreneurship-supporting channels such as the KSU Entrepreneurship Institute [41] and Badir Technology Incubator [42]. It is anticipated that many successful stories will emerge in the near future from the ideas that were born in this hackathon to become real products that empower the healthcare system around the country.

Conclusion

Due to the national transformation initiatives empowered by the Saudi government to achieve Vision 2030, the healthcare transformation strategy is the main methodology for improving healthcare services. E-health is a critical enabler to the proposed MoC systems and necessary to enforce health system quality and safety practices. Connected health can enable virtual academies that build the skills and knowledge necessary to deliver the new MoC. It also facilitates the implementation of data quality programs and clinical coding practice and provides access to high-quality data to improve policymaking and medical research. These data can also help in developing disease prediction tools.

To ensure the future success of various connected health technologies, the KSA must increase awareness through workshops, seminars, campaigns, and conferences. Developed tools should be associated with easy-to-use interfaces that minimize system misuse and enhance its benefits. Policymakers across all sectors should be encouraged to integrate health in all policies and optimize the already available resources that support connected health services, such as networking, research centers, and investments. Technology, computational power, mobile devices, the Internet, and big data analysis must be utilized to improve quality and build a powerful and adaptable health system. To keep pace with future breakthroughs, distributed governance systems, information systems, accounting systems, and communication practices should also be enabled.

KSA investments in connected health will lead to more effective and safer services along with integrated and efficient systems. Connected health will increase the productivity of healthcare and create new knowledge industries. Thus, future development is required, and the new MoC must be implemented correctly.

References

1. Khalil MK, Al-Eidi S, Al-Qaed M, AlSanad S. The future of integrative health and medicine in Saudi Arabia. Integr Med Res. 2018.
2. MoH. Annual report of the Ministry of Health. 2017. https://www.moh.gov.sa/Ministry/About/Documents/MOH_INFO_GRPH_2017%20FINAL.pdf

3. Dawoud A, Althbiti AAJ, Al Khatib FM, AL-Ghalayini NA. Telemedicine: between reality and challenges in Jeddah hospitals. Egypt J Hosp Med. 2017;68(3).
4. Caulfield B, Donnelly S. What is connected health and why will it change your practice? QJM Int J Med. 2013;106(8):703–7.
5. Al Kuwaiti A, Al Muhanna FA, Al AS. Implementation of Digital Health Technology at Academic Medical Centers in Saudi Arabia. Oman Med J. 2018;33(5):367.
6. Sayedalamin Z, Alshuaibi A, Almutairi O, Baghaffar M, Jameel T, Baig M. Utilization of smart phones related medical applications among medical students at King Abdulaziz University, Jeddah: a cross-sectional study. J Infect Public Health. 2016;9(6):691–7.
7. Alajmi D, Khalifa M, Jamal A, et al. The role and use of telemedicine by physicians in developing countries: a case report from Saudi Arabia. Transforming Public Health in Developing Nations: IGI Global; 2015. pp. 293–308.
8. Nasser H. Assessment of telemedicine by physicians at Prince Sultan Military Medical City. J Nutr Hum Health. 2017;1(1):1–10.
9. Alaboudi A, Atkins A, Sharp B, Alzahrani M, Balkhair A, Sunbul T. Perceptions and attitudes of clinical staff towards telemedicine acceptance in Saudi Arabia. Paper presented at: 2016 IEEE/ACS 13th international conference of Computer Systems and Applications (AICCSA) 2016.
10. Taylor K. Connected health: how digital technology is transforming health and social care. London: Deloitte Centre for Health Solutions; 2015.
11. Ahmed ME, Aldosh M. Telemedicine and teleradiology in Saudi Arabia. IOSR J Dent Med Sci. 2014;13(2).
12. World Health Organization. Telemedicine: opportunities and developments in member states: report on the second global survey on eHealth. World Health Organization 2010: http://www.who.int/goe/publications/goe_telemedicine_2010.pdf
13. Kvedar J, Coye MJ, Everett W. Connected health: a review of technologies and strategies to improve patient care with telemedicine and telehealth. Health Aff. 2014;33(2):194–9.
14. Fronczek AE. Nursing theory in virtual care. Nurs Sci Q. 2019;32(1):35–8.
15. National Transformation Program Office. National transformation program: delivery plan 2018–2020.2018.: https://vision2030.gov.sa/sites/default/files/attachments/NTP%20English%20Public%20Document_2810.pdf
16. MoH. Health sector transformation strategy. Vision 2030. vol. 3. Saudi Arabia 2018: https://www.moh.gov.sa/en/Ministry/vro/Pages/Health-Transformation-Strategy.aspx
17. Alaboudi AA, ATKINS A, Sharp B. A holistic framework for assisting decision makers of healthcare facilities to assess telemedicine applications in Saudi Arabia. 2015.
18. Alaboudi A, Atkins A, Sharp B, Balkhair A, Alzahrani M, Sunbul T. Barriers and challenges in adopting Saudi telemedicine network: the perceptions of decision makers of healthcare facilities in Saudi Arabia. J Infect Public Health. 2016;9(6):725–33.
19. King Faisal Specialist Hospital & Research Centre. New and Advanced Centre for Telemedicine at KFSH&RC is Launched. 2016. https://www.kfshrc.edu.sa/en/home/news/1756. Accessed 2019.
20. MoH. All the kingdom will be covered by telemedicine in two months. 2018. https://www.moh.gov.sa/en/Ministry/MediaCenter/News/Pages/news-2018-03-06-006.aspx. Accessed 2019.
21. MoH. MOH Apps for smartphones. 2019. https://www.moh.gov.sa/en/Support/Pages/MobileApp.aspx
22. KFSH&RC. Health outreach. 2019; https://www.kfshrc.edu.sa/en/home/aboutus/healthoutreach
23. KFSH&RC. E-Services. 2019; https://eservices.kfshrc.edu.sa
24. International Communication Center. Saudi Arabia to transform Hajj with cutting-edge technology. 2018. https://cic.org.sa/2018/10/saudi-arabia-to-transform-hajj-with-cutting-edge-technology/. Accessed 2019.
25. Atallah N, Khalifa M, El Metwally A, Househ M. The prevalence and usage of mobile health applications among mental health patients in Saudi Arabia. Comput Methods Prog Biomed. 2018;156:163–8.

26. Alenazi H, Alghamdi M, Alradhi S, Househ M, Zakaria N. A study on Saudi diabetic patients' readiness to use mobile health. Stud Health Technol Inform. 2017;245:1210.
27. Jusoh S. A survey on trend, opportunities and challenges of mHealth Apps. Int J Interact Mob Technol. 2017;11(6):73–85.
28. Aldosari B. Patients' safety in the era of EMR/EHR automation. Inform Med Unlocked. 2017;9:230–3.
29. Alotaibi M. A social robotic obesity management and awareness system for children in Saudi Arabia. Int J Online Eng. 2018;14(09):159–69.
30. Alghamdi K, Alsalamah S, Al-Hudhud G, Nouh T, Alyahya I, AlQahtani S. Region-based bed capacity mHealth application for emergency medical services: Saudi Arabia case study. eTELEMED. 2018;2018:114.
31. Al-Humaimeedy AS, Almozaini R, Almansour L, Alaqeely K, Almutairi A, Alolayan A. So'rah: an Arabic mobile health application for Saudi dietary evaluation. eTELEMED. 2018;2018:139.
32. Abdelsamee NM, Algarni A. IOT based solution for teleconsulting cardiac patients in Saudi Arabia. Paper presented at: 2018 21st Saudi Computer Society National Computer Conference (NCC) 2018.
33. Zhong X. A queueing approach for appointment capacity planning in primary care clinics with electronic visits. IISE Trans. 2018;50(11):970–88.
34. Anderson KA. The virtual care farm: a preliminary evaluation of an innovative approach to addressing loneliness and building community through nature and technology. Act Adapt Aging. 2019:1–11.
35. Al Otaibi MN. Internet of Things (IoT) Saudi Arabia healthcare systems: state-of-the-art, future opportunities and open challenges. J Health Inform Dev Countries. 2019;13(1).
36. Aldahmash AM, Ahmed Z, Qadri FR, Thapa S, AlMuammar AM. Implementing a connected health intervention for remote patient monitoring in Saudi Arabia and Pakistan: explaining 'the what' and 'the how'. Glob Health. 2019;15(1):20.
37. Gubin TA, Iyer HP, Liew SN, et al. A systems approach to healthcare innovation using the MIT hacking medicine model. Cell Syst. 2017;5(1):6–10.
38. Cell Press. Healthcare hackathons: model for success. 26 July 2017. www.sciencedaily.com/releases/2017/07/170726132118.htm
39. MIT Hacking Medicine. Saudi Arabia Hack. 2018:2018.. http://admin.mithackmed.com/event/saudi-arabia-hack-2018/
40. Badir. Health hackathon puts digital health under the microscope. 2019. https://www.badir.com.sa/en/node/183
41. King Saud University. Entrepreneurship Institute. 2019. https://alriyadah.ksu.edu.sa/en
42. Badir. Badir technology incubators and accelerators program. 2019. https://www.badir.com.sa/en/
43. Ibn Khaldun Fellowship for Saudi Arabian Women. MIT Hacking Medicine Riyadh - An initiative of KACST, Badir and the MIT-IBK Society. 2018: https://ibk.mit.edu/news-events/news/mit-hacking-medicine-riyadh-initiative-kacst-badir-and-mit-ibk-society. Accessed 2020.

Chapter 6: Simple Technology for Menstrual Hygiene Management: A Case Study from Northern Ethiopia

Shewaye Belay, Freweini Mebrahtu, Anne Sebert Kuhlmann, Amanuel Haile, and L. Lewis Wall

Introduction

Menstruation is part of human eutherian mammalian physiology [1]. Human females, like most other placental mammals, bear live young, carrying them inside the uterus where they are nourished through a placenta until they are born. Menstruation occurs when the engorged endometrial lining of the uterus is shed 2 weeks after ovulation if the ovulated egg is not fertilized or if blastocyst implantation to produce a placenta does not occur successfully after fertilization. In normally cycling females of reproductive age, menstruation occurs every 21–35 days. A girl's first menstrual period (menarche) is a developmental hallmark, normally occurring during adolescence within 2–3 years after the development of breast buds (thelarche). Most well-nourished girls in industrialized countries experience menarche between the ages of 12 and 13, and 98% of girls will have their first menstrual period by age 15 [2].

Although the biology of menstruation is now well studied and well understood by scientists and clinicians [3] and the relationship of menstruation to the

S. Belay
Institute of Biomedical Sciences, College of Health Sciences, Mekelle University, Mekelle, Ethiopia

F. Mebrahtu
Mariam Seba Sanitary Products Factory, Mekelle, Ethiopia

A. Sebert Kuhlmann
College of Public Health and Social Justice, Saint Louis University, St. Louis, MO, USA

A. Haile
College of Health Sciences, Mekelle University, Mekelle, Ethiopia

L. L. Wall (✉)
Departments of Anthropology and Obstetrics & Gynecology, Washington University in St. Louis, St. Louis, MO, USA
e-mail: walll@wustl.edu

© Springer Nature Switzerland AG 2020
P. Murthy, A. Ansehl (eds.), *Technology and Global Public Health*,
https://doi.org/10.1007/978-3-030-46355-7_11

beginnings of potential reproductive life is recognized in all cultures around the world, most people in the general population of most countries do not have a good scientific understanding of this important aspect of human biology. Misconceptions and false beliefs concerning menstruation are common. Folk understandings of menstruation are based upon inaccurate assumptions concerning the nature of menstrual bleeding and interpretations of what this bleeding means [4, 5]. Many of these beliefs, including those found in ancient religious texts, originated in the distant past, before the biology of menstruation had been investigated in detail [6].

Challenges for Girls and Women

Irrespective of their biological understanding of menstruation, girls and women have always faced the challenge of managing their menstrual flow. Why does this bleeding arise? What does it mean? What should be done about it? What social or hygienic problems arise from the presence of menstrual blood on clothing or in the local environment? How can the bleeding be contained and controlled? In the absence of accurate biological understanding, more fanciful explanations have arisen in various cultures that are detrimental to the well-being of girls and women. The association between sexuality and the genital bleeding of menstruation often causes discussion of menstruation to be relegated to the margins of social discourse, where it is hidden behind a veil of embarrassment and shame [7–10]. In many cultures, such barriers even make mothers reluctant to talk about these issues with their daughters. The hesitancy to discuss menstruation is not confined to poor developing nations. Even in resource-rich Western countries, many girls reach menarche and experience their first menstrual periods without adequate instruction in what to expect, what it means, and how to manage it [11, 12]. For some, menarche is a frightening and emotionally unsettling experience that further complicates the practical problem of menstrual hygiene management.

In northern Ethiopia, these problems are common [13]. In the Tigray Region, the people live mainly in rural areas where they engage in subsistence agriculture. The climate is dry, rainfall is seasonal and sporadic, and water is a scarce commodity that often must be hauled several miles to homes from the nearest water source. Schools generally have no running water and often do not have a water source of any kind on site. In Tigrayan culture, menstruation is an embarrassing subject that is not spoken of openly, even among close friends and family members. Within the Ethiopian Orthodox Church (the predominant religion in the region), menstruation is believed to make girls and women ritually unclean, preventing them from entering churches or attending religious services during the time of their flow. Similar beliefs are also prevalent among local Muslims. Commercially produced menstrual hygiene products are scarce, and if they can be found at all, they are usually available only in cities or larger towns at relatively high cost. As a result, most Tigrayan women make their own menstrual pads out of old mattress covers, discarded clothing, or *natellas* (the ubiquitous lightweight shawl worn by most Tigrayan women).

In discussing menstruation generally (and menarche specifically) in local focus groups, we have encountered numerous stories of the shock experienced by girls at the time of their first menstruation. Many girls had no knowledge whatsoever that menstruation was something that would normally occur to them some day, and they were panicked when they unexpectedly began bleeding while at school. Many girls have recounted how they made excuses about suddenly being ill, then ran home, where they frantically hid their soiled clothing from their parents and stuffed old rags between their legs to contain the bleeding, while worrying about what this meant or what they had done to cause it. We have also encountered a belief in some quarters that menstruation does not begin until a girl has sexual intercourse, which has resulted in some young girls being beaten by their fathers for alleged sexual misbehavior at the time of menarche. The bewilderment, emotional pain, and family turmoil created by such incidents are hard to imagine. Such incidents could be prevented completely through appropriate biological and health education in schools and family discussions at home.

Even after the initial experience of menarche has been navigated successfully, the monthly recurrence of menstrual bleeding poses a continuing challenge for adolescent school girls. The culturally shameful connotations associated with menstruation and the personal embarrassment of a menstrual hygiene accident are omnipresent worries for girls in school. Each month, they worry about 3–5 days of potential shame and embarrassment if they are caught unawares and unprepared for the start of their menstrual periods. Focus-group participants have recounted numerous stories of girls standing in front of classrooms to write on the chalkboard with visible menstrual staining on their clothing and remorseless teasing by mean-spirited students (often, but not always, male) that subsequently cause them to stay home during menstruation, change schools, or stop their education altogether. Older women tell similar stories from their adolescence in which the presence of menstruation would keep them house bound and curtail their social activities for fear of embarrassment and ridicule. Even after menopause, such childhood experiences are vividly remembered and recounted with sadness.

Menstrual Hygiene

Adequate menstrual hygiene management is defined by the United Nations as "women and adolescent girls using a clean menstrual management material to absorb or collect blood that can be changed in privacy as often as necessary for the duration of the menstruation period, using soap and water for washing the body as required, and having access to facilities to dispose of used menstrual management materials" [14]. Throughout developing countries generally – and certainly within Ethiopia specifically – most girls and women do not have ready access to adequate menstrual hygiene management [10].

Advocacy Efforts

Freweini Mebrahtu is an Ethiopian woman who was born and raised in a large family in Adigrat in northern Ethiopia. Her experience with menarche and menstruation growing up in this region was difficult, but typical of the experiences of Tigrayan adolescents. She vividly remembers the struggles she had in coping with the needs of menstrual hygiene. An excellent student throughout high school, she was admitted to Prairie View A&M University just outside of Houston, Texas, in the United States. It was her first time outside of Ethiopia. One of her earliest and most vivid memories after arriving in the United States was going to a local drug store to look for menstrual hygiene supplies and being overwhelmed by the sheer quantity, quality, and variety of sanitary products available. She never forgot that moment.

After graduating from college with a degree in chemical engineering, she worked for over a decade in the United States before returning to Ethiopia. When she went back to Tigray after nearly 15 years away, she was shocked to discover that nothing about menstrual hygiene management had changed during her absence. Armed with her engineering education, bolstered by her work experience, confident in her abilities, and adamant that things had to change, she set out to make a difference. Given the resource constraints in the local economy, what seemed most logical was the creation of a locally produced, reusable menstrual pad. She created a workable design and was awarded a patent on her product by the Ethiopian government. She successfully applied for a business loan from the Development Bank of Ethiopia (unusual for a woman) and built a factory named after her daughter to produce the pads. She hired local girls and women, trained them, supervised them, and began producing menstrual hygiene pads in Mekelle at the Mariam Seba Sanitary Products Factory in 2009.

Mariam Seba sanitary pads (Fig. 1) have a waterproof backing to prevent external leakage. They have a soft inner lining, underneath which are eight layers of absorbent cotton batting that contain the menstrual blood. The pads are held in place by a simple, single button, which secures the two sides of the pad around the crotch of a pair of underwear, keeping it in the proper position to receive the menstrual flow. If cared for properly, each menstrual pad will last 18 months or longer. Used pads are cleaned by soaking them in a basin of water for an hour, after which they are gently washed with normal laundry detergent, rinsed free of residual soap, and air-dried in the sun. The ultraviolet solar rays in Tigray produce rapid drying and have a reliable bacteriostatic action. Reusable Mariam Seba pads offer numerous advantages over disposable menstrual hygiene products (Table 1). They are locally produced, comfortable, effective, affordable, and discrete. Because they are reusable, they do not produce large volumes of disposable waste, which can clog school latrines and cause environmental contamination, particularly in the context of very limited municipal sanitation systems. Both the economic and social benefits of Mariam Seba sanitary pads flow directly to women.

The development of the reusable sanitary pad and the opening of the factory to produce them was the first step in the creation of a social enterprise to benefit

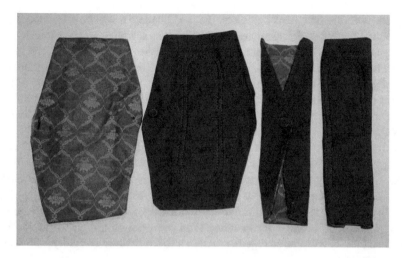

Fig. 1 Reusable Mariam Seba sanitary pads. From left to right: outer covering of pad showing waterproof backing; inner lining of pad; underside of pad folded over and secured with a single button; absorbent side of pad as it would be folded over the crotch of a pair of underwear. (Photo by L. Lewis Wall)

Table 1 Characteristics of Mariam Seba reusable menstrual hygiene pads

Feature	Comments
Environmentally friendly	Reusable pads do not produce the type or quantity of waste generated by disposable pads, which clog latrines and pose an increasing environmental burden, particularly in areas with marginal sanitation systems.
Affordable	Reusable pads cost 80–90% less than disposable pads for equivalent menstrual protection.
Locally produced	Pads are produced in a locally owned and operated factory in Mekelle, Ethiopia, providing local jobs and supporting the local economy.
Comfortable and effective	Mariam Seba pads are well designed and well accepted by local women.
Discrete	An individual menstrual pad folds into a small, compact bundle that can be carried easily and discretely.
Female empowering	The pad was designed by a woman. The factory is owned and operated by a woman. The employees are women and are given 1 month of paid training before they start work, earn a competitive salary in the local economy, and are given health insurance and 12 weeks of paid maternity leave. The factory has also opened a daycare center for young children so that new mothers can continue to work, contribute to their family economy, and enjoy the social interaction of the workplace. These are all unusual and unique characteristics for a factory within the Ethiopian economy.
Complete	Each menstrual hygiene kit contains four reusable pads and two pairs of underwear for use with the pads. Many girls and women, especially in rural Ethiopia, lack underwear, without which menstrual pads are difficult to use.

women. With the first steps complete, the next challenge was how to implement a program to expand social awareness of the problems surrounding menstrual hygiene management and to help communities understand the substantial barrier to regular school attendance that menstrual hygiene management presents for adolescent girls in Ethiopia. Part of this awareness was to get parents generally (and fathers specifically) to understand that menstrual hygiene supplies are basic necessities for girls and women and that their lack has negative social, psychological, and economic consequences for women and the wider society in which they live.

In January 2014, Dr. Lewis Wall and his wife, Helen, arrived in Mekelle on a Fulbright Scholarship to the College of Health Sciences at Mekelle University and Ayder Comprehensive Specialist Hospital. Dr. Wall is an obstetrician-gynecologist and medical anthropologist with a long history of working in Africa. Beginning with an introduction to Freweini and her work from a colleague in the School of Public Health, he began corresponding with her prior to his arrival in Mekelle. Based on their collaboration together, within a few months the Dignity Period project was created.

Dignity Period was created as a nonprofit corporation in the U.S. state of Missouri and received its designation as a not-for-profit, tax-exempt charity from the United States Internal Revenue Service in 2014. The name, Dignity Period™ is also a registered U.S. trademark. After thoughtful consultations and discussions with Dr. Kindeya Gebrehiwot, president of Mekelle University, a tripartite partnership was created to advance the promotion of better education concerning menstruation and improved menstrual hygiene management in northern Ethiopia. The Dignity Period project operates as a community service project through Mekelle University. Money to support the project is raised by Dignity Period in the United States through solicitation of funds from individuals and corporations and by grant applications to foundations and charities in the United States and other countries. The money is transferred as a grant to the Dignity Period project office at Mekelle University to fund specific components of the initiative. Menstrual hygiene kits, consisting of four reusable pads and two pairs of underwear, are purchased at cost by Mekelle University from the Mariam Seba Sanitary Products Factory for distribution in local schools. The project also distributes a bilingual menstrual education pamphlet, in English and Tigrigna, called *Growth and Changes* written by Marni Sommer and Dana Smiles of the Columbia University Mailman School of Public Health in New York City, purchased from the local publisher, Shama Books, in Addis Ababa [15].

The Dignity Period Project

The Dignity Period project operates throughout Tigray via the local schools and, as of 2017, in Afar, with plans to expand to other parts of Ethiopia. The Dignity Period team makes contact with local schools through the regional bureau of education, targeting grades 5 and higher. The schools are selected through a multistage process in which the zones and districts are purposely selected to ensure representation across the region and to give the project the widest possible spread throughout the areas in which it operates. After preliminary selection, the project team visits the local education bureau and the school to check the suitability of the site, to confirm the willingness of the community to participate, and to ensure that other menstrual hygiene education projects are not already being carried out in the area. Once the initial screening and agreement to participate has been completed, the team schedules a visit to the school to provide a menstruation education program and to demonstrate the use and care of the reusable pads. At this initial visit, the educational pamphlet *Growth and Changes* is distributed to all boys and girls in grades 5 and higher. The provision of menstrual education to males as well as females is a critical component of the program's success.

The program gains acceptance and legitimacy by operating through the local school system. By making menstruation and menstrual hygiene subjects of discussion in school, these culturally sensitive and embarrassing topics are pulled into the public arena, where they become an acceptable topic of conversation. The pamphlet provides basic biological and hygiene information about menstruation to all students, male and female, and opens up the subject for further dialogue. One school even created a contest open to all students to see who could achieve the highest score on an examination based on the material covered in *Growth and Changes*. The students take this booklet home, where its presence opens the door to further discussions with parents and siblings about menstruation, creating a "ripple effect" of menstrual awareness throughout the community.

Depending on the logistics of any given community, the Dignity Period team returns in roughly 2 weeks to distribute the menstrual hygiene kits. Distribution of the kits takes place through the school. The kits are handed individually to each female student in grades 5 and above who sign for the kit in a ledger to document the distribution process. This mechanism not only highlights menstrual hygiene education within the schools but also ensures that the kits actually reach those students for whom they are intended and are not diverted for other purposes. The community response to this program has been overwhelmingly positive, particularly in remote rural areas.

Prior to beginning large-scale distribution of pads and pamphlets throughout Tigray, the Dignity Period team undertook two important preliminary research efforts. First, a cross-sectional community survey of beliefs, attitudes, and practices was carried out in 5 rural and 5 urban subdistricts in 4 zones throughout Tigray, involving 428 households [13]. Interviews were carried out in local languages by native speakers. The survey documented a generally low level of scientifically accurate knowledge about the biology of menstruation among both females and males throughout Tigray, as well as many misconceptions about reproductive biology. The belief that menstruation makes women ritually unclean was widespread, and 22% of males and 11% of females held that menstruating girls should not attend school [13]. These survey findings were confirmed by a detailed ethnographic study based on 40 focus-group discussions with premenarchal girls, menstruating adolescents, women of reproductive age, postmenopausal women, adolescent boys, and married men, as well as 64 in-depth interviews with key informants (teachers, school directors, priests, imams, nurses, and menstruating adolescents) through which important menstrual motifs were identified. Recurrent themes identified by focus-group participants included the importance of menstruation for reproductive health, the psychosocial trauma of menarche, the burden of menstrual restrictions (particularly ritual uncleanliness in Christian and Muslim religious traditions), the widespread prevalence of unmet menstrual hygiene needs (including lack of access to sanitary pads and toilet/washing facilities at schools), and the stigma and shame associated with menstrual hygiene accidents by girls at school [16].

The Dignity Period project's underlying assumptions are (1) that better understanding of the biology of menstruation and access to high-quality menstrual hygiene products will improve the quality of life for girls and (2) that by providing accurate education and reliable menstrual hygiene supplies, a barrier to school attendance for adolescent girls will be eliminated. It is hoped that better female school attendance will eventually result in more girls getting advanced education and that this, in turn, will improve their abilities to be economically productive and to be better mothers to their children.

The Dignity Period project carried out a pilot study to test these two assumptions before scaling up the interventions to large numbers of schools. A total of 15 schools (2 urban and 1 rural) in 5 districts (*weredas*) in Tigray were chosen for a pilot project. A total of 8839 students participated in the study. School attendance was tracked by age and sex in grades 7–12, both retrospectively using school records for the year prior to the intervention and then prospectively during the intervention year. We purposefully restricted the pilot evaluation to grades 7–12 to ensure that most girls had already reached menarche and therefore were more likely to have school attendance affected by access to menstrual hygiene supplies. The intervention, as noted earlier, consisted of distribution of the educational pamphlet, demonstrations on the proper use of menstrual pads, and subsequent delivery of the menstrual hygiene kits to girls in school. There was no change in school attendance by male students during the pilot study, but school absences among females decreased by 24% compared to males after the intervention took place [17]. We regard this as a robust proof of concept for the assumptions underlying the Dignity Period program.

Conclusion

The Dignity Period project is an example of effective social entrepreneurship, carried out in partnership by educational institutions (Mekelle University and local schools), charitable nongovernmental organizations (Dignity Period), and socially aware business enterprises (Mariam Seba Sanitary Products Factory). The project is effective at raising awareness about menstruation, which is a universal female health concern, and promoting improved menstrual hygiene, which enhances the psychosocial well-being of girls, improves school attendance, and promotes greater gender equity. As these benefits become more widely appreciated throughout the region, it is likely that this will increase the demand for more and better menstrual hygiene products, which in turn should stimulate commercial interest in meeting women's ongoing menstrual needs. The development of a robust local industry devoted to providing high-quality menstrual hygiene supplies at an affordable price will produce continuing social and economic benefits that can only improve the quality of life for people in local communities. Replication of similar projects in other parts of the world could be expected to produce similar benefits elsewhere.

References

1. Vitzthum VJ. The ecology and evolutionary endocrinology of reproduction in the human female. Yearb Phys Anthropol. 2009;52:95–136.
2. American College of Obstetricians and Gynecologists. Committee Opinion 651. Menstruation in girls and adolescents: Using the menstrual cycle as a vital sign. Obstet Gynecol. 2015;126:e143–6.
3. Jabbour HN, Kelly RW, Fraser HM, Critchley HOD. Endocrine regulation of menstruation. Endocr Rev. 2006;27:17–46.
4. Buckley T, Gottlieb A, editors. Blood magic: the anthropology of menstruation. Berkeley: University of California Press; 1988.
5. Van de Walle T, Renne EP, editors. Regulating menstruation: beliefs, practices, interpretations. Chicago: University of Chicago Press; 2001.
6. Meachem T. An abbreviated history of the development of the Jewish menstrual laws. In: Wasseefall R, editor. Women and water: menstruation in Jewish life and law. Hanover: Brandeis University Press; 1999. p. 23–39.
7. McMahon SA, Winch PJ, Caruso BA, et al. 'The girl with her period is the one to hang her head': reflections on menstrual management among schoolgirls in rural Kenya. BMC Int Health Hum Rights. 2011;11:7.
8. El-Gilany AH, Badawi K, El-Fedawy S. Menstrual hygiene among adolescent schoolgirls in Mansoura, Egypt. Reprod Health Matters. 2005;13(26):147–52.
9. Sommer M. Where the education system and women's bodies collide: the social and health impact of girls' experiences of menstruation and schooling in Tanzania. J Adolesc. 2010;33:521–9.
10. Kuhlmann AS, Henry K, Wall LL. Menstrual hygiene management in resource-poor countries. Obstet Gynecol Surv. 2017;72:356–76.
11. Farage MA, Miller KW, Davis A. Cultural aspects of menstruation and menstrual hygiene in adolescents. Expert Rev Obstet Gynecol. 2011;6:127–39.
12. Koff E, Rierdan J. Early adolescent girls' understanding of menstruation. Women Health. 1995;22:1–19.
13. Wall LL, Belay S, Bayray A, Salih S, Gabrehiwot M. A community-based study of menstrual beliefs in Tigray, Ethiopia. Int J Gynecol Obstet. 2016;135:310–3.
14. Sommer M, Cherenack E, Blake S, Sahin M, Burgers L. WASH in schools empowers girls' education: proceedings of the menstrual hygiene management in schools virtual conference 2014. New York: United Nations Children's Fund and Columbia University; 2015.
15. Somer M, Smiles D, Berhanu A. Growth and Changes. Addis Ababa: Shama Books; 2015.
16. Wall LL, Teklay K, Desta A, Belay S. Tending the 'monthly flower:'A qualitative study of menstrual beliefs in Tigray, Ethiopia. BMC Women's Health (2018) 18:183. https://doi.org/10.1186/s12905-018-0676-z.
17. Belay S, Kuhlmann AS, and Wall LL. Girls' attendance at school after a menstrual hygiene intervention in northern Ethiopia. Int J Gynecol Obstet 2020;149(3): https://doi.org/10.1002/ijgo.13127.

Chapter 7: Technology and the Practice of Health Education in Conflict Zones

Kamiar Alaei and Arash Alaei

Introduction: Education in Conflict Zones

According to UNICEF, in 2017, 27 million children were out of school in conflict zones such as Syria, South Sudan, Iraq, and Yemen, and in areas divided by religion and resources, such as Nigeria and Niger [1, 2]. Based on data from the Institute for International Education (IIE) in 2017, 120,000–140,000 of internally displaced persons (IDPs) in Syria are students who are qualified to attend university [3]. Human rights organizations have long identified education as a fundamental basic need, one that all people ought to be able to access. However, in 2011, the UN's definition of basic needs was amended to include Internet access. The increasing importance of technology in functioning and communicating with the world necessitated this change [4]. Furthermore, access to the Internet has been found to be extraordinarily useful in providing other basic needs, including education and, in turn, healthcare access.

Children in emergency countries, countries affected by conflict and disaster, are disproportionately likely to be out of school. Furthermore, the percent of out-of-school children rises significantly with age. According to the UN, 20% of primary school–aged children in emergency countries are out of school, but that number rises to 43.8% in upper secondary school–aged children [5]. Despite these rates, primary and secondary education is still more resilient during conflict than tertiary

K. Alaei (✉)
Health Science Department, California State University Long Beach, CA, USA

Global Health Diplomacy, Diplomatic Studies Program, Department of Continuing Education, University of Oxford, Oxford, UK

The Institute for International Health and Education (IIHE), Albany, NY, USA
e-mail: kamiaralaei@gmail.com

A. Alaei
The Institute for International Health and Education (IIHE), Albany, NY, USA

© Springer Nature Switzerland AG 2020
P. Murthy, A. Ansehl (eds.), *Technology and Global Public Health*,
https://doi.org/10.1007/978-3-030-46355-7_12

111

education. Institutions of higher learning are the most impacted by conflict. A lack of funding and emphasis on the importance of tertiary education is a direct cause of this. A 2005 report found that the World Bank education sector gave over three times as much funding for primary education as tertiary education to postconflict countries [6].

While tertiary education does require greater financial support, its need for skilled labor and sophisticated management in order to maintain the more complex education system is also a potential cause for lack of resiliency. Additionally, higher education is most strongly affected by the isolation caused by conflicts. An inability to communicate with the outside academic world causes a marked decline in educational quality, even when schools can remain open. Tertiary educational institutions are also set back by the systemic lag of primary and secondary educational institutions because they are unable to exist without them.

The Dire Need for Medical Education in Conflict Zones

Despite these setbacks, it is critical for conflict zones to maintain access to tertiary education. Maintaining proper health education is of vital importance. This is needed, not only to maintain education levels, but to create a new generation of doctors in areas already suffering from doctor shortages. For example, the conflict in Syria has resulted in the deaths of over 800 medical personnel [7]. Additionally, over 15,000 medical professionals in Syria have relocated to other countries. As a result, only 45% of their hospitals still maintain full function. In Aleppo in 2014, there were only approximately 40 physicians present in the city at any time, treating a city of 300,000 residents. In Raqqa, Syria, alone, 590,000 people were in need of medical assistance [8].

This clear shortage of medical professionals has caused many health crises. In Syria, this has included a sharp decline in vaccination rates, from 90% before the war down to 52% in 2014. The result has been a rapid rise in typhoid and measles cases, with measles now the deadliest disease for Syrian children [9]. Additionally, the lack of medical care has resulted in the maternal mortality rate in Syria rising for the first time. In 2015, the World Health Organization found the rate to be 68 deaths per 100,000 live births, up from 49 in 2010 [10].

The need for more medical professionals in conflict zones, such as Syria, is undeniable. However, the rapid decline of access to healthcare education is exacerbating this situation. By 2017, one quarter of medical students at the University of Damascus, one of Syria's largest medical schools, were forced to leave the school. A 2018 study following 128 medical students in 7 conflict zones found that 55% of the medical schools in Libya, Palestine, Syria, Venezuela, and Yemen were forced to shut down. Furthermore, all medical schools in Libya and Yemen were forced to close at some point during the conflicts in those countries. While medical schools are shutting down and medical students are leaving, even students that stay in open schools receive poorer education. In Syria, 20% of all medical students who took their national, standardized exams in 2017 did not pass [11].

To maintain the number of medical students in conflict zones such as Syria, there is a need to improve the quality and accessibility of medical education. One of the most efficient ways to do this is through e-learning. These online education platforms would allow students in conflict zones to continue their education, even if their schools become damaged, inaccessible, or unsafe. This technology has already become essential for many students throughout the Middle East, including medical students in Palestine, Iraq, and Syria.

Barriers Faced by Internally Displaced Students and Refugees Seeking or Continuing Higher Education in Conflict Zones

While several barriers stem from a lack of resources, cultural differences between displaced people and their host country can also represent a major obstacle. Furthermore, students and faculty must feel safe in their school, and therefore a lack of safety in higher educational institutions is a significant barrier that must be overcome in conflict zones.

Barriers Caused by Shortage of Financial and Educational Resources

1. **Financial resources and budgets** for primary, secondary, and tertiary levels of education drop dramatically in conflict zones.
2. **Lack of in-depth educational curricula and materials** is often caused by the destruction of libraries and laboratories during conflicts. Additionally, access to online materials is especially minimal in conflict zones, and, as a result, students cannot easily access the necessary educational material.
3. **Lack of human resources, such as teachers and school counselors,** is one of the most dire consequences of war, causing a significant shortage of human resources in conflict zones.
4. **Lack of universal school and university qualification certificates** makes it difficult for students to provide proof of their learning achievements, especially for students who study in a setting that does not meet the criteria of the ministry of national education of their host country.
5. **Low access to technology,** such as shortage of electricity, access to the Internet and computers, places an extra burden on students in conflict zones in terms of accessing educational materials.

Barriers Caused by Cultural Differences

1. **Language and cultural barriers** can prevent refugee children and adolescents from gaining access to the educational system of their host countries and to adjusting to their new living environment.
2. **Unstable, unfamiliar living arrangements and the long journey to school** contribute greatly to the high student dropout rate in conflict zones.
3. **Xenophobia, exclusion, and stigmatization** can create an unsafe environment for children and adults seeking to join a new school or university system.

Barriers Caused by Insufficient and Inadequate Policies and Laws

1. **Low prioritization of higher education**, despite its being a basic human right, results in a significant dearth of resources targeted at maintaining higher education. Education is a human right; it gives hope and resilience. Furthermore, it is required for the long-term maintenance and growth of communities and to protect children and young adults from discrimination in society. Yet there is no mention of the role of tertiary education in the future of children and young adults by humanitarian organizations in conflict zones. When these countries eventually stabilize, they will need skilled young adults, with higher education, to rebuild their country – physically, intellectually, and emotionally.
2. **Legal barriers** exist in many host countries that do not recognize the rights of undocumented migrants to enter or use the school or university system.

Barriers Caused by Lack of Safety

1. **Despite the lack of safety at schools and universities in conflict zones,** many schools and universities may still function, but the ongoing violence and instability make it more difficult for students to keep up with their studies. As a result, the number of students enrolled in schools and universities has decreased significantly [12].
2. **Destruction of university and school property** can result in a lack of safe and accessible space for students to continue their education.
3. **Gender-based violence and lack of safety** for girls and women contribute to gender inequity in education access in conflict zones. According to a report from UNICEF in 2017, girls are 2.5 times more likely to be out of school than boys in conflict regions [13]. Women and girls are more prone to gender-motivated abuse and sexual violence in conflict settings, making it more challenging for them to continue their education.

Using Technology to Overcome Barriers to Delivering Health Education in Conflict Zones

As mentioned previously, several barriers must be overcome to provide health education in conflict zones. However, case studies of previously implemented projects have shown that it is possible to overcome these obstacles using technology. E-learning platforms provide a unique way to deliver education that can minimize the cultural barriers to education. Furthermore, e-learning can be utilized in conflict zones with fewer physical resources needed than in a physical school while also allowing students to work in a safe location, as opposed to a school to which it may be difficult or dangerous to travel. This section will emphasize the importance of technology in conflict zones by illustrating its use in providing health care education, using the case study of an online higher education medical program for internally displaced Syrian medical students. This health care education access is imperative, not only to allow students to meet a need as basic as education but also to be able to increase the number of potential health care providers. This in turn will improve healthcare access in conflict zones.

E-Learning Models Delivering Higher Medical Education in Conflict Zones

Overview

To overcome the challenges faced by internally displaced students and refugees to continue higher education, programs need to be able to address the aforementioned barriers and to provide young, aspiring internally displaced and refugee students with educational materials and skills that can assist them in continuing their education and in finding jobs, as well as contribute to their own family and society. While e-learning platforms are a relatively new technology, many different organizations have utilized these platforms to provide education to students in conflict zones around the world. War Child Holland, a nongovernmental organization NGO based in the Netherlands, created E-Learning Sudan, a program that uses tablets to provide informal education to out-of-school Sudanese children in remote villages. The Can't Wait to Learn program similarly employs tablets and web-based learning (WBL) to provide children in Sudan, Lebanon, Uganda, and Jordan with education access [11]. Although there are e-learning programs around the world targeted at a range of educational levels, the following three case studies will specifically discuss the role of WBL in providing health education in conflict zones in the Middle East.

Medical Education for Palestinian Medical Students, Developed by OxPal MedLink in Partnership with Oxford University in 2012 [12]

For decades, Palestinian medical students have been dealing with a lack of resources, funding, collaborative opportunities, and access to medical literature. As a result, the rate and quality of healthcare and educational development have suffered. International organizations have noticed this crisis and begun to work toward a solution. In 2012, OxPal MedLink was established to partner medical students and faculty in Palestine with clinicians at Oxford University Hospitals. Inspired by Medicine Africa, a similar e-learning platform utilized in Africa, OxPal utilizes WizIQ, a virtual-classroom technology, to allow tutors in Oxford to video conference with medical students in Palestine. By April 2013, OxPal had recruited and educated around 40 students through the Foundation for Al-Quds University Medical School in East Jerusalem. Subsequently, the program was expanded to include approximately 120 students at other medical schools as well, including Islamic University in Gaza and Al Azhar University.

This deliverance of real-time, case-based learning across a variety of medical specialties has allowed medical students to improve their clinical skill set while also practicing applications of their classroom knowledge to a patient-centered setting. Furthermore, the program is focused on the types of cases that future doctors serving the Palestinian population ought to be most prepared to see. WizIQ allows for a multimedia classroom, synthesizing audio learning, text-based chat, and interactive whiteboards into one platform. A vital aspect of WizIQ is that the application only requires a very low-bandwidth Internet connection, allowing for OxPal MedLink to minimize costs while increasing accessibility for its students.

Technology-Enhanced or Web-Based Learning (TEL or WBL) for Clinical Training of Iraqi Psychiatrist, Developed by MedicineAfrica and OxPIO in 2016 [13]

Iraq suffers from education difficulties similar to those in other conflict zones, including difficulty in collaborative educational opportunities. Additionally, Iraq has a greater shortage of psychiatrists than other medical specialties. Therefore, a WBL program was designed for Oxford physicians to train Iraqi psychiatrists.

MedicineAfrica and OxPIO created a WBL program for Iraqi psychiatrists. The two organizations connected psychiatrists in Oxford University's Medical Education Fellowship who had previously worked in Iraq with Iraqi psychiatry trainees. Then the trainees' needs were assessed by Iraqi Board of Psychiatry supervisors. The team of ten Iraqi psychiatry trainees and five British senior psychiatrists was formed. Unlike most e-learning methods, this program was focused on feedback, assessment, and discussion, as opposed to a lecture-based format. This allowed for accessible, immediate discussion and training opportunities. However, there were logistical and financial difficulties, including the expenses of the required technology, online learning templates, and technical support.

Feedback from both the Iraqi trainees and the UK supervisors was positive. While improvements in clinical skills and knowledge was evident, all the psychiatry trainees also received certificates for participation in the tutorials, supporting their portfolio development.

Development, Implementation, and Importance of Online Education for Displaced Syrian Medical Students (OEDSS), Developed by State University of New York (SUNY) at Albany in 2016

Part 1: Situation Analysis and Need Assessment by OEDSS Program

The current conflict in Syria has similarly impacted the country's medical education. Overall, around 200,000 displaced Syrian students that were qualified for higher education were unable to attain it, due to physical, financial, language, and technological barriers. As previously stated, the healthcare crisis in Syria is startling, and active medical schools are essential for building Syria's next generation of doctors. Medical schools in Aleppo and Damascus have already suffered attacks, causing many students to be too afraid to attend school. Professors and students have held underground classes, with lectures delivered in secret locations and safe houses. However, e-learning platforms could provide a safe, widely accessible alternative, as shown by Table 1.

Part 2: Implementation

Doctors Arash and Kamiar Alaei have been at the forefront of e-learning platforms for medical students in Syria. Their mission was to develop an educational platform that did not require the physical presence of students, while ensuring that it would be available and accessible to all students, regardless of the barriers they faced. Their steps to develop this program, as outlined in what follows in Table 2, first began in 2014. From 2014 to May 2016, in collaboration with several universities in Turkey, Council of Higher Education in Turkey, State University of New York (SUNY) at Albany, and several funders, Doctors Arash and Kamiar Alaei were able to develop their project for internally displaced medical students in Syria in non-government-controlled areas. These students were previously forced to discontinue their education, either because their universities were destroyed or their faculty members fled the country or died. They are able to provide continuity in education,

Table 1 Online Education for Displaced Syrian Medical Students (OEDSS) removes barriers faced by students in conflict zones

Barrier	OEDSS Approach	Notes
1. Physical	Distance learning program	This approach removes physical barriers and benefits **students** and **internally displaced persons (IDPs)** who live in areas, such as conflict zones, where accessing physical schools and universities is difficult or impossible.
2. Gender-based inequality	E-learning virtual platform	This approach addresses **gender-based inequality** in pursuing higher education in conflict zones by removing potential discomfort or inaccessibility that could arise from an in-person, mixed-gender classroom setting. This is especially true for settings where female students are hindered from attending universities and pursuing higher education.
3. Financial	Offering programs free of charge	The IIHE is aware of the lack of budget and financial resources for educational purposes in conflict zones, so programs and training are offered to students free of charge.
4. Educational	Developing in-depth curriculum	**In-depth curriculum in medicine removes educational barriers** that hinder young students and IDPs from continuing their education. This can eventually contribute to the revival of the currently poorly structured health system in Syria.
5. Technological	Using smartphone apps	**Using technology such as smartphone applications removes the technological barriers** that prevent young refugee students and IDPs from accessing educational materials and acquiring knowledge and skills. This is especially vital in conflict zones, where access to the Internet is limited or nonexistent.
6. Language	Offering intensive English language program (IELP)	The **English program** will teach medical terminology as well as conversational English through lessons and assignments aimed at enhancing students' reading, writing, and speaking skills in English. In the long term, this method can connect the target population both to other available online programs and to the international community at large.

at no cost, to students who would not otherwise be able to complete their medical education.

This platform designed in such a way that medical students can use educational material and discuss their questions with their mentors via smartphone. It was found that the availability of smartphones among medical students was higher than other devices, and due to lack of access to a permanent Internet connection, we needed to develop a platform that would allow the educational material to be available offline as well.

To make the program accessible to Arabic-speaking Syrian students, professors from Yale University, SUNY Albany, and Syria all volunteered to record their lectures. These lectures were transcribed and translated into Arabic. They then recruited

Table 2 Evolution of OEDSS program since inception

First step (2014 to May 2016)	Outreach to universities in Turkey Discussions with Turkish Higher Education Council Discussions with SUNY branches and faculty members Meetings with funders
Second Step: 2-day workshop at Yale University (May 2016)	Brainstorm and discussion, Skype meeting with displaced Syrian students at Yale University in May 2016 320–400 health science students have been targeted 50:50 female-male ratio

Third Step (June–September 2016)	Enroll 330 students:
	    Deliver online genetics course
	Offer English language proficiency exam to 400 students and faculty
	    Enroll 35 students qualified for upper-intermediate level of intensive English language program

Fourth Step (January–May 2017)	Delivery of medical terminology Delivery of head and neck anatomy Delivery of biochemistry Delivery of microbiology Delivery of intermediate intensive English language program (IELP)
Fifth Step (June 2017–June 2018)	Total of 525 students

bilingual instructors to teach live sessions and utilized mobile apps to relay their information to medical students. Working with Yale students, they were able to acquire free access to an app that allows students to study human anatomy in full color. It was ensured that the courses would be completely accessible through a smartphone app and that much of it would be accessible offline, since few students had computer access or reliable Internet access. The already available apps were not accessible most of the time, so an app was developed at the University of Albany, called SHABAN, which allows for live, virtual classroom sessions and is accessible both online and offline. Additionally, it only requires minimal Wi-Fi connection to function.

Once this preparation was complete, the program was presented in two parts. The online academic courses allowed for teaching medical courses that were accessible to Arabic speakers, while the intensive English learning program (IELP) taught the medical students English, with volunteers across the globe acting as teaching assistants and providing live language sessions. Students were given daily homework assignments, meant to enhance their reading, writing, and speaking skills, and attendance was taken during live sessions in order to emphasize communication.

The program has been successfully implemented, and over 500 students have enrolled in it in the last two and a half years, with hundreds on the waiting list. In 2018, the program had its first virtual graduation ceremony, held for students who completed their advanced English class, and aims to improve, expand, and scale up in the near future in a different part of the world, especially in conflict zones.

Part 3: Data Analysis and Evaluation

The first year of the OEDSS program can be considered a success in three areas: gender balance, dropout rates, and course completion. The program was consciously designed to be equally accessible to both female and male students, so half the students are female and half are male. In addition, the dropout rate has been extremely low, about 3%. Finally, approximately 70% of all students successfully passed their exams and obtained credit for their courses. For upper-intermediate IELP, 89% of students passed the course while approximately 66% passed the intermediate-level IELP. Grades were based on daily homework assignments that included tasks to enhance reading, writing, and speaking skills. Furthermore, attendance at live sessions was required to emphasize listening, speaking, and communication. Following the second phase of program delivery, OEDSS conducted a survey of participating students. The sample size was 231 students. A total of 113, or 49%, identified themselves as female, while a total of 98, or 42%, identified themselves as male. Twenty respondents (9%) did not list a gender. The age distribution of the group ranged from 17 to 30, with most students listing their age as 19, 20, or 21 (Fig. 1).

The data revealed interesting patterns in the use of online courses. Most (73%) students who responded had never taken an online course before. Both male and female students expressed more comfort with online classes including both genders as compared to in-person classes including both genders (Fig. 2).

The data also reveal an interesting gap between the online learning tools students are comfortable with using and the tools that are actually available to them. For example, while most (70%) students are comfortable using laptops to access online courses, only 9% actually had access to laptops, and while 65% of students had access to smartphones, only 20% of students felt comfortable using them to take online courses (Fig. 3).

In terms of Internet access, 73% had access, 24% did not, and 3% had access some of the time. If Internet access was available, most students had variable access or access between 1 and 6 h per day. Only about 25 students, or 11%, reported Internet access between 19 and 24 h per day. Interestingly, only 6% of students were able to access the Internet free of charge, while 97% reported that they had to pay for access (Fig. 4).

Interviews with students reflect what the data showed, a picture of general satisfaction with the offerings and appreciation for the opportunity, coupled with an outline of the main challenges related to such factors as Internet access and electricity. For example, below is feedback obtained by interviewing two students who participated in OEDSS program, via Skype:

> Hello, I am a student. I want to thank you for giving us this great opportunity. The Genetics course has been very useful. The way the course presented is helpful and easy to understand. However, we face some technical challenges especially in communicating with our professors and other students due to limited internet access. We are trying to cooperate as students to overcome these challenges. The university tries to help as well by providing internet access to students on campus. Also, this semester, we have heavy course loads. Next semester, we will be able to manage the course load better. Thank you again.

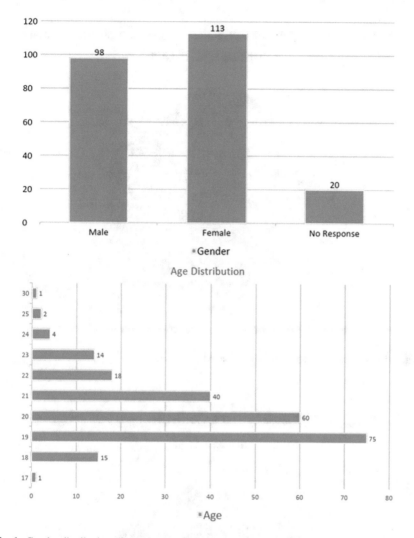

Fig. 1 Gender distribution of sample size_(left); age distribution of sample size (right)

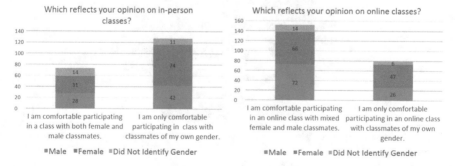

Fig. 2 Opinion about on-campus coeducational classes (left); opinion about online coeducational classes (right)

Which devices are available for you to access online course materials?

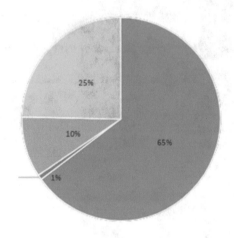

25%

10%

65%

1%

■Smartphone ■Desktop computer ■Laptop ■Tablet

Fig. 3 Comparison of usage by device for online education

Is internet connection available in your physical location?

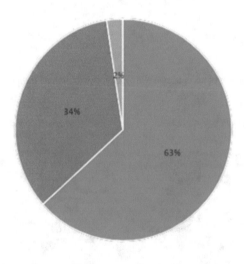

2%

34%

63%

■Yes ■No ■Sometimes

Fig. 4 Availability of Internet access among cohort

Hi, I am a first year student in medical school. I am taking the Genetics course. The course is presented wonderfully, and is useful for the students. The course provides a comprehensive approach that helps students understand the content of the course. The videos are very helpful in facilitating and explaining some of the difficult parts of the course content. During the weekly live session, we are able to discuss all questions students have related to that week's lectures.

The students are appreciative of the fact that the courses are being made available to them, pointing out the benefit of live sessions with instructors and students and the clear manner in which the courses are taught. However, they also pointed out key flaws in the program. Technical challenges, such as Internet access, remain. Additionally, it is often difficult for students to adapt to the heavy course load, especially when dealing with the burden of living in a conflict zone. These challenges and potential solutions will be discussed in greater detail in the following section.

Part 4: The OEDSS Program's Key Challenges and the Potential Solutions

Despite the advances that this program has made, difficulties still arise. This program in Syria exemplifies many of the challenges of developing online education programs in conflict zones. This highlights several key challenges in providing online medical education to displaced Syrian students.

We must recognize that many of the barriers faced by medical students within Syria are physical impediments to accessing education, whether it is access to physical classrooms or to electricity and Internet connection; when electricity is simply not available, then the choice of platform or device to access online learning seems almost irrelevant. Some students' smartphones are not compatible with SHABAN, and often their Internet connection is not reliable enough for the app to work properly. Although the courses themselves are free to students, the cost of Internet access represents a great burden. While 73% of students had Internet access, only 11% reported having more than 19 h of access per day, and 97% of students had to pay for Internet access. Although offline access to the program is particularly helpful to these students, lack of Internet access is still a hindrance to their education. One student remarked on this concern in his feedback about the program, stating, "We face some technical challenges especially in communicating with the professors and other students due to limited Internet access." For students in a conflict zone, this is particularly challenging to overcome, so using and installing satellite technology in the future has the potential to remove the technological barriers that prevent young Syrian students and IDPs from accessing educational materials by broadening access to the Internet in regions in Syria, especially in conflict zones, where there is no or very limited access to the Internet.

Some students feel the work load of the course is difficult and fast-paced, and this points to the challenge that IDP students face in pursuing education via online programs. Among the participants, 30% did not pass their English course, and interviewed students stated that the course load felt heavy. Therefore, it may be helpful to have a longer transition period for these students to allow for more time to adjust to being back in a class, completing assignments, and taking exams.

The OEDSS program is at the intermediate level, based on the curriculum of SUNY Albany, and delivered to students at various academic levels. To make it better suited to the academic background of students, the current curriculum must be further tailored and revised.

The IELP part of the OEDSS program was developed on the basis of general English language proficiency; however, the target students need to learn medical content and terminology in addition to conventional English; therefore, to benefit medical students, the IELP has been specifically adjusted to teach medical terminology as opposed to teaching only conversational English.

Practice Recommendations and Lessons Learned to Improve Programs Such as OEDSS

In addressing the challenges faced by medical students and IDPs in Syria, we have learned many lessons from the past 3 years of using the OEDSS program for medical students. The key lessons, presented in what follows, are to inform other programs such as the OEDSS, as well as to inform policy and practice for medical education in conflict settings:

1. In conflict zones, online learning platforms are a revolutionary way to provide medical education to displaced students. However, these programs are exceedingly rare. These programs additionally need constant feedback, monitoring, and adjustment in order to optimize their potential. Few programs provide accredited medical education, especially in the students' own language and country. The low dropout rate of the program in Syria, 3%, reflects the value students see in this program. This was frequently stated by the participants, and it encourages the development of additional such programs in the near future for displaced students in conflict zones as well as refugees wishing to pursue higher education.

2. Constant adjustment by in response to the frequent input and feedback received from faculty members and students in Syria is key improving and maintaining programs such as the OEDSS. For example, we had to try a few different approaches to get the Arabic accent right or to make female students more comfortable attending these courses. We always encourage participants to attend classes on a regular basis to maximize the efficacy of the program. Before moving on to the next session, we make sure that all the students understand the academic material thoroughly and are able to ask whatever questions they may have.

3. The value of human interaction and volunteerism should not be underestimated. Informal and personal contact with students, as well as ongoing communication between Syrian students and volunteers in the U.S. and other countries, was critical to giving students hope under terrible circumstances and the feeling that they

were moving forward, despite daily challenges. Live sessions were important, as was the participation of more than 16 faculty members, graduate students, and administrators as volunteers.

4. To facilitate external evaluation and expand the network of volunteer (faculty and staff) and overall support for the program, in February 2017, Global Institute for Health and Human Rights (GIHHR) invited experts from Yale University, the University of South Carolina, and the Harvard Humanitarian Initiative to form the Collaboration for Health Education in Conflict (CHEC). The purpose of this partnership is to share experiences and resources and improve the overall quality of the program. Furthermore, CHEC will analyze the existing project to assess strengths and weaknesses in order to scale up and be applicable to conflict zones in other parts of the world. CHEC findings are in process and will be incorporated into future program plans.

Conclusion

Higher education is no longer a priority in conflict zones, causing a sharp drop in financial resources and budgets for the education sector. A lack of safety, electricity, and water at schools and universities, the lack of in-depth educational curricula and materials, the destruction of university and school property, libraries, and laboratories, limited or poor Internet access, technology and geographical barriers, and a lack of human resources, teachers, and staff to teach – all have contributed to this dire situation. There is an urgent need for innovative programs such as OEDSS to be implemented in conflict zones. This initiative has overcome physical, financial, linguistic, and cultural barriers and even offered advantages over traditional medical training. For example, female students were able to interact with, and learn alongside, male classmates and peers.

By constantly improving upon and expanding OEDSS, medical students in conflict zones can attend medical school and pursue higher education at a rate previously unseen within conflict zones.

Acknowledgements We would like to thank all the volunteers who, in varying capacities, helped develop and deliver the OEDSS program. We are grateful to all of those in Syria and other partner institutions with whom we have had the pleasure to work during this program. Special thanks go to our IIHE team members – Mansoureh M. Karimi, Mahtab Naji, and Afaf Moustafa – who assisted us with the literature review and drafting and editing the chapter.

The names of the students who provided feedback on the program have been removed and their feedback anonymized for privacy.

We also express our gratitude to the previously mentioned team members for their assistance on the figure captions and credit lines for all included figures and on the drafting and editing of the chapter.

References

1. Edwards A. Forced displacement at record 68.5 million. UNHCR. 2018. https://www.unhcr. org/news/stories/2018/6/5b222c494/forced-displacement-record-685-million.html. Accessed 1 Apr 2019.
2. 27 million children out of school in conflict zones – UNICEF. 2017. Unicef.org. https:// www.unicef.org/press-releases/27-million-children-out-school-conflict-zones. Accessed 1 Apr 2019.
3. AlAhmad M. The crisis of higher education for Syrian refugees. Brookings. 2016. https:// www.brookings.edu/blog/education-plus-development/2016/06/17/the-crisis-of-higher-education-for-syrian-refugees/. Accessed 1 Apr 2019.
4. Jackson N. United Nations declares internet access a basic human right. The Atlantic. 2011. https://www.theatlantic.com/technology/archive/2011/06/united-nations-declares-internet-access-a-basic-human-right/239911/. Accessed 1 Apr 2019.
5. A future stolen: young and out of school. UNICEF. 2018. https://data.unicef.org/wp-content/uploads/2018/09/Out-of-school-children-Fact-Sheet-individual-pages.pdf. Accessed 1 Apr 2019.
6. Reshaping the future education and postconflict reconstruction. Siteresources.worldbank.org. http://siteresources.worldbank.org/INTCPR/Resources/Reshaping_the_Future.pdf
7. Maternal mortality in 1990–2015. Who.int. 2015. https://www.who.int/gho/maternal_health/countries/syr.pdf?ua=1
8. *Syria's Medical Community Under Assault*. Physicians for Human Rights. 2015. https://s3.amazonaws.com/PHR_other/Syria%27s-Medical-Community-Under-Assault-February-2015.pdf. Accessed 1 Apr 2019.
9. Sedlak M. Medical Education is #NotATarget! International Federation of Medical Students' Associations (IFMSA). 2018. https://ifmsa.org/2018/04/21/medical-education-is-notatarget/. Accessed 1 Apr 2019.
10. Ibrahim M. Education USA Syria: An Update | NAFSA. 2016. Nafsa.org. https://www.nafsa. org/Professional_Resources/Browse_by_Interest/International_Students_and_Scholars/Network_Resources/International_Enrollment_Management/EducationUSA_Syria__An_Update/. Accessed 1 Apr 2019.
11. The history of War Child. 2019. Warchildholland.org. https://www.warchildholland.org/history/. Accessed 1 Apr 2019.
12. Ali MA, Penfold RS, Patel I, MacGregor T, Cahill TJ, Ali AM, Shankar S, Nguyen M, Finlayson AET, Mahmud I. The Palestinian territories: barriers to healthcare and medical education and the strategic role of distance-learning partnerships in education systems strengthening. Med Confl Surviv. 2014;30(1):11–8. https://doi.org/10.1080/13623699.2014.873644.
13. Hameed Y, Al Taiar H, O'Leary D, Kaynge L. Can online distance learning improve access to learning in conflict zones? The Oxford psychiatry in Iraq (Oxpiq) experience. Br J Med Pract. 2018. http://www.bjmp.org/files/2018-11-2/bjmp-2018-11-2-a1114.pdf.

Chapter 8: Law, Technology, and Public Health

Denise Scotto

Background

The Sustainable Development Goals (SDG) that the 70th session of the United Nations General Assembly adopted in September 2015 provide member states with a blueprint for action to improve many of our world's pressing challenges. SDG number three (SDG 3) concerns health insofar as governments have agreed to ensure healthy lives for their people and to promote well-being for everyone at all phases of an individual's life cycle [1].

While the level and degree of a nation's development impacts the kinds of health policies, programs, treatment, services, and education it provides to its people, technological innovation has influenced the health sector globally, so much so that less economically developed countries are able to provide health information and, in some instances, health services to a significant portion of its population.

Drones transport medicine and blood samples, computer Internet connections link doctors with patients to schedule appointments, exchange information including medical test results, and conduct virtual appointments. Cell phones provide patients with health reminders from medical providers, bridging great distances between provider and client, and, Fitbit monitors a person's vital signs and provides information on wellness.

This article explores some of the key legal issues relating to global health in the context of technological innovation from a variety of perspectives. The practice of medicine, the reimbursement and coverage for health services, patient privacy, and patient safety have all been areas of concern for years. With widespread new technology including wireless devices and social media, these matters have grown in scope and, along with it, emerging issues. The ability to transcend boundaries

D. Scotto (✉)
International Policy Advisor, New York, NY, USA
e-mail: denise.scotto@gmail.com

© Springer Nature Switzerland AG 2020
P. Murthy, A. Ansehl (eds.), *Technology and Global Public Health*,
https://doi.org/10.1007/978-3-030-46355-7_13

through information and communications technology (ICT) has the potential to create a unified, borderless world in the context of health systems and healthcare delivery. As a consequence, a myriad of stakeholders in the international community need to join with one another to create a coherent, workable, and equitable system for all countries.

Definitions and Examples

According to the World Health Organization (WHO), telehealth involves using telecommunications and virtual technology to deliver healthcare beyond traditional healthcare facilities. Telehealth, which requires access only to telecommunications, is the fundamental element of eHealth, which uses a broader range of ICT. An example of virtual healthcare is when a chronically ill or elderly person receives guidance while at home [2].

According to the European Commission (EC), eHealth refers to tools and services using ICT that can improve health prevention, diagnosis, treatment, monitoring, and management. It includes information and data sharing between patients and health service providers, hospitals, health professionals and health information networks, electronic health records, telemedicine services, portable patient-monitoring devices, operating room scheduling software, robotized surgery, and research on the virtual, physiological human [3].

A noteworthy 2010 WHO report described telemedicine as "*healing from a distance*," which reaches back to the mid-1800s. It has evolved particularly since the 1960s and 1970s through initiatives involving the military and aerospace industries. The WHO explained that telemedicine narrows services performed by physicians, whereas telehealth expands delivery to include nurses, pharmacists, and other healthcare personnel. While the two terms may at times be used interchangeably, there is a consensus that telehealth is broader because it encompasses continuing medical education, professional healthcare training, and the use of technology for medical billing, scheduling, and holding administrative meetings. It is widely agreed that telemedicine is not a separate medical specialty [4].

According to the American Telemedicine Association (ATA), telemedicine is used in various ways. Networked programs link hospitals and clinics with outlying clinics and community health centers in rural or suburban areas through high-speed lines or the Internet for telecommunication between sites. Point-to-point connections using private, high-speed networks are used by hospitals and clinics that deliver services directly or outsource specialty services to independent medical service providers. Monitoring center links are used for cardiac, pulmonary, or fetal monitoring, home care, and related services that provide care to patients at home. Web-based eHealth patient service sites provide direct consumer outreach and services over the Internet [5].

Within telehealth there are four recognized applications. One is live, two-way interactive videoconferencing, which is known as synchronous. A second is the electronic transmission via secure e-mail of medical information such as documents and images – X-rays, MRIs, photos – and is known as asynchronous. Another is the remote monitoring of personal patient medical and health data through observation of daily living routines, usually through sensors from a person in one location sent electronically to a person in a second location. A fourth is mobile, or *mHealth*, where public healthcare and education are supported by mobile communication and wireless devices such as cell phones, smartphones, portable monitoring sensors, tablet computers, wireless devices, and special software including "apps." This includes text message appointment reminders, recordkeeping/data collection, and the growing number of wearable devices that allow people to track their own health and wellness and become more responsible for it [6]. mHealth encompasses numerous market participants, consumers, compatibility of systems, varied regulatory compliance, and a high degree of coordinated efforts. Wireless and Internet service providers, technology manufacturers, software specialists, and start-ups are also crucial actors.

According to a Global Health: Science and Practice article of 2013, mHealth is a health systems strengthening tool where mHealth strategies are seen as integrable systems that fit into existing health system functions and complement the eHealth system goals of health service provisions; a well-performing health workforce; a functioning health information system; cost-effective use of medical products, vaccines, and technologies; and accountability and governance. The article describes 12 common mHealth and ICT applications, ranging from client education and behavior change communication to registries and vital-event tracking. This is in addition to data collection and reporting to electronic decision support (information, protocols, algorithms, checklists) to provider-to-provider communication (user groups and consultation) to supply chain management to financial transactions and incentives [7].

Health information technology (HIT) involves the design, development, implementation, and maintenance of an array of information systems used in the healthcare industry. Examples of HIT include administrative billing, electronic prescribing or ePrescribing, electronic health records, mobile medical carts, and e-mail communication with patients [8].

In discussing technological innovation, a core principle is interoperability – the ability of different information technology systems and software applications to communicate, exchange data, and use the information that has been exchanged or, to put it more simply, to share a common operating platform. Interoperability is a critical piece of facilitating health information exchange, for example, a specialist using an eHealth record from a primary care physician [9].

Growth of Telehealth

There is no doubt that telemedicine is a global industry that is explosively expanding. Cross-border activities in healthcare in the European market are growing, with many of them related to eHealth. In 2010 the global telemedicine market reached

$9.8 billion; in 2011, it rose to $11.6 billion and is expected to triple to $27.3 billion by 2016 [10]. In the U.S., in 2013, the market for telehealth generated annual revenues of $9.6 billion, a 60% increase from 2012 [11]. The World Bank reported that there were more than 500 mobile health projects in 2011 alone [12].

Teleservice expansion can be attributed to its benefits. Given provider shortages around the world in rural and urban areas, telehealth is uniquely suited to increase service to millions of new patients. In the U.S., 59 million people reside in Health Professional Shortage Areas. Telehealth has been shown to reduce the cost of healthcare and increase efficiency through better management of chronic diseases, shared health professional staffing, reduced travel times, and fewer or shorter hospital stays. In the U.S., chronic disease accounts for roughly 75% of all healthcare costs and contributes to an estimated 70% of deaths in the country [11]. The quality of healthcare services is as good as those given in traditional in-person consultations. In mental health and intensive care unit care, it delivers superior services with greater outcomes and patient satisfaction. It is convenient for consumers with studies showing high patient satisfaction and support for these services [11].

In support of the WHO's Global Action Plan for the Prevention and Control of Noncommunicable Diseases (NCDs) and in response to the 2011 United Nations Political Declaration on NCDs, in October 2012, the International Telecommunications Union (ITU), together with the WHO, launched the global mHealth program Be He@lthy, Be Mobile. This program specifically targets NCDs using mobile phone technology to influence behaviors that can help control the world's biggest killers. Underlying the program is the acknowledgement that 90% of the world's population was already covered by a mobile cellular network and that by the end of 2014, mobile cellular subscriptions reached close to 7 billion [13].

Given the continually increasing use of mobile technology, the WHO convened a group of global experts working at the intersection of mHealth research and program implementation called the mHealth Technical Evidence Review Group (mTREG) in order to assess the need for guidelines for the reporting of evidence on the effectiveness of mHealth interventions. In 2016, the review resulted in the creation of the mHealth evidence reporting and assessment (MERA) checklist [12].

Telehealth in the European Union

An outgrowth of the EC's 1999 "e-Europe initiative" led naturally to the Health Online Action. The Health Online Action, combined with rapid technological progress, resulted in the development of a high-level committee on health that formed a Working Group on Health Telematics. The working group reviewed specific applications of ICT in health such as health cards, virtual hospitals, and provision of health-related information concerning health professionals and patients [14].

In 2004, the EC designed the first Action Plan for a European eHealth Area. In a report issued in December 2007, the EC named eHealth as one of the six leading markets in Europe. In November 2008, it issued a communication on telemedicine for the benefit of patients, healthcare systems, and society. By the end of 2011, member states were called upon to complete a review of their national regulations providing greater access to telemedicine services in the areas of accreditation, liability, reimbursement, privacy, and data protection. By the end of 2011, several other significant steps were undertaken to further eHealth. The eHealth Network, the main governance body at the EU level relating to the interoperability of cross-border eHealth services, was born, a directive on the application of patients' rights in cross-border healthcare was issued, and the eHealth Action Plan for 2012–2020 was concluded [14].

In a statement dated October 25, 2013, to mark the entry into force of the directive concerning patients' rights in cross-border healthcare, Health Commissioner Tonio Borg stated, "...EU law in force enshrines citizens' right to go to another EU country for treatment and get reimbursed for it. From today, all EU countries should have transposed the Directive...adopted 30 months ago, into their National law" [15].

Legal and Market Concerns in the European Union

A key aim of the eHealth Action Plan 2012–2020 – Innovative Healthcare for the Twenty-First Century – is to create favorable legal and market conditions for developing eHealth products and services. Noteworthy European legal accomplishments that apply to eHealth are the Data Protection Directive, Ecommerce Directive, Medical Device Directive, and Directive on Distance Contracting. Legal obstacles that have diminished growth are the absence of interoperability between eHealth solutions, the lack of legal clarity for health and well-being mobile applications, the nonexistence of transparency regarding data collected by them, and inadequate or fragmented legal frameworks, including the lack of reimbursement mechanisms for eHealth services and liability issues [10].

Given that European Union (EU) use of electronic health platforms and electronic health records continues to rise, ICT specification standardization is of prime importance with regard to necessitating measures for interoperability. Much has been undertaken to facilitate cross-border interoperability specifications on the eHealth Interoperability Framework. Guidelines on minimum/nonexhaustive patient summary data sets for electronic exchange in accordance with the Cross-Border Directive were adopted in 2013 [16]. Guidelines known as the ePrescription Dataset for Electronic Exchange Under Cross Border Directive were adopted in 2014 [17]. Both sets of guidelines aim to provide safe and quality healthcare with a high level of trust and security. These guidelines, therefore, govern technical specifications such as software engineering, coding and document design, and hosting institutions and, at the same time, take into account the need for confidentiality of sensitive patient information and data security [16, 17].

Other legal aspects that are dealt with in the guidelines relate to eDispensing, ePrescription, clinical coding systems, health professional liability, uniform identification of medical products and substitution of medicines/drugs, minimum technical requirements with regard to data security and trusted third parties to registered system users, logging of transactions, user system authentication, accidental or unlawful destruction or accidental loss of personal data, and storage periods of eRecords.

Encryption of data is one of the most common ways to ensure eHealth data protection. Yet confidentiality goes well beyond encryption and takes on a whole new dimension with the development of eHealth. Suitable and more specific legal regulations generally related to the processing and sharing of personal health data, as well as for purposes far broader in scope than health treatment, such as research and quality review, require harmonized rules for health data processing [14].

Patient privacy and patient consent are cornerstones of the legal basis for processing health data and providing medical treatment. Usually, informed consent (obtaining patient permission prior to creating health documents or providing health services) ensures the right to privacy and that the patient understands the course of treatment with possible adverse effects. The EU is no exception in this understanding. Under EU regulations, appropriate rules to achieve a maximum level of personal data protection need to be provided. However, regulations on patient consent to create eHealth records, as well as to share them and transmit them across borders, vary among member states, as do rules for identification and authentication by health professionals [18].

The European Health Telematics Association issued its 2008 revised version of a patients' charter for eHealth information systems. It places front and center the protection of patients' individual rights in various contexts, such as electronic health records, home care and home monitoring, and patient safety. In doing so, it also supports the EC Guidelines for Quality Criteria for Health-Related Websites. Essentially, it calls on national healthcare authorities across the EU to adopt a patient-centered approach to formalizing and harmonizing guidelines related to the use of eHealth systems and the processing of electronic health records [19].

An emerging issue is the use of human tissue and genetic data. eHealth is enhancing the use of human tissue and genetic data, as human tissue, as well as the blood from the genetic data derived from tissue, is increasingly being used and stored for treatment and other purposes, especially research. Regulations already in place are vague and do not provide healthcare systems clear and detailed rules on the further use of genetic data and tissue [14].

Pursuant to the April 2015 report from the EC to the Parliament and Council regarding the reimbursement for cross-border healthcare, the directive on telemedicine has led to confusion, where some member states reimburse or provide consultations with general practitioners at a distance, while others do not. The report further notes how the directive gives effect to mutual recognition of medical prescriptions between member states, and, an implementing directive provides measures to assist member states in making it operational [19].

A paramount concern is physician liability for a telemedical transaction. Two issues for evaluation are whether a telemedical appointment is the best approach for a given patient's treatment and whether telemedicine poses an increased risk for the patient. A telemedical session may not be the best method of healthcare delivery [14].

Liability questions arise again in the instance of telemonitoring, where medical devices are implanted to monitor and follow the patient such as in the case of heart conditions. Putting the issue of product liability aside, a question about physician liability arises if doctors do not respond immediately to messages received during their absence. Doctors are obligated to ensure the continuity of care for any treatment undertaken, and, they are expected to inform their patients of absences [14]. Another question that arises is whether a suitably competent colleague who is covering for the original doctor is permitted to access the professional mailboxes of the original physician to retrieve the electronic messages. These scenarios point to providing patients with more information and broadening the scope of patient consent [14].

A larger variety of people will be held liable if something goes wrong during a telemedical appointment. The technical failure of some devices used during a session can lead to claims against software producers or Internet providers. As liability relates to a defective medical device, the Product Liability Directive is applicable and generally sets forth that a manufacturer is responsible for damages when the product does not provide the safety that person is entitled to expect, taking all circumstances into account, including the presentation of the product, the use to which it reasonably could be expected to be put, and the time at which the product was released to the public [14].

France and Belgium have no-fault liability for healthcare, while other member states do not. No-fault means that if a patient is harmed, that patient is compensated regardless of the intent or negligence of the healthcare practitioner. The issue of no-fault liability as an EU-wide mechanism must be settled because a situation of differing rules for liability among member states does not serve patients, physicians, or insurers. When deciding the issue of no-fault, regulations should extend to damage caused by a tele-expert located in a country different from the patient.

Telehealth in the Developing World

The WHO established the Global Observatory for eHealth to review benefits that ICTs can bring to healthcare and patients' well-being. The 2009 second global survey on eHealth found that in developing countries, major impediments to telemedicine include resource allocation for the high cost of developing the necessary technical infrastructure absence a dearth of technical expertise [20].

The survey revealed that in low-income countries and in regions with limited infrastructure, telemedicine applications are primarily used to link healthcare providers with specialists, referral hospitals, and tertiary care centers. While these are low-cost, feasible, useful, and sustainable, they are not being adopted on a larger scale due to a plethora of factors [20].

Infrastructure in developing countries is insufficient and unable to accommodate the most up-to-date Internet technologies. This insufficiency, combined with the absence of access to computing facilities, poses significant obstacles. The instability of electrical power supplies, widespread unavailability of Internet connectivity beyond large cities, unreliable connectivity, limited bandwidth, computer viruses, and ICT equipment that is not appropriate for tropical climates are other challenges [20].

Some healthcare workers resist adopting new methods that differ from traditional approaches or indigenous practices. Others lack ICT literacy, while still others face language-related problems. A lack of computer-literate workers with expertise in managing computer services, combined with the lengthy process required to master computer-based peripheral medical instruments, can hinder expansion. Meeting local education needs can also be difficult due to differences in the diagnostic and therapeutic resources available as well as the literacy and language skills across multiple sites [20].

Simple low-cost, low-bandwidth solutions have proven to be successful for delivering telemedicine. Store-and-forward e-mail has shown to be a low-cost and beneficial use of telemedicine in a variety of specialties and international contexts not bound by bandwidth limitations [20]. A noteworthy venture developed for family planning being used in Kenya, Rwanda, and Tanzania is Mobile for Reproductive Health (mRH). It is an automated, interactive, and on-demand text message system (SMS) that provides essential facts about contraception; at the same time, it addresses common misconceptions and allows users to locate nearby family planning clinics [21].

Another effective venture in Senegal also uses SMS to inform communities of the availability and benefits of maternal and neonatal health services at their local healthcare facilities. A separate component targets pregnant women and new mothers, advising them about the importance of antenatal care visits, delivery with a skilled birth attendant, and postnatal care [22]. In India, Nutrition Day Care Centers mobile device (mNDCC) allows for the generation of a monitoring and evaluation feedback loop between local and state-level actors through mobile-based management information, client-wise tracking of nutrition and health behavior change, and action to be taken locally through software-generated alerts [23].

Notwithstanding the above referenced successful projects, legal issues in this context are major obstacles to expanding telemedicine. Some of the key challenges here are the same as those noted earlier in the context of the EU: the nonexistence of an international legal framework to allow health professionals to deliver services in different jurisdictions and countries; lack of policies governing patient privacy and confidentiality relating to data transfer, storage, and sharing between health professionals and jurisdictions; and health professional authentication and the risk of medical liability for health professionals offering telemedicine services. Again, other legal barriers relate to technological challenges [20].

One method to enhance the growth of teleservices in the developing world is by arranging projects between developed nations and developing ones. Joint partnerships with multiple countries with varying specialties could prove beneficial to all parties. One collaboration project already under way is between the Ghanaian Ministry of Health and the Millennium Villages Project relating to the use of mobile phones for data collection in connection with maternal health [24]. Another initiative brings the government of Pakistan, Indus Hospital, Johns Hopkins School of Public Health, and openXdata.org of Norway together to improve vaccine immunization in Pakistan through SMS reminders and a lottery system with cash prizes for participants [25].

The use of telemedicine services in developing countries has been questioned from an ethical perspective. Using it to increase access to care brings great benefits, yet the question remains as to whether this is the most effective use of scarce resources not only in terms of money but also in terms of electricity or medicines [20]. Given these concerns, the question of partnerships becomes even more relevant and meaningful.

Telehealth in the United States

The Food and Drug Administration, the Federal Trade Commission (FTC), the Federal Communications Commission (FCC), and the Department of Health and Human Services (HHS) in the U.S. all have some jurisdiction regarding telehealth governance. Individual states also regulate various aspects of telehealth. Consequently, there is no uniform legal approach, which itself poses pressing challenges to telehealth's growth.

The HHS issued a report to Congress in 2016 on telehealth noting that it can increase access to care with better health outcomes and reduce costs. Roughly 61% of healthcare institutions and between 40 and 50% of all U.S. hospitals engage in some form of telehealth already [11].

As noted earlier, 59 million Americans live in places that experience shortages of primary care providers, and in rural areas where access to medical specialists, such as oncologists, is limited. Telehealth appears to be particularly effective in chronic disease management. This is significant because in the U.S., about 50% of adults live with at least one chronic illness that contributes to almost 70% of all deaths. Chronic illness accounts for close to 75% of healthcare costs – a staggering amount of money. Aside from its application in the area of mental health, the majority of telehealth provided for chronic conditions has, thus far, been limited to asynchronous monitoring [11].

The HHS report demonstrated in detail that current policy challenges include reimbursement for services, including coverage by Medicare, state medical licensing, and lack of infrastructure with the absence of high-speed broadband connections to rural hospitals and clinics [11].

Under Medicare's fee-for-service program, reimbursement for telehealth services in 2015 has been small, equaling less than 0.01% of total healthcare spending. Medicare Advantage plans cover telehealth services that the fee-for-service program provides, yet these plans are slated to expand their coverage even moreencouraged to go further. In 2016, two of the largest insurers started offering remote access technology services to Medicare Advantage enrollees across multiple states [11].

Reimbursement for telehealth by Medicaid and private insurers varies greatly across the U.S. (state governance), as do the kinds of services covered. For example, 48 state Medicaid programs provide some type of telehealth reimbursement, 22% of large employers in 2014 covered telemedicine consultations, and more than 68% were expected to do so by 2017. Moreover, 32% of states have enacted telehealth parity laws, which require private insurers to reimburse telehealth services at the same rate as in-person consultations. While states have enacted telehealth parity laws, telemedicine coverage differs in each state [11]. A key question to ask in connection with increasing telehealth services is how hospitals can encourage states to enact full parity laws that require private health insurers to pay for services provided via telehealth the same way in-person services are paid [26].

Additionally, each state has the responsibility to regulate the practice of medicine within its borders and to grant medical licenses allowing doctors to practice medicine. Licensing includes the use of telehealth services, with the majority of states currently requiring out-of-state clinicians providing telehealth services to be licensed in the state where the patient resides. This requirement serves as an obstacle to telehealth expansion [11].

The adoption of the Model Policy for the Appropriate Use of Telemedicine Technologies in the Practice of Medicine by the Federation of State Medical Boards in April 2014 is one important initiative to remove state hurdles while protecting public well-being. Physicians using telemedicine technologies must take suitable steps to establish the physician-patient relationship and conduct all appropriate patient evaluations and case histories consistent with traditional standards of care for the particular patient presentation [27].

The Model Policy clarifies that the practice of medicine occurs at the patient's location at the time of the telemedical session, that patient informed consent for the use of telemedicine technologies needs to be obtained and maintained, and ePrescribing of medications must uphold patient safety [27]. Similarly, credentialing and privileging refers to a hospital's responsibilities for verifying doctors' qualifications in order to use its facilities and for defining the scope of services they are able to render. While the hospital closest to the patient would seem to have the ultimate decision-making authority regarding privileging for telehealth service delivery, concerns linger about telehealth among specialists who object to the idea that an originating site should have the ability to limit their authority or scope of practice [11]. Another question of primary importance concerns the changes in state insurance, state medical board, or Medicaid policies that are needed to allow clinicians in addition to physicians, such as advanced practice nurses and physician assistants, to provide telehealth services [26]. Two other areas of liability that may not immediately come to mind yet are important in the telemedical context include physician/provider liability concerning fraud and abuse.

The Interstate Medical Licensure Compact goes beyond the Model Policy to offer an expedited and streamlined licensing process for physicians interested in practicing medicine in multiple states. It also safeguards public welfare by enhancing the ability of states to share investigative and disciplinary information. As of June 2016, only 17 states had adopted compact legislation [28].

In 2010, in conjunction with the signing of the Affordable Care Act into law, a new and revised Health Insurance Portability and Accountability Act (HIPAA) and a Patient's Bill of Rights were formulated. HIPPA was enlarged to include telehealth companies, increased maximum penalties for negligence, strengthened data breach notification requirements, and set down new instructions for using patient information for fundraising and marketing purposes [29]. The Patient's Bill of Rights provides patients with the right to be informed about their condition, treatment, and confidentiality. It guarantees a patient the right to access all healthcare records and stipulates that healthcare professionals, insurers, and suppliers are to refrain from discussing a patient's health story with employers or anyone else unless they have permission to do so, except if the exchange of information is necessary for care and, in some cases, where the law or public health is implicated [30].

It is estimated that each year, 400 million procedures in the U.S. require at least one medical imaging study. Along with the increasingly huge numbers of medical images comes accountability to share, manage, and maintain them in a safe way because the security of a patient's data is paramount. Cyberattacks, which entail breaches of security by outside actors, are real threats in our technological era. Cybersecurity has become an important field in its own right and has given rise to a multitude of companies and specialists. Firewalls, user access controls and monitors, secure event management tools, data encryption, and disaster recovery are all methods being used to protect health information. Some network and security companies are also utilizing third-party audit services to test and validate the adequacy of security and to identify areas for improvement [31].

The Common Security Framework was designed in consultation with U.S. stakeholders in healthcare, business, technology, and information security. It is an information security framework that harmonizes rules of existing standards and regulations including federal (HIPAA), third-party, and government (FTC) for the implementation and maintenance of an information security management system with high-level controls. While it has been widely adopted, it has not yet achieved universal recognition [32].

The Centers for Medicare and Medicaid Services (CMS) eHealth initiative aligns health information technology and electronic standards programs. It includes electronic health records, ePrescriptions (eRx), hospital and physician quality reporting systems, and administrative simplification (health plan identifier, electronic funds transfers). The CMS acknowledges, much like that in E.U., that eHealth is dependent on access to technology and interoperability [33].

In some areas in the U.S., especially in rural areas and on tribal lands, either there is no broadband connectivity or technology is lagging and unable to keep up with the demands of today's high-quality video, graphics, and data offerings. The FCC reports that 53% of rural Americans, around 22 million people, lack access to benchmark services (25 Mbps/3 Mbps). Another challenge is that the price of broadband services can be three times higher in rural areas. Finally, a sizeable portion of older Americans do not use the Internet (an estimated 40% in 2015). All of these factors are barriers to telehealth service growth [11].

Large health IT companies have stepped into the telemedicine market, including IBM, McKesson, Honeywell Life Care Solutions, GE Healthcare, Cerner, and Philips Healthcare. Other providers started in the urgent care market such as CVS and Walgreens. In response to the larger number of telemedicine providers and start-ups that have achieved market access, the ATA launched its Accreditation for Online Patient Consultations [34]. As of April 2016, roughly 300 organizations have registered for the program [35].

Numerous legal issues arise relating to business and contract law, including anti-trust concerns, as demonstrated in the case of Teladoc's lawsuit against the Texas Medical Board. Teladoc claimed the Medical Board promulgated antitelemedicine legislation since the board was composed of practicing doctors who had a financial incentive to minimize telemedicine, thereby violating antitrust laws. The Medical Board filed a motion to dismiss, responding that state supervision of the board would qualify it as a state agency immune to lawsuits. The judge denied the motion and the board appealed the dismissal. In September 2016, a number of briefs were filed with the appellate court, including one from the U.S. and the FTC in support of Teladoc. Overall, the FTC's position is that the appeal is inappropriate because the court does not have jurisdiction. Addressing the merits of the case, the FTC brief notes how the state action doctrine does not shield the board's rules from federal review because the board did not demonstrate active supervision. The FTC's argument described how no evidence was produced showing any state official reviewed the board's rules to decide whether they advanced state regulatory policy rather than doctors' private interests [36]. At the time of publication, no decision has been issued by the appellate court.

Trends

The global telemedicine market is expected to expand at a compound annual growth rate of 14.3% through 2020, eventually reaching $36.2 billion [37].

In September 2016, AT&T announced its latest technological innovation, called AirGig. It delivers high-speed connections without burying wires in the ground or building towers. Instead, using a mounted plastic antenna, it delivers overpower lines without tapping into them. A company representative, John Donovan, stated that the technology is applicable in urban and rural areas and has the capability to transform Internet access worldwide [38]. This revolutionary device's potential effects on the telehealth industry is a key to and holds great promise for telehealth's continued explosive expansion.

Already over 200 U.S. academic medical centers offer video-based consulting globally. This trend will persist with an ever-increasing number of U.S. hospitals and healthcare providers forging alliances with overseas medical facilities. These cross-border ventures will deliver services to an ever larger number of patients and create new revenue streams, thereby bolstering international brands [37].

At the same time, the growing purchasing power of middle-class populations in countries such as China provides the means and fosters opportunity to pursue treatment from Western medical institutions. Both for-profit and nonprofit models for international telemedicine are emerging whereby hospitals in the developed world are partnering with organizations in the developing world to broaden healthcare availability or are offering commercial care to customers in nations with areas of concentrated wealth but lacking the capabilities and access of Western healthcare [37].

In the U.S., Congress has proposed a number of telehealth-related bills that deal with reimbursement and coverage. Similarly, during the 2015 legislative session, over 200 bills of telemedicine-related legislation were introduced into 42 states. Federal and state governments will continue to propose bills in support of telehealth in these two very important areas [38].

Telemedical services offered by health insurers got off to a slow start. Aflac expanded teleservices to its group critical-illness plans in November 2015, and before that, in 2014, Blue Cross Blue Shield Association, together with Anthem Inc., united with American Well to offer telehealth services to an estimated 3.5 million of its members. Other health insurers are expected to join with teleservice providers, thereby enlarging its use [39].

Another growth area is the rise of Compacts relating to licensure. Aside from that of physicians, mentioned earlier, nurses, psychologists, physical therapists, counselors, and emergency medical service personnel are some of the groups evaluating compact models [38].

As an increasing number of start-ups and businesses enter the telehealth field, accreditation programs will also soar. In addition to the previously mentioned ATA accreditation process, URAC, a longstanding accrediting organization, recently started a telehealth accreditation program of its own [38].

Already, over 35% of employers with onsite health facilities offer telemedicine services, and an additional 12% plan to add these services within 2 years. Studies suggest that around 70% of employers will offer telemedicine services as an employee benefit by 2017 [36]. According to the National Business Group on Health, 74% of large employers are expected to offer telehealth services in 2016 compared to 48% in 2015 [38].

Personal wearable devices are flooding the market, and their use is anticipated to continue expanding rapidly. According to Soreon Research, the wearable health market is projected to reach $41 billion by 2020, with diabetes, obesity, sleep disorders, and cardiovascular disease as the largest growth segments [38].

Widespread popularity of easy-to-wear devices is partly due to FCC policy that allows for more intensive use of a spectrum by Medical Body Area Network (MBAN) devices. These are miniaturized body-worn sensors that collect patient-specific information, including electrocardiogram readings and respiratory functions [29]. Statistics reveal that 32% of consumers have at least one health app on their phone, a 16% gain from 2013 [40].

Similarly, health industry technology is also improving. One example of this is how clinical apps for physicians are becoming more adaptable. Another example relates to HIT, and how the use of a telemedicine app by Teladoc quadrupled its membership to more than 8 million users since 2013, which contributed to the company's going public [40]. As the use of apps continues to proliferate, cybersecurity in the context of teleservice apps and medical devices is becoming a prime concern and growth areas.

According to the big telemedicine companies such as Teladoc, MDLive, and American Well, upcoming directions for telehealth service delivery include addiction (to aid in quitting smoking) and other mental health issues. Walgreens signed an agreement earlier in 2016 to provide its customers with access to 1000+ licensed therapists and psychiatrists through a partnership with Breakthrough, a subsidiary of MDLive.[41]

Conclusion

Telehealth is increasing beyond the stage of infancy, and its continued surge seems undeniable. Spreading teleservices depends on various factors and requires many actors. The law is an essential tool in facilitating its spread. Public protection and welfare is a central component, so regulation in this area must remain an underlying principle of growth policy.

References

1. About the Sustainable Development Goals – United Nations. https://www.un.org/sustainabledevelopment/sustainable-development-goals/. Accessed 20 June 2019.
2. Telehealth – WHO. https://www.who.int/sustainable-development/health-sector/strategies/telehealth/en/. Accessed 20 June 2019.
3. Overview | Public Health. https://ec.europa.eu/health/ehealth/overview_en. Accessed 20 June 2019.
4. Wicklund E. Is there a difference between telemedicine and Telehealth? June 2019. Is there a difference between telemedicine and telehealth. Accessed 20 June 2019.
5. Download book PDF. https://link.springer.com/content/pdf/10.1007%2F978-3-319-08765-8.pdf. Accessed 20 June 2019.
6. Telehealth Resource Center. http://www.telehealthresourcecenter.org/sotes/main/files/file-attachments/telehealth_definitions_framework_for_trcs_1.pdf. Published June 20, 2019. Accessed 20 June 2019.
7. Labrique AB, Vasudevan L, Kochi E, Fabricant R, Mehl G. Global health: science and practice 2013, volume1, number 2, technical concept, mHealth innovations as health system strengthening tools: 12 common applications and a visual framework. June 2019;1.
8. GlobalMed. https://www.globalmed.com/. Accessed 20 June 2019.
9. Interoperability – Wikipedia. https://en.wikipedia.org/wiki/Interoperability. Accessed 20 June 2019.

10. Communication From the Commission to the European Parliament, The Council, The European Economic and Social Committee of the Regions, eHealth Action Plan 2012–2020-Innovative healthcare for the 21st Century. June 2019.
11. United States Department of Health and Human Serves Report to Congress on E-heath and Telemedicine. August 2016.
12. Guidelines for reporting of health interventions using mobile phones: mobile health (mHealth) evidence reporting and assessment (mERA) checklist. 2016.
13. Be He@lthy, Be Mobile – 2013-2014 Annual Report. https://www.itu.int/en/ITU-D/ICT-Applications/eHEALTH/Be_healthy/Documents/Be_Healthy_Be_Mobile_Annual_Report%202013-2014_Final.pdf. Accessed 20 June 2019.
14. Callens S. The EU Legal Framework on E-Health. In: 573–587.
15. European Commission - PRESS RELEASES – Press release. http://europa.eu/rapid/press-release_MEMO-13-932_en.htm. Accessed 20 June 2019.
16. Guidelines on Minimum/Non-Exhaustive Dataset for Electronic Exchange in Accordance with the Cross-Border Directive. November 2014.
17. Guidelines on ePrescriptions Dataset for Electronic Exchange under Cross-Border Directive. In: 2014.
18. Overview of the national laws on electronic health records in the EU. July 2014. https://ec.europa.eu/health/sites/health/files/ehealth/docs/laws_report_recommendations_en.pdf.
19. 52015DC0421 – EN – EUR-Lex – EUR-Lex. https://eur-lex.europa.eu/legal-content/EL/TXT/?uri=CELEX:52015DC0421. Accessed 20 June 2019.
20. TELEMEDICINE.   https://www.who.int/goe/publications/goe_telemedicine_2010.pdf. Accessed 20 June 2019.
21. https://apps.who.int/iris/bitstream/handle/10665/112318/WHO_RHR_14.06_eng.pdf;jsessionid=F54182BE04501058AFC38A62B0037B6D?sequence=1. Published 2014.
22. Improving access to maternal health care in Senegal: WAHA International's mHealth programme.   https://apps.who.int/iris/bitstream/handle/10665/184985/WHO_RHR_14.32_eng.pdf?sequence=1&isAllowed=y. Published 2014.
23. Improving maternal and child health in India – SERP's Nutrition Day. http://apps.who.int/iris/bitstream/10665/192494/1/WHO_RHR_13.27_eng.pdf. Accessed 20 June 2019.
24. Ghanaian health workers use mobile phones to collect real-time. https://www.who.int/newsroom/feature-stories/detail/ghanaian-health-workers-use-mobile-phones-to-collect-real-time-maternal-health-data. Accessed 20 June 2019.
25. Small incentives improve vaccine coverage in Pakistan. http://apps.who.int/iris/bitstream/10665/92806/1/WHO_RHR_13.16_eng.pdf. Accessed 20 June 2019.
26. The Promise of Telehealth for Hospitals, Health Systems, and Their Communities. January 2015.
27. Model Policy for the Appropriate Use of Telemedicine Technologies. https://www.fsmb.org/siteassets/advocacy/policies/fsmb_telemedicine_policy.pdf. Accessed 20 June 2019.
28. Day J. Digital health law update, an overview of notable happenings affecting digital health, Mobile Health and Telemedicine June 2016;2:3.
29. Trends in Telehealth, Making healthcare more collaborative, affordable and effective. 2014.
30. http://www.healthsouorceglobal.com/docs/Patient%20Bill%20of20Rights_Merged.pdf.
31. Healthcare Under Cyber-Attack: The New Normal See page 6. http://hfmanj.org/images/news/2016Summer_.pdf.   http://hitrustalliance.net/content/uploads/2014/05/HITRUST_CSF__v6_2014.pdf.Accessed June 20, 2019.
32. The CMS eHealth Initiative. https://www.cms.gov/eHealth/downloads/eHealth-Fact-Sheet.pdf. Accessed 20 June 2019.
33. 32 things to know about telemedicine. https://www.beckershospitalreview.com/healthcare-information-technology/32-things-to-know-about-telemedicine.html. Accessed 20 June 2019.
34. FTC weighs in on Teladoc's side in ongoing antitrust case. https://www.mobihealthnews.com/content/ftc-weighs-teladocs-side-ongoing-antitrust-case. Accessed 20 June 2019.

35. Five Telemedicine Trends Transforming Health Care in 2016. https://www.foley.com/en/insights/publications/2015/11/five-telemedicine-trends-transforming-health-care. Accessed 20 June 2019..

36. AT&T might have just complicated the future of internet - Dallas. https://www.bizjournals.com/dallas/blog/techflash/2016/09/at-t-might-have-just-complicated-the-future-of.html. Accessed 20 June 2019.

37. Green E Becker. The Telehealth Outlook for 2016, Blog TechHealth perspectives. http://wwwtechhealthperspecitvecom/2015/12/22/the-telehealth-outlook-for-2016/ Published 22 Dec 2015.

38. A Reliable Approach for Sustainable Telehealth Partnerships Bryan. https://telehealthandmedicinetoday.com/index.php/journal/article/download/91/79/. Accessed 20 June 2019.

39. Top 5 Telemedicine Trends – MedCity News. https://medcitynews.com/2016/05/top-5-telemedicine-trends/. Accessed 20 June 2019.

40. http://www.forbes.com/sites/brucejaen/2016/06/30/telemedicinee-companies-see-mental-health-as-the-next-frontier/#4c01c03d95ac.

Chapter 9: mHealth for Better Quality of Life, Healthier Lifestyles, and More Meaningful Lives

Aishwarya Narasimhadevara and Renuka Rambhatla

Introduction

Health is an essential aspect of a person's well-being and is synonymous with quality of life. Industrialisation, followed by globalisation, has given rise to a sedentary modern lifestyle, which represents a shift from the ancestral hunter-gatherer subsistence. The Global Burden of Disease study highlights that the period 2005–2015 saw a 14.1% increase in mortality attributable to non-communicable diseases (NCDs), including, but not limited to, cancer, ischemic heart disease and cirrhosis. Ischemic heart disease, stroke and diabetes were underscored as the chief burden among various populations [1]. The Tracking for Universal Health Coverage report, published by the World Bank and the World Health Organisation (WHO), discusses the stark reality that 400 million people worldwide have no access to basic healthcare due to socio-economic factors and geographic barriers [2]. Universal health coverage (UHC) refers to the concept that all individuals should have access to essential healthcare without financial hardship [2, 3]. This notion is further endorsed by the United Nations, through its Sustainable Development Goals, a set of goals set forth by member states pertaining to education, poverty, health, gender equality, and climate change. The third goal is to "ensure healthy lives and promote well-being for all at all ages". The specific target 3.8 is to "Achieve universal health coverage", which enters into the realm of human rights as well [4]. To achieve universal access to health coverage, innovative measures, including electronic health (eHealth), have been implemented by civil society, governments and the private sector.

A. Narasimhadevara (✉)
University of Kent-Brussels School of International Studies, Brussels, Belgium

Chulalongkorn University, Bangkok, Thailand
e-mail: aishu@aol.com

R. Rambhatla
University of Sydney, Sydney, NSW, Australia

© Springer Nature Switzerland AG 2020
P. Murthy, A. Ansehl (eds.), *Technology and Global Public Health*,
https://doi.org/10.1007/978-3-030-46355-7_14

The concept of eHealth refers to the use of information and communications technology (ICT) to provide health services and has been incorporated by members of civil society, governments and the private sector [5]. Mobile health (mHealth) is a division of eHealth, whereby medical and public health practices are enabled by mobile technology [6]. Health services can be delivered through mobile phones, patient monitoring devices and other wireless solutions [7].

Mobile phones have risen in popularity, with 90% of the world connected by a cellular signal [8]. Many mobile subscribers reside in low- to middle-income countries, where Internet usage is consistently high. The market share for mHealth was estimated at USD10.5 billion in 2014. Globally, this is projected to rise exponentially to USD58.8 billion [9].

The use of mobile technology to disseminate health-related information for analysis from various biomedical systems facilitates healthcare delivery in low resource settings [10].

This chapter will discuss the significance of mHealth in strengthening health systems and managing disease burdens and its relevance in international sustainable development. Global perspectives will be provided in the form of case studies, explored across the spectrum of low- to high-income countries. Furthermore, the sustainability implications of mHealth and its significance will be discussed. Technology has made the world more connected, and mHealth will enable healthier future generations. Projects pertaining to mHealth include child and maternal health and reducing the effects of illnesses associated with poverty, HIV/AIDS, malaria and tuberculosis (TB) management [10].

Types of mHealth

The dynamic nature of populations, coupled with emerging health issues, has resulted in a metamorphosis from traditional archetypes of health service delivery. The methods of delivery can be through an application, a software application installed on mobile devices, Short Message Service (SMS), Multimedia Messaging Service (MMS), voice calls and video conferencing or automated sensing systems that interface with other electronic devices to analyse data [10].

Labrique and colleagues identified the areas in which mHealth strategies can be utilised, including behaviour change, point-of-care diagnostics, health registries, data collation and reporting, electronic patient records, electronic decision support, provider-to-provider communication, provider work planning and scheduling, provider professional development, human resource management, supply chain management and financial management, including incentives [11]. Furthermore, interventions are adaptable across the management of communicable diseases and NCDs and non-specific conditions.

The explosion of mobile technology available has unlocked unprecedented opportunities for innovations in health service delivery in the following areas [12] (Fig. 1):

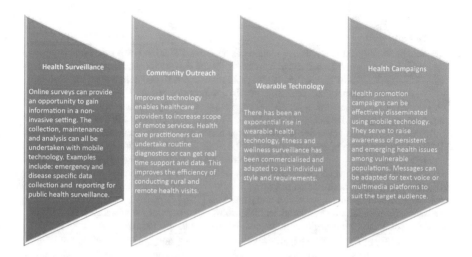

Fig. 1 mHealth impact in health service delivery

Novel approaches have also been developed to capture the interest of the public, achieved through social media, the gamification of health, and decision-making or behaviour change applications. This variety enables individuals to self-monitor their health status and transmit data to healthcare providers as needed. The potential for mHealth is immense, and the evolving architecture and software of mobile technology can serve as a catalyst for quality and low-cost healthcare [11].

Health System Integration

Mobile information, communication and technology can be integrated into global health systems, transcending geographical barriers and enhancing healthcare. A collaboration between the technology and health sectors will be beneficial for global health systems, creating mechanisms for health service improvements.

Because technology evolves rapidly, national health systems need to be equally robust to seamlessly integrate with these new innovations in healthcare. The principal pillars of a health system include health financing, health information systems, sound leadership and governance, stable human resources and universal health coverage [3]. Mobile technology can be adapted across all dimensions of a health system to achieve equilibrium between expanding health service provision and quality healthcare. The upstream and downstream factors surrounding health need to be acknowledged, in particular at the user level, where the social determinants of health play a critical role in overall well-being and healthy behaviours [12].

In addition to making the technology available, the following facets of a health system need to be considered (Table 1):

Table 1 Facets of a health system

Human Resources:

The ratio of workforce to national population has been calculated, and over time three key thresholds have emerged globally. The first, set by the 2006 *World Health Report*, highlights a minimum requirement of 22.8 skilled health professionals per 10,000 population [13]. Currently, 44.6%, or 83 out of 186, of analysed countries do not meet the criteria. The second threshold of 34.5 skilled health professionals per 10,000 population was set by the International Labour Organisation [13]. Figures indicate that 9.1%, or 17 out of 186, do not reach this threshold. Lastly, the WHO, in collaboration with the United States Agency for International Development (USAID), references an updated threshold of 59.4 skilled health professionals per 10,000 population, where 9.7%, or 18 out of 186, countries have maintained this [13]. Data modelling has been utilised to predict a global 12.9 million skilled health professional shortfall by 2035 [13]. The largest gaps were evident in low- to middle-income countries across South-East Asia and Africa, including nurses, midwives and physicians [13]. Maintaining workforce equilibrium is a topic of contention in considering health finances and quality of workforce. These statistics provide a solid basis for capacity building and redesigning the health workforce.

The stark reality of the frontline health workforce strengthens the case for the utilisation of technology in health services to decrease the burden whilst not compromising on patient care. In light of the brain drain occurring in many low- to middle-income countries or regions impacted by conflict, mHealth can assist in filling the healthcare gaps.

Governance:

Governance incorporates policy setting, advocacy, trend analysis and standards monitoring. Good governance is required to advance the cause of equitable and universal access to healthcare. Elements include advocating for health and setting sustainable strategies, followed by standards development, implementation and evaluation [3]. Regulation is a key factor of governance that ensures that scarce resources will be equally distributed and monitoring from the point of health financing to the end user. Additionally, priority setting for mobile health services is integral for long-term sustainability. A policy commitment from national governments and peak health bodies is required, in addition to standards and practical codes of practices. Access, quality and costs are the three key facets of healthcare [3]. Public-private partnerships established between healthcare and telecom providers enhance public health services.

Health Financing:

Acute health issues and emergencies arise constantly, so the financing and allocation of resources are critical. Current finance models for mHealth are centred around grants or short-term funding [14]. A cost–benefit analysis can shed light on whether mHealth can be sustainable as a long-term solution. Research into the mHealth market is on the rise, and a report published in 2016 highlights that mHealth has the potential to save up to USD370 billion in healthcare spending globally by the end of 2017 [15]. Consumers face several challenges, including high out-of-pocket expenditures, and mHealth can close the gap in service provision and costs.

Universal Health Coverage:

Access to quality healthcare is a challenge in rural and remote environments. Some of the existing barriers to healthcare include lack of facilities per capita and inadequate health infrastructure. Setting up mHealth services, with point-of-care diagnostics, can bridge the gap in healthcare [2, 3].

Health Information Systems:

Technology can provide the foundations for an efficient and functioning health information system. Critical health messages can be integrated into the architecture of mobile systems. Technology can be used effectively in the areas of provider–client or provider–provider communication and consultation, client education and behaviour modification, vital event tracking, or point-of-care diagnostics [11, 12].

Global Applications of mHealth

Health service delivery across the world is multifaceted and contingent on the strength of national health systems, in addition to the socio-political climate. Mobile technology has the capacity to alter the landscape of healthcare delivery, whereby immediate and preventive resources are available at the point of care [11]. An awareness of the current global integration and trends in mHealth provides insight into future acceptance, adoption and scale-up of services. To understand the vast potentials in healthcare, four case studies across the world will be presented.

Health Promotion in India

A healthy nation is a catalyst for social and economic development. India is currently classed as a low middle-income country, and data indicate that in 2011, 21.9% of Indians lived below the national poverty line [16]. The dilemma faced by the Indian government is providing equitable access to essential healthcare for 1.3 billion people [16]. There exists an intricate interplay between financing and maintaining human rights, along with equity for sustainable development. The complexities of the Indian healthcare system can accommodate pragmatic and innovative technological solutions.

The following solutions revolve around health promotion and point-of-care diagnostics (Table 2):

HIV and AIDS Management in Africa

Africa is a continent steeped in rich tradition and diversity. External influences, including widespread poverty and volatile socio-political intricacies, have served to destabilise the health systems of some countries across the continent.

Human immunodeficiency virus (HIV) and acquired immunodeficiency syndrome (AIDS) have collectively strained the public health system and society for decades.

The United Nations has developed the UNAIDS 2016–2021 Strategy [20], which is a global call to action, to bridge the current gaps in treatment of HIV/AIDS. The UNAIDS 2016–2021 Strategy sets out the targets, goals, and vision to be achieved by nations globally.

The key principles of the strategy, to be achieved by 2020, include [20] the following (Fig. 2):

These targets aim to accelerate progress towards meeting the strategy's goals, which are also aligned with the Sustainable Development Goals, specifically Goals 3, 5, 10, 16, and 17 [4]. Smartphone-based technology has been harnessed across

Table 2   mHealth applications for health promotion and point-of-care diagnostics

mDiabetes:

Arogya World collaborated with Nokia Life to launch the national public health campaign mDiabetes in 2011. The mobile-based application has since been hailed as the largest mobile-based prevention plan worldwide. Post-intervention research conducted by Ipsos, on a sample of around 1000 people, revealed a positive impact on the cohort that was involved with the mDiabetes campaign. Pfammatter and colleagues reported that over a million Indian participants received free health messages, twice per week and over a 6-month period, in 2012. The 56 SMSs were evidence based, developed in partnership with Emory University and translated into 12 Indian languages. The outcomes were statistically significant, indicating improvements across exercise patterns and uptake of fruits and vegetables [17].

Swasthya Slate:

Government commitment and governance are keys for the success of mHealth programmes. The Public Health Foundation of India and the Affordable Health Technologies division has invested in Swasthya Slate, a suite of applications that interfaces with an Android tablet or phone to deliver 33 medical diagnostics [18]. Evaluation has been validated through field tests in Punjab and Andhra Pradesh; other countries utilising these services are Peru and Timor-Leste. The overall framework of Swasthya Slate operations involves diagnostic devices interfaced via Bluetooth between patients and health practitioners [18]. Actions include motivating women to give birth in hospitals, bringing children to immunisation clinics, encouraging family planning (e.g. surgical sterilisation), treating basic illnesses and injuries with first aid, keeping demographic records and improving village sanitation. It is beneficial in following up for primary healthcare services, whereby mobile technology serves as a gatekeeper and leads to less hospitalisation and reduced chances that patients will be subjected to additional health interventions.

ResApp:

ResApp has been used to identify lower respiratory tract disease, particularly bronchitis, bronchiolitis and pneumonia. Evaluations reveal an accuracy level exceeding 90% with the ResApp diagnostic algorithms in distinguishing between lower (LRTD) or upper respiratory tract diseases (URTD) and infections. This is vital in treatment and patient management. Furthermore, 99% accuracy was attained when distinguishing between individuals with a LRTD and individuals with no disease. This diagnostic tool supersedes the labour-intensive steps of chest auscultation using a stethoscope and observations for oxygen saturation, followed by a chest x-ray and blood and sputum tests. It makes it possible to avoid preventable deaths among those who may face delays or barriers to diagnosis. Its use in field tests has yielded clinical results and it has been deployed in low-resource settings [19].

Africa, and several companies are working collaboratively with the health sector to reduce the morbidity and mortality associated with HIV/AIDS. The *Global AIDS Update 2019* provides progress towards these targets. UNAIDS analysis has highlighted the following: people living with HIV who know their status is 79%; people living with HIV on treatment is 62%; and people living with HIV who are virally suppressed is 53% [21]. Data from 2018 reveals that 23.3 million out of 37.9 million people living with HIV worldwide were accessing treatment, a threefold increase from 2010 [21]. This greater access to treatment has contributed to a decline in deaths, an estimated 770,000 deaths, down from 1.7 million in 2004 [21]. The UNAIDS targets are also aligned with the Sustainable Development Goals,

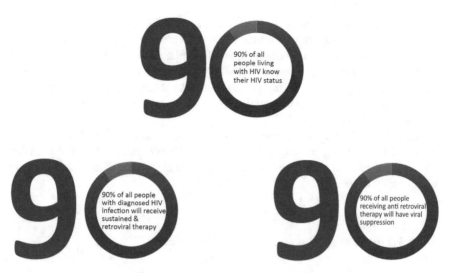

90% of all people living with HIV know their HIV status

90% of all people with diagnosed HIV infection will receive sustained & retroviral therapy

90% of all people receiving anti retroviral therapy will have viral suppression

Fig. 2 Visualisation of key targets of UNAIDS 2016–2021 strategy

Table 3 mHealth applications for HIV/AIDS patients

Aviro Health:
Identified as a medicine, design and technology organisation, Aviro Health operates to offer unique solutions to the health issues faced in Africa. The Aviro HIV/AIDS Med Mentor application is a complementary service which aids nurses and healthcare workers to provide critical medical and psychological support for people living with HIV/AIDS. The platform provides education and resources for healthcare workers, based on South African national guidelines for HIV diagnosis, eligibility, and planning for antiretroviral therapy. The service is extended to include a referral system and an HIV hotline to enhance patient care. In Africa, Aviro Health has developed a suite of tools for self-care in supporting people living with HIV/AIDS [22].
TextIT:
Kenya has been listed by UNAIDS as a priority for support in HIV services (UNAIDS strategy report). The Kenya Medical Research Institute (KEMRI) launched the Texting to Improve Testing (TextIT) campaign to provide HIV health promotion in Nyanza, Kenya, and encourage people to seek adequate medical care. TextIT features include interactive messaging for HIV-positive pregnant women or among healthcare practitioners or to access peer support through mentor mothers and hospital-trained women who have lived the experience of HIV. The aim is to promote clinic attendance for postpartum checks for mothers and their infants [23, 24].

specifically goals 3, 5, 10, 16, and 17 [4]. Smartphone-based technology has been harnessed across Africa, and several companies are working collaboratively with the health sector to reduce the morbidity and mortality associated with HIV/AIDS.

Below is a list of applications designed to HIV/AIDS-assist patients in Africa (Table 3):

Kazi and colleagues evaluated the feasibility of SMS-based mHealth for antenatal care and immunisation in northern Kenya. A survey was conducted among 284 pregnant women or carers living in central highlands and northern arid lands in Kenya. The outcomes revealed that 92% of participants who had access to mobile phones found it beneficial to receive weekly text messages from their maternal or child health clinics [25]. More studies need to be conducted for evidence-based scale-up of mHealth services.

Transformative mHealth projects in Africa have created a robust healthcare service and provides a patient-centric experience. People living with HIV or AIDS have a litany of daily challenges, and these applications serve to immensely improve their quality of life.

Zika Virus Prevention in Brazil

Mobile health has hastened the prevention of epidemics by containing viruses and is at the forefront of disease control. A recent example includes the outbreak of the Zika virus, which challenged governments and civil society to curtail the effects of the illness. The world has been interconnected through the advent of modern technology, and globalisation has contributed to creating an ecosphere of progressive collaboration. Increased global travel opportunities have also enabled diseases to be spread rapidly among populations. Hence, it is imperative to prevent viruses becoming a global pandemic.

The Zika virus is a disease-causing pathogen that is triggered by an *Aedes* mosquito bite. Characteristic symptoms include fever, headache, muscle and joint pain, and microcephaly in infants. Expectant women are advised to be cautious as the foetus may develop microcephaly [26]. The WHO has confirmed the Zika virus causes birth defects, such as microcephaly, where the head size is smaller than average [27]. The disease is contagious and people are able to contract it through bodily fluids, including sweat or saliva, for example. The treatment for the Zika virus is to rest, stay hydrated and use common medicines for fever. Currently, there is no vaccine, but prevention is a solution to combat the virus. What follows is a table of the states most affected by the virus during Epidemiological Week 33 of 2017 in Brazil (Table 4):

The vast majority of cases were in the north and central-western regions of the country.

The outbreak of the Zika virus in Brazil in 2016 caused worldwide concern. Many babies were born with microcephaly, and the number of cases of people contracting the virus increased from 2015 to 2016. The Zika virus in Brazil was first discovered in 2014 in the north-east region [29]. The international community was concerned about travel to Brazil in connection with contracting the virus. Furthermore, Brazil hosted the 2016 Summer Olympics. To contain the virus, the Brazilian Ministry of Health, the Skoll Global Threats Fund, and the Brazilian eHealth startup Epitrack [30, 31] launched an application, Guardiões da Saúde (Guardians of Health), to monitor the virus and to report symptoms [32]. The application is available on the Internet

Table 4 Brazilian regions affected by Zika during Epidemiological Week 33 in 2017

State:	Number of Cases (per 100,000 persons):
Mato Grosso	714
Rio de Janeiro	419
Bahia	349
Alagoas	208
Tocantins	208
Goiás	204

Source: Brazil Ministry of Health [28] Reproduced by: Pan-American Health Organisation (PAHO)/WHO https://www.paho.org/hq/dmdocuments/2017/2017-phe-zika-situation-report-bra.pdf

and on iOS and Android systems. The application asks users questions with regard to symptoms, including cough, fever and diarrhoea. It is available in Arabic, Chinese, English, French, Russian, Spanish and Portuguese and allows users to report their health. The application has a feature called Health Map which traces the locations of the Zika virus [32]. This will alert users to avoid areas where the virus is widespread. Information with regard to health services, pharmacies, Zika virus, prevention and treatment is also provided. The application has an interactive interface that enables users to submit information and view data. The application assisted the Centre for Integrated Health Operations in the Ministry of Health in controlling the virus [30]. The results are shown in real time, which can prevent the illness from spreading. The data collected from the application are to be released by the Ministry of Health. There have been at least 60,000 downloads of the application, and it serves as a model in the field of mHealth and public health.

Guardiões da Saúde received the Best Mobile Government Service award at the World Government Summit in Dubai, United Arab Emirates, in 2017 [32]. In addition, Brazil declared an end to the Zika virus emergency in May 2017 as the number of cases of the illness had dropped by 95% from January to April 2017 compared to the same period in 2016 [33]. The Brazilian government also developed a mosquito eradication programme which involved health workers fumigating breeding areas for mosquitoes. The Pan-American Health Organisation/WHO and the Brazilian International Health Regulations (IHR) National Focal Point (NFP) shared information and improved knowledge transfer during the Olympics to further assist in these efforts. The Zika virus has been contained in Brazil, and it is important to be vigilant to prevent the spread of the virus. The WHO also developed an application for healthcare workers, responders and the public to monitor the Zika virus on mobile phones. The WHO Zika app provides the latest information on the virus and the organisation's technical guidance [34]. Guardiões da Saúde has contributed to Brazil's success in managing the virus and is an innovative solution to prevent outbreaks and global pandemics. Through collaboration with the private sector, the Brazilian government and civil society, diseases and epidemics can be prevented so that all individuals can lead healthy lives and the third Sustainable Development Goal can be achieved.

Cardiovascular Disease in Europe

Mobile health has also been a catalyst in the presentation of illnesses and educating people on health. Cardiovascular diseases (CVDs) are any disorder of the blood vessels and include coronary heart disease, cerebrovascular disease, peripheral arterial disease, rheumatic heart disease, congenital heart disease, deep vein thrombosis and pulmonary embolism [35].

Cardiovascular disease is a widespread illness in Europe that accounts for half of all deaths in the region and is responsible for more deaths than HIV/AIDS, tuberculosis and malaria combined across the continent [36]. There are 11,000,000 new cases of CVDs every year in Europe, and some of the contributing factors include smoking, alcohol consumption, diet, genetics and lack of exercise [36, 37]. According to the WHO report on the global tobacco epidemic, Europe had the highest rate of smoking, 28%, in 2015 [38]. The WHO *Global Status Report on Alcohol and Health 2014* states Europe's rate of pure alcohol consumption was at 10.9 l per capita (15+ years) [39]. It is imperative for people to take measures to reduce their risk of developing CVDs. Quitting smoking, leading a healthy lifestyle and exercising are some methods for reducing the risk of CVDs.

Mobile health is a catalyst in reducing the risk of CVDs because it empowers people to lead healthier lifestyles. The European Union developed a plan for eHealth from 2010 to 2020 that reiterated the importance of ICT in improving people's health and increasing the efficiency of the healthcare system. Projects including the 2011 directive on the application of patients' rights in cross-border healthcare and the development of an eHealth network are part of the initiative. The European Society of Cardiology (ESC) has also initiated eHealth projects, including electronic medical records, e-referrals and teleconsultation [40]. Some applications that will reduce the risk of cardiovascular disease include the following.

Cardiio
The smartphone application determines a person's cardiovascular health and heart rate fitness using a camera to take measurements.

Blood Pressure Companion
The application records the user's heart rate and blood pressure and stores it in a special database. The application also reminds users if a reading is overdue.

Healthy Heart Meal Planner
The application enables users to create weekly meal plans that are healthy and balanced. Furthermore, there is advice on the types of food to consume.

Atherosclerotic Cardiovascular Disease Risk Estimator
This application assists in assessing risks for atherosclerotic cardiovascular disease, which is an illness where plaque builds up inside arteries [41]. A person's weight, blood pressure, age, and lifestyle habits are indicators of the illness and the application uses them to measure the user's risk. There are two risk categories, which include lifetime risk and risk within the next decade.

AliveCor ECG Heart Monitor
This application records electrical patterns in the heart and notifies users of any irregularities.

iBP Blood Pressure
This is an application that monitors the user's blood pressure and indicates if it is normal, high or hypertensive. An interactive graph records the results and indicates lows, highs and averages on a long-term basis, which assists in managing conditions.

Source: NueMD and PwC Analysis [42, 43].

The aforementioned applications serve to warn people about heightened risk levels of developing cardiovascular disease and take appropriate measure. They provide information that allows people to lead healthier lives and that can lead to reduced alcohol consumption and smoking rates in Europe. The European Society of Cardiology and the European Heart Network conducted a project known as EuroHeart from 2007 to 2010, which focused on reducing cardiovascular disease rates in Europe. Some of the objectives included increasing support for cardiovascular health promotion and cardiovascular disease prevention and entailed analysing national plans and policies to support the initiative, focus on cardiovascular disease-related issues for women and improving prevention practices at the primary care level [44]. Mobile health initiatives also have the same objectives as EuroHeart and focus on prevention to encourage people to lead healthier lives.

There are 17,600,000 people in the European Union at risk of developing CVD. Of the 48,800,000 smokers in the European Union, 3,900,000 can quit through the use of mHealth applications. Furthermore, mHealth can reduce the risk of CVD for 833,000 people of the 8,300,000 people who use the applications [43]. Furthermore, obesity affects 29,100,000 people and through mHealth applications, 9,900,000 people are able to lose weight without additional treatment [43]. Through awareness and monitoring, mHealth can prevent cardiovascular disease and extend people's lives.

The four cases presented from around the world serve to highlight the potential and breadth of services that can be provided by mHealth in dealing with both communicable and non-communicable diseases. This global commitment ultimately reflects the values and attitudes of modern society in terms of desiring to shape a world in which the spread of preventable diseases is halted.

Monitoring and Evaluation of Mobile Health

Public health impact is assessed by a combination of factors, such as the efficacy and reach of a strategy. The following table presents some advantages and disadvantages of mHealth [10–12, 15] (Table 5).

Table 5 mHealth advantages and disadvantages

Advantage	Barriers
mHealth is transformative for both patients and practitioners.	Barriers to system-wide implementation and adoption.
The technology empowers individuals to self-manage and monitor their health status, whilst enabling practitioners to provide more effective and timely services.	Reliance on technology and inadequate infrastructure.
mHealth has the potential to fill gaps in health systems, including human resources and inventory management.	Supply chain barriers, such as treatment required from skilled practitioners once mHealth diagnosis is made, coupled with unassigned health system responsibilities.
Specific and targeted interventions can be cost effective.	Lack of financing and limited evidence for intervention cost-effectiveness.
Bridges geographic distances.	Quality assurance for mHealth programmes and lack of auditing in some areas.
Strengthens surveillance and feedback systems.	Need for standardised privacy laws surrounding data collation and maintenance.

Evidence Base

Key factors in the sustainability of mHealth in global communities include local government commitment, affordability, accessibility and end user adoption. These have been identified through pilot programmes and stakeholder involvement. Furthermore, conducting a local needs assessment is critical in the initiation phase, followed by an outcome evaluation appropriate to the strategy. Studies available, though limited, on mHealth reveal positive outcomes on both a macro system-wide level and a micro client level [10, 12, 15].

Hall et al. analysed 76 papers to determine concrete health outcomes across low- to middle-income countries. They found evidence for the efficacy of mHealth interventions which focused on improving patient treatment and appointment compliance, data collation and the creation of support networks for health practitioners [12]. However, they noted that the quantity and quality of the evidence remain inadequate and call for more rigorous experimental studies in the field. This notion of limited studies for generalisability is concurred by other investigators into mHealth.

Coughlin and Stewart conducted a review of 274 articles to determine whether consumer wearable devices encouraged healthy behaviours. They found a small sample of positive results. However, a limited number of studies focused on the effectiveness of wearable technology in encouraging active and healthy lifestyle choices [45].

Gamification for health and wellness has been applied in various contexts to enhance mental health support, physical activity promotion or chronic disease rehabilitation. The approaches have provided short-term gains for patients, but they require more development based on psychological theories and impact on behaviour modification. Empirical evidence is required for the scale-up of game mechanics and software [46].

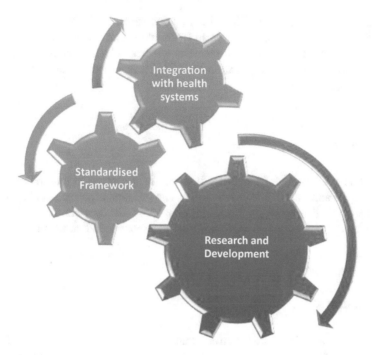

Fig. 3 mHealth recommendations

Recommendations

The core nature of mHealth leads to decentralising healthcare, so robust quality-monitoring systems must be implemented for a sustainable mHealth system (Fig. 3).

Research and Development

It is important not to generalise research findings in mHealth; thus, more targeted and gold standard research will be required in future. Future studies will need to highlight the benefits and challenges based on cost, quality and health equity.

Standardised Framework

Monitoring the quality of devices, technology and services is key to continuous improvement in the health sector. Currently, a robust global framework is needed to evaluate health outcomes related to the use of mobile information, communication and technology. Agarwal et al. identify the applicability of the mHealth evidence reporting and assessment (mERA) checklist developed by the WHO. The 16-point checklist focuses on mHealth content and technology and endeavours to standardise the reporting of mHealth interventions. The widespread adoption of standard measures supports the future replication of mHealth interventions and improves the evidence base [47].

Integration

mHealth is not a standalone solution; it should be incorporated into the continuum of healthcare and sustainable development. The primary advantages and challenges of mHealth shed light on its future developments. The barriers identified can be overcome through effective auditing, risk assessment and mitigating strategies [48, 49].

Conclusion

Mobile health is an innovative platform that provides effective access to healthcare, facilitating collaboration between governments, the private sector and civil society. Various applications in mHealth are dedicated to prevention, disease control, health education and increasing access to health services. The field of mHealth is a catalyst for achieving universal healthcare access, reducing the global morbidity and mortality associated with communicable and non-communicable diseases.

Different types of mHealth have enabled medical practices and healthcare systems to assist people in an efficient manner. The case studies presented in this chapter illustrate the importance of mHealth across low- to high-income countries. In Africa, Aviro Health has developed a suite of tools for self-care to support people living with HIV/AIDS. mHealth has enhanced the quality of life for people living with chronic conditions in India, reducing preventable burdens of disease through diagnostic support and remote care. The application Guardiões da Saúde was used to prevent the Zika virus from spreading during the Rio Olympics, which showcased its significance in disease control. CVD applications for smartphones have enabled people to lead healthier lifestyles. Governments are also devising plans to incorporate mHealth to provide access to quality healthcare.

The achievement of the third Sustainable Development Goal can be accomplished through innovative approaches in mHealth. Attaining the third goal will pave the way achieving other goals on the 2030 Agenda for Sustainable Development.

The adage "health is wealth" is the cornerstone of mHealth, and a consistent state of well-being is essential for enhancing the quality of life and empowering people to lead meaningful lives.

References

1. GBD 2015 Mortality and Causes of Death Collaborators. Global, regional, and national life expectancy, all-cause mortality, and cause-specific mortality for 249 causes of death, 1980–2015: a systematic analysis for the global burden of disease study 2015. Lancet. 2016;388(10053):1459–544.
2. World Health Organization. Tracking for universal health coverage. Geneva: World Health Organization; 2015.
3. World Health Organization. Key components of a health care system. Geneva: World Health Organization; 2010.
4. Goal 3: Ensure healthy lives and promote and well-being for all at all ages. UN.org. http://www.un.org/sustainabledevelopment/health/. Published 2015. Accessed 19 Sept 2016.
5. World Health Organization, International Telecommunication Union. National eHealth strategy toolkit. Geneva: World Health Organization/International Telecommunication Union; 2012.
6. Istepanian RSH, Laxminarayan S, Pattichis C, editors. M-Health: emerging mobile health systems. New York: Springer Science+Business Media, Inc.; 2006.
7. Adibi S, editor. Mobile health: a technology road map. Cham: Springer International Publishing; 2015.
8. International Telecommunication Union. The world in 2010: ICT facts and figures: International Telecommunication Union; 2010.
9. Global mHealth Market (Devices, Services, Application, Stakeholders and Geography)–Industry analysis, market size, share, growth, company profiles, demand, insights, opportunities, trends and forecast, 2014–2020. LeadingMarketResearch.com http://www.leadingmarketresearch.com/global-mhealth-market-devices-services-application-stakeholders-and-geo. Published May 1, 2015. Accessed 8 June 2017.
10. World Health Organization. mHealth: New horizons for health through mobile technologies: second global survey on eHealth. Geneva: World Health Organization; 2011.
11. Labrique AB, Vasudevan L, Kochi E, Fabricant R, Mehl G. mHealth innovations as health system strengthening tools: 12 common applications and a visual framework. Glob Health Sci Pract. 2013;1(2):160–71.
12. Hall CS, Fottrell E, Wilkinson S, Byass P. Assessing the impact of mHealth interventions in low- and middle-income countries – what has been shown to work? Glob Health Action. 2014;7(1):25606.
13. Global Health Workforce Alliance, World Health Organization. A universal truth: no health without a workforce. Geneva: World Health Organization; 2014.
14. Health Alliance, Vital Wave Consulting. Sustainable financing for mobile health (mHealth): options and opportunities for mHealth financial models in low and middle-income countries: mHealth Alliance and Virtual Wave Consulting; 2013.
15. The mHealth (Mobile Healthcare) Ecosystem: 2017–2030 – Opportunities, challenges, strategies & forecasts. SNSIntel.com. http://www.snsintel.com/the-mhealth-mobile-healthcare-ecosystem-2017-2030.html. Published 2016. Accessed 14 July 2017.
16. India. WorldBank.org. http://data.worldbank.org/country/india?view=chart. Published 2016. Accessed 8 June 2017.
17. Pfammatter A, Spring B, Saligram N, et al. Eysenbach G, ed. mHealth intervention to improve diabetes risk behaviors in India: a prospective, parallel group cohort study. J Med Internet Res. 2016; 18(8):52–63.
18. Panchal H. Recent advances in mobile diagnostics. IPHIndia.org. https://iphindia.org/recent-advances-in-mobile-diagnostics/. Published August 22, 2015. Accessed 11 May 2017.
19. Abeyratne UR, Swarnkar V, Setyati A, Triasih R. Cough sound analysis can rapidly diagnose childhood pneumonia. Ann Biomed Eng. 2013;41(11):2448–62.
20. UNAIDS. UNAIDS 2016–2021 strategy: on the fast-track to end AIDS. Geneva: UNAIDS; 2015.

21. UNAIDS. The global AIDS update 2019. UNAIDS Joint United Nations Programme on HIV/AIDS; 2019.
22. Aviro Health App. AviroHealth.org. http://www.avirohealth.com/projects/med-mentor/. Published 2015. Accessed May 25, 2020.
23. Odeny TA, Newman M, Bukusi EA, McClelland RS, Cohen CR, Camlin CS. Developing content for a mHealth intervention to promote postpartum retention in prevention of mother-to-child HIV transmission programs and early infant diagnosis of HIV: a qualitative study. PLoS One. 2014;9(9):e106383.
24. World Health Organization. Text messaging to improve early infant testing for HIV in Kenya: KEMRI's TextIT: World Health Organization; 2014.
25. Kazi AM, Carmichael J-L, Hapanna GW, et al. Assessing mobile phone access and perceptions for texting-based mHealth interventions among expectant mothers and child caregivers in remote regions of Northern Kenya: a survey-based descriptive study. JMIR Public Health Surveill. 2017;3(1):e5.
26. Zika Virus. WHO International. http://www.who.int/mediacentre/factsheets/zika/en/. Updated September 6, 2016. Accessed 22 May 2017.
27. Zika Virus and Complications: Questions and answers. WHO International. https://www.who.int/features/qa/zika/en/. Updated March 10, 2017. Accessed 27 May 2017.
28. Brazil Ministry of Health. Boletim Epidemiológico. 2017; 48(26):1–9. Quoted by: Pan American Health Organization/World Health Organization. *Zika-Epidemiological Report Brazil*. Washington D.C.: Pan American Health Organization/World Health Organization; March 2017. https://www.paho.org/hq/dmdocuments/2017/2017-phe-zika-situation-report-bra.pdf. Accessed 9 Jan 2020.
29. Heukelbach J, Alencar CH, Kelvin AA, de Oliveria WK, de Góes Cavalcanti LP. Zika virus outbreak in Brazil. J Infect Dev Ctries. 2016;10(2):116–20.
30. Brazilian Ministry of Health. Preventing health epidemics with crowdsourced data. Social Tech.org.uk. http://www.socialtech.org.uk/projects/guardioes-da-saude/. Published September 19, 2016. Accessed 23 May 2017.
31. Abu-Eid H. Guardiões da Saúde (Guardians of Health) receives recognition at the World Government Summit. Skollglobalthreats.org. http://www.skollglobalthreats.org/2017/02/27/guardioes-da-saude-guardians-of-health-receives-recognition-at-the-world-government-summit/. Published February 27, 2017. Accessed 2 June 2017.
32. Mack H. Brazil health authorities launch app to map Zika during 2016 Olympics. MobiHealthNews.com. http://www.mobihealthnews.com/content/brazil-health-authorities-launch-app-map-zika-during-2016-olympics. Published July 20, 2016. Accessed 23 May 2017.
33. Phippen J. Brazil declares an end to its Zika health emergency. Theatlantic.com. https://www.theatlantic.com/news/archive/2017/05/brazil-ends-zika-emergency/526509/. Published May 12, 2017. Accessed 3 June 2017.
34. WHO Zika App. WHO International. http://www.who.int/risk-communication/zika-virus/app/en/. Published 2017. Accessed 28 June 2017.
35. Cardiovascular Diseases. Euro WHO International. http://www.euro.who.int/en/health-topics/noncommunicable-diseases/cardiovascular-diseases/cardiovascular-diseases2. Published 2017. Accessed May 31, 2017.
36. Data and Statistics. Euro WHO International http://www.euro.who.int/en/health-topics/non-communicable-diseases/cardiovascular-diseases/data-and-statistics. Accessed 31 May 2017.
37. Wilkins E, Wilson L, Wickramasinghe K, Bhatnagar P, Rayner M, Townsend N, Leal J, Luengo-Fernandez R, Burns R. European cardiovascular disease statistics 2017 edition. Brussels: European Heart Network; 2018.
38. Data and Statistics. Euro WHO International. http://www.euro.who.int/en/health-topics/disease-prevention/tobacco/data-and-statistics. Published 2017. Accessed 20 June 2017.
39. World Health Organization. Global status report on alcohol and health 2014. Luxembourg: World Health Organization; 2014.

40. Cowie M, Bax J, Bruining N, Cleland J, Koehler F, Malik M, Pinto F, van der Velde E, Vardas P. e-Health: a position statement of the European Society of Cardiology. Eur Heart J. 2015;36(1):63–6.. http://www.efsma-scientific.eu/wp-content/uploads/2016/01/eurheartj-avg-2015-e-health-position-statement-ESC.pdf. Accessed 2 June 2017
41. What is Atherosclerosis?. Nhlbi.nih.gov. https://www.nhlbi.nih.gov/health/health-topics/topics/atherosclerosis. Accessed on June 3, 2017.
42. McCarthy K. 5 of the best smartphone apps for heart disease patients. NueMD.com. https://www.nuemd.com/news/2016/06/29/5-best-smartphone-apps-heart-disease-patients. Accessed on 2 June 2017.
43. PwC India. Socio-economic impact of mHealth: an assessment report for the European Union. India: PwC India; June 2013. https://www.pwc.in/publications/publications-2013/socio-economic-impact-of-mhealth-an-assessment-report-for-the-european-union.html. Accessed 10 Mar 2020.
44. EuroHeart: European heart health strategy. Ehnheart.org. http://www.ehnheart.org/projects/euroheart/about.html. Accessed on 2 June 2017.
45. Coughlin SS, Stewart J. Use of consumer wearable devices to promote physical activity: a review of health intervention studies. J Environ Health Sci. 2016;2(6)
46. Sardi L, Idri A, Fernández-Alemán JL. A systematic review of gamification in e-Health. J Biomed Inform. 2017;71:31–48.
47. Agarwal S, LeFevre AE, Lee J, L'Engle K, Mehl G, Sinha C, et al. Guidelines for reporting of health interventions using mobile phones: mobile health (mHealth) evidence reporting and assessment (mERA) checklist. Br Med J. 2016;352:i1174.
48. World Health Organization. Global diffusion of eHealth: making universal health coverage achievable: report of the third global survey on eHealth. Geneva: World Health Organization; 2016.
49. Ali EE, Chew L, Yap KY-L. Evolution and current status of mHealth research: a systematic review. Br Med J Innov. 2016;2(1):33–40.

Chapter 10: Digital Health Transforming Health Care in Rural and Remote Australia

Christine C. Bennett and Uma Srinivasan

About Rural and Remote Australia

Australia is the largest country in Oceania with a vast geographic landmass – the world's sixth largest country by total area. The Australian population of approximately 25 million people is highly urbanized, with 70% living in metropolitan areas, particularly on the eastern seaboard, and over seven million living in regional, rural, and remote locations spread across this vast continent. The "remote" definition alone covers 85% of the Australian landmass. Delivering timely, appropriate, and high-quality care in rural and remote environments is challenging for a number of logistical reasons, including geographic spread, low population density, workforce availability, limited infrastructure, and the significantly higher costs of rural and remote healthcare services [1].

Australians generally enjoy one of the longest life expectancies in the world, ranked fifth among 35 of the Organization for Economic Co-operation and Development (OECD) countries [2]. The Commonwealth Fund describes the Australian Health System as one of the best in the world, and expenditures on health and aged care services are about 10% of GDP, at the OECD average [3].

However, even though Australia is a high-income, politically stable country with a "health system" that looks after most of the people very well most of the time, there are hidden areas of significant inequality and inequity.

C. C. Bennett (✉)
School of Medicine, Sydney, The University of Notre Dame Australia, Chippendale, NSW, Australia

Digital Health Cooperative Research Centre, The Rocks, NSW, Australia
e-mail: christine.bennett@nd.edu.au

U. Srinivasan
School of Business, Western Sydney University, Sydney, NSW, Australia

© Springer Nature Switzerland AG 2020
P. Murthy, A. Ansehl (eds.), *Technology and Global Public Health*,
https://doi.org/10.1007/978-3-030-46355-7_15

Aboriginal and Torres Strait Islanders – Australia's first nations peoples – people living in rural and remote areas, and refugees experience poorer access to care and health outcomes. Gaps in care, including dental care, mental health services, and inadequate care and support of people with disabilities, are also of concern.

Gender inequality in healthcare is perhaps not as significant and widespread as in other countries. However, it is the case in Australia that women and girls face specific challenges in terms of their wellbeing, such as domestic and family violence, poor access to maternity care in rural and remote areas, and relative economic disadvantage and vulnerability, particularly among older women [4]. Living in a rural area adds significantly to the risk of inequality – often increasing with level of remoteness.

Rural Australia

regional – nonurban centers with populations over 25,000;
rural – nonurban localities with populations under 25,000; and
remote – communities with fewer than 5000 people who have very little access to services.

About 2% of the Australian population lives in remote or very remote locations. Our rural and remote communities support important industries, including agriculture and mining. These communities tend to be culturally diverse with significant migrant and refugee populations. These settlements and individual rural properties can be hours of driving from any services and with no alternative transportation.

Health Disparities in Rural and Remote Australia

Australians who live outside of urban areas face significantly poorer outcomes than their city counterparts [5]. They have shorter lives and higher levels of illness. Of particular concern, the life expectancy of Aboriginal and Torres Strait Islander people is significantly shorter than that of the nonindigenous population [6]. Also, the health of older people in rural and remote areas is generally poorer than that of older people living in metropolitan areas.

Women and girls living in rural settings in Australia face a number of health challenges and inequalities [7, 8]. Some notable issues are as follows:

- *Maternity services* have halved over the last 20 years with small maternity units closed, allegedly owing to low patient numbers (<50–100 births annually) and safety concerns. Importantly, it's not just the birthing services that have been impacted by closures, but also reduced access to prenatal care [4].

- Indigenous women have the added concerns of wanting to birth "on country" with family and on their ancestral lands. Many do not present for *prenatal care* for fear of being transferred.
- They have higher rates of *obesity* and health risk factors such as *smoking and drinking to risky levels.*
- *They have higher mortality rates* for lung cancer, chronic obstructive pulmonary disease, and ischemic heart disease [9].
- *Osteoporosis* is at a lower rate in rural areas, but this may be related to underdiagnosis owing to a lack of access to bone densitometry.
- *Surgical procedures* are less than for women in urban areas, except for hysterectomy.
- *Fetal alcohol spectrum disorder* is higher in these populations and increases with remoteness.
- *They have poor access to specialist services* and to women general practitioners (GPs) in some areas.
- *Screening and prevention* for breast and cervical cancer rates are comparable, although services are more difficult to access, but *national bowel cancer screening is less prevalent.*

There are several measurable positive predispositions of women in rural areas: they tend to be more resilient and happy and have higher levels of neighborhood satisfaction and social support. Life satisfaction and optimism are greater and increase with remoteness; interestingly, short sightedness is less frequent [10].

Huge distances, poor roads, social isolation, and sparsely distributed services contribute to poor access. Additionally, in small communities, fear of stigma, shame, and gossip may deter women from seeking help from local health professionals on sensitive issues such as domestic violence or drug and alcohol addiction out of fear of breaches of privacy [11].

The health disparities are a consequence of several challenges in rural and remote Australia:

- *Shortages of health professionals*: Shortages of doctors, nurses, allied health professionals, pharmacists, and dentists become more pronounced with remoteness. There are challenges in attracting and retaining health professionals in rural and remote areas, particularly in specialty fields [12].
- *Lack of equitable access to care*: Access to quality care in rural areas is impacted by factors such as the standards of clinical and cultural safety and quality of rural and remote services, the alignment of services provided with local needs, including language needs, and the availability and sustainability of an appropriately trained and skilled workforce. Access to primary care, dental care, and allied health and specialist services is more difficult in rural areas. People frequently need to travel great distances to access basic services, a problem compounded by expenses for travel and accommodation, lost work productivity, and social disruption [13].

- *Uncertain funding and poor infrastructure*: Unpredictable service funding arrangements and shifting political priorities impact health service infrastructure in rural and remote areas. Health-related activity is limited and being further eroded by a lack of ongoing investment [13]. The viability of many rural hospitals is uncertain, and there has been a serious loss of capacity for maternity services and other procedural healthcare in rural areas.

Policy Context and the National Strategic Framework for Rural and Remote Health

The need for a specific policy approach addressing the health needs of rural and remote Australians was recognized with the launch of the first National Rural Health Strategy, which was endorsed by health ministers in March 1994. In 1999, the Healthy Horizons Framework 1999–2003 was developed in collaboration with the National Rural Health Alliance, and is acknowledged as contributing to increasing effort and resources towards rural and remote health at the time. This was followed by the release of *Healthy Horizons Framework: Outlook 2003–2007 (Healthy Horizons 2003–2007). A Healthier Future for All Australians: The Final Comprehensive Report of the National Health and Hospitals Reform Commission (2008/2009)* included a focus on facing inequities in rural Australia. Thereafter the new National Strategic Framework for Rural and Remote Health was released in November 2011 [1].

The National Strategic Framework for Rural and Remote Health identified systemic issues that require most attention to improve health outcomes for rural and remote Australians, such as access, appropriate models of care, a sustainable workforce, embracing new technology, the development of collaborative partnerships and governance approaches, and ensuring that differences between health services and communities are respected and without impeding local planning.

Further challenges to our health system stem from its traditional focus on reactive, acute care in hospital settings. Over time, our disease burden has shifted toward chronic conditions, often with multiple comorbidities that require out-of-hospital management. Over 10% of Australians live with asthma, 7% with high cholesterol, and 5% with diabetes, and the leading causes of death are heart disease, dementia, and cancer [2]. Moreover, four million Australians – nearly 16% of our population – have experience living with mental or behavioral conditions. As a result, there is a need to shift the health paradigm to a more proactive, prevention-focused system that can foster good health and deliver quality care and management of health risk and disease in the community.

Data and Digital Health – A Policy Priority

Australia needs a healthcare environment that prevents, predicts, and supports early intervention and delays the onset of chronic and long-term diseases; eliminates low-value care and other forms of waste; and constantly evaluates pharmaceuticals, treatments, diagnostics, and medical devices to ensure that they are delivering value and are in the best interests of patients. *Prevention at both a population and individual level, and precision-personalized medicine* are at the very center. Data and sophisticated data analytics are vital to achieving these objectives.

However, according to Australia's Population Health and Research Network, "no single data collection" is sufficient to "allow an understanding of the complex pathways that result in health or disease" or to determine "whether Australia's health and social systems work in optimal ways" [14].

As highlighted in the recent report *Flying Blind: Australian Researchers and Digital Health*, the more data sets researchers are able *to link* together, the more complex and *valuable* are the questions that they can hope to solve [15]. Linking numerous different sources of data can help shed light on the complex interplay of factors that lead to different diseases. This information can be used to identify health risks and predict the onset of morbidities in individuals and to provide clinicians with the ability to target interventions. Such approaches can lead to better health, improving patient quality of life and reducing demand for health services over their lifetime. Figure 1

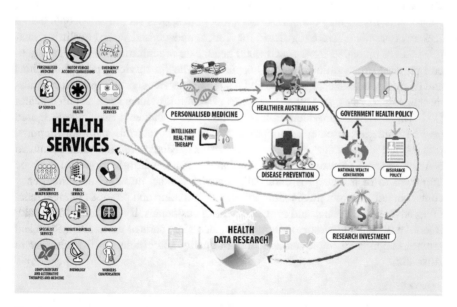

Fig. 1 Virtuous Research Cycle. (Source: *Flying Blind: Australian Researchers and Digital Health, Volume 2: Health Data Series, p. 10.* © CMCRC Limited and Digital Health Cooperative Research Centre, Sydney Nov. 2018. Retrieved from https://flyingblind.cmcrc.com/files/cmcrc_flying_blind_vol_2_web4.pdf)

illustrates a virtuous research cycle that can be integrated into policy and service delivery. Effective prediction can be particularly valuable in rural areas where access to care is limited, compromising early intervention and health risk management. The unique challenges and issues in rural and remote areas require innovative models of care and approaches to health service delivery supported by data and applied data science technologies.

Innovations in Digital Health Technologies in Rural and Remote Australia

Digital healthcare is disrupting the health industry with the promise of delivering an enhanced patient journey, better health outcomes, and better value for the health dollar [16]. The following discussion highlights some innovative examples of digital health to demonstrate the possibilities for applying these practices to improve challenges in rural and remote healthcare.

My Health Record

The national My Health Record system is currently being rolled out for all Australians, unless they opt out. As of October 2018, over six million people (about 25% of Australians) were registered for clinical updates and shared health summaries that are uploaded from over 14,000 healthcare organizations that include general practice organizations, public hospitals and health services, private hospitals and clinics, pharmacies, aged care and residential services, pathology and diagnostic imaging services, and other categories of health providers such as allied health [17]. These various providers upload a variety of documents that include shared health summaries, discharge summaries from hospitals, referrals, pathology reports, prescription documents, immunization registers, Medicare, and pharmaceutical benefits reports. Consumers can also share additional information that may be important to their care providers. This includes contact numbers and emergency contact details, current medications, allergy information and previous allergic reactions, advance care plans, and contact details of custodians. By 2022, the My Health Record will constitute a core system that connects key parts of the health system and provides significant improvements in both quality and efficiency of healthcare in Australia.

Telehealth Services

A recent review of telehealth services in Australia provides a description of the services in Australia and describes the factors influencing success and sustainability [18]. Videoconferencing continues to be the technology used in the majority of cases. Although telehealth can effectively improve access to healthcare for people living in rural and remote areas of Australia, the services are not mainstream or routinely available in many rural and remote locations. Innovative approaches and collaborations can allow a blending of different technologies that can be leveraged for comprehensive healthcare solutions.

Besides healthcare audio or video conferencing facilities, *telelearning* can be used for distance-based education, offering options for training health professionals or consumers in rural and remote areas. A 2010 rapid review and evidence check indicated that telelearning can be as effective as or equivalent to face-to-face learning in terms of outcomes [19].

A few illustrative case studies are presented as examples of innovation and service enhancement.

Case Study: Northern Territory Telehealth Project
The provision of telehealth services to deliver outpatient appointments was assessed at three Northern Territory sites between 2014 and 2015: Alice Springs, Katherine, and Tennant Creek. The evaluation demonstrated that increasing telehealth use in these locations (more than sevenfold in Tennant Creek, fourfold in Alice Springs, and a doubling in Katherine) led to reductions in travel, with patients in Tennant Creek more likely to use telehealth than to travel. The "Did Not Attend" (DNA) rate for appointments decreased significantly. The estimated cost savings of the project for participants was on the order of $1.189 million [20]. Surveys indicated high levels of support for telehealth from participating patients and a strong desire to use telehealth in the future. Clinicians had similar attitudes in their endorsement of telehealth, reporting an improvement in continuity of care for their patients and that they would be likely to use telehealth in the future and recommend it to colleagues.

Case Study: Royal Far West – Telecare for Kids

Children in "the bush" often struggle to access the support that they need to develop, learn, and meet their potential due to geographic isolation and chronic gaps in local health services. Children who need ongoing and regular therapy to address speech, movement, behavior, or anxiety, for example, face difficulties accessing sustained services, which in turn affects their development, education experience, and life outcomes. In 2013, in response to this issue, Royal Far West began developing a telehealth capability, using its highly specialized, multidisciplinary team in Sydney to fill gaps in pediatrics and allied health services for children in rural and remote Australia [21]. The aim was to improve health and education outcomes for country children by providing the right development care at the right time. Starting with a small telespeech therapy pilot, Royal Far West has now developed a full assessment and therapy service called Telecare for Kids, covering speech therapy, occupational therapy, clinical psychology, and developmental pediatrics. In 2017/18, Royal Far West delivered nearly 7000 telecare sessions into New South Wales (NSW), Queensland, and remote parts of Western Australia (WA), working collaboratively with parents/caregivers, schools, and local communities. Sessions are tailored to each child and delivered directly at school or in the home, with around 500 children participating in a telecare session each month.

Royal Far West continues to expand its telehealth services through new partnerships, innovative technology, new delivery methods, and a research and advocacy agenda focused on the important role of telehealth in ensuring that country children have the same access to the standard of health and well-being as their city counterparts.

https://www.royalfarwest.org.au/our-story/

Case Study: Communicare by Telstra Health

Communicare is Telstra Health's leading, fully-integrated clinical and practice management solution specially designed for community health. It supports multidisciplinary health services, allied health providers, and community services in delivering care and improving patient outcomes across the communities they serve, no matter where they are based.

Founded in 1994, it has serviced remote communities using light aircraft. A wide range of healthcare providers use Communicare, which supports a holistic-care model for Aboriginal and Torres Strait Island people's health and is currently Australia's leading health record system supporting indigenous and remote populations.

Communicare includes a comprehensive electronic health record for recording a patient's demographics, adverse reactions, social and family history, medications, and clinical history. A follow-up system that enables manual and automatic recalls and reminders can be configured according to the service's requirements. A secure messaging system allows efficient and secure sharing of documents, such as hospital discharge summaries, outgoing and incoming referrals, and radiological images. It includes electronic claims/billing for both Medicare and private patient claims, with alerts for invalid or expired cards and rejected claims.

The service is fully integrated with the Australian My Health Record. Communicare has recently been installed as a state-wide system for Western Australian Country Health Service community centers. Soon to be released in WA is the Maternity Notifications Solution, which will ensure proper postnatal care for young mothers in remote communities.

https://www.communicare.org.au/

Case Study: Pop-Up Model of NSW Paediatric Palliative Care Programme

The NSW Paediatric Palliative Care (NSWPPC) Programme provides care and support to children or young people who have a life-threatening illness and their families [22]. The aim of the program is to ensure that every child in NSW has access to appropriate, high-quality, coordinated, and culturally appropriate palliative care that meets their physical, psychological, social, and spiritual needs. To achieve these outcomes, specialist pediatric palliative care services are dependent on the mobilization of multidisciplinary teams that provide timely, well-coordinated support to children and their families across the hospital and community health sectors and throughout the duration of the child's illness, including into bereavement for families. Specialist pediatric palliative care services within the NSWPPC Programme are delivered by the Sydney Children's Hospitals Network (SCHN) – Sydney Children's Hospital (SCH) and Sydney Children's Hospital Westmead (CHW) – and John Hunter Children's Hospital (JHCH).

The program continues to support an increased number of patients being cared for by each site, facilitating a pop-up model of care enhanced by ongoing telehealth access. The pop-up model relies on the multidisciplinary specialist palliative care service at SCH, CHW, and JHCH to provide responsive and well-coordinated palliative care and in-time training/education to local health providers (including GPs, pediatricians, and community nursing services) using telehealth support.

https://www.caresearch.com.au/caresearch/tabid/2979/Default.aspx

Artificial Intelligence in Health

Combining machine learning and artificial intelligence (AI) allows faster and more accurate diagnosis of health conditions. The demonstration of the use of AI in the diagnosis of disease received global media attention in 2016, when IBM's AI system Watson could use genetic data from a leukemia patient in Japan and cross reference the data with its own database to detect mutations in the patient's DNA, and thereby detect a different type of leukemia to the one that she had been treated for. Watson could do this in 10 min, whereas it would have taken human scientists over 2 weeks.

Cancer remains the number one disease-related cause of death in children despite significant improvements in survival rates over the last three decades. The Zero Childhood Cancer campaign led by SCH is an initiative applying AI technologies on diverse data sets.

An excellent overview of the potential role of AI in healthcare can be found in the JASON report [23]. The role of AI in health, along with discussions on areas where much progress is expected in the short to medium terms, is discussed in a recent report by Federico Girosi, Chief Scientist of the Digital Health Cooperative Research Centre (DHCRC) [24].

Case Study: Zero Childhood Cancer Program
The Zero Childhood Cancer program is Australia's first ever personalized medical program for children with high-risk cancer. The program uses state-of-the-art genome sequencing and other so-called *omic* platforms to better understand what is driving growth of each individual child's cancer in order to provide potential new treatment options.

Data synthesis and interpretation is coordinated using digital technologies and enhanced with machine learning to facilitate engagement and collaboration of clinical and research communities. This approach ensures rapid translation of bench-to-bedside breakthrough treatments and equitable access for patients regardless of geographic location.

http://www.zerochildhoodcancer.org.au/

Analyzing large amounts of digital health data and extracting meaningful patterns, AI can remove some of the uncertainty that is so pervasive in healthcare and enable physicians to make informed decisions guided by clinical decision support systems. These systems combine existing medical knowledge and patient observations, often integrated with electronic health records, that can assist the clinical decision-making process at the point of care [25, 26].

An important application of AI is in the risk assessment of both individuals and populations. For example, by combining individual health data with expert opinion and applying machine learning and predictive modeling techniques, AI systems can be used to identify individuals and populations at high risk of developing a chronic condition or experiencing an adverse event or recovering poorly from an injury. To understand the variation in health indicators at a geographical level, the Capital Markets Cooperative Research Centre (CMCRC) and Western Sydney University researchers have developed a framework to group homogeneous socioeconomic areas and detect variations in health indicators [27]. This foundational piece of work can enable informed resource allocation decisions for health services in rural and remote geographical regions.

Case Study: Using Administrative Data Sets to Predict Chronic Disease and Avoid Potentially Preventable Hospitalizations

The Australian Institute of Health and Welfare (2018) [2] defines a potentially preventable hospitalization (PPH) as an admission to hospital that might have been prevented had there been appropriate individualized preventive health-care or early disease management – usually delivered in primary care and community-based care settings. In 2015–2016, residents of remote and very remote areas had the highest rates of PPHs across all PPH categories. Key contributing factors for adults were cardiovascular disease, the leading cause of indigenous mortality and disease burden, and diabetes, in particular a very high prevalence of type 2 diabetes (T2D).

Researchers from the University of Sydney and the CMCRC have used 4 years of hospital administrative data and applied network analysis and predictive modeling techniques to examine the progression of T2D. They have been able to identify a series of common comorbidities that predicted the onset of T2D well before it had manifested, allowing them to identify individuals at risk of T2D with 86% accuracy [28]. This research can be applied to populations in rural and remote areas to identify individuals at high risk for T2D, enabling clinicians to target interventions and avoid potentially preventable hospitalizations.

Case Study: Accident and Injuries in Rural and Remote Areas – Utilization Patterns and Risk Profiles

People in rural and remote areas are significantly overrepresented in the number of deaths and serious injuries on our roads. Country people are three times more likely to die as a result of a transport accident than their city counterparts [29]. The National Rural Health Alliance (the Alliance) has found little or no information available on crash injury risk factors such as road condition, intoxication, relative safety of vehicles in each area, or number of car occupants in each crash [30]. Many of these data are likely to be available but do not appear to have been used to explore why death rates and injury are much higher in rural and remote areas and why crashes involving indigenous people in remote areas more often result in fatalities. Researchers from DHCRC and University of Technology Sydney have used a machine learning approach on de-identified transport accident data and identified clusters of user groups with varying utilization patterns and risk profiles [31]. This work, when applied to rural remote areas, could be used for appropriate resource planning and service provision as well as to shape policy in this area, thereby benefitting the health and wellbeing of people living in rural and remote areas.

AI solutions have the potential to communicate with patients via chatbots and to extract valid patient-reported outcome measures (PROMs) from analyses of text gathered via SMS, e-mail, or social media. Chatbots are designed to simulate conversation with human users. For example, they can facilitate automation of remote health worker or physician inquiries and routing them to the proper specialists when necessary.

Australian Examples of Chatbots

A chatbot forms part of Healthdirect Australia's innovation strategy to improve access to health services and information through a range of different channels, such as social media [32]. It also represents a significant technical innovation by linking a chatbot to the clinically validated decision management system that also powers the Healthdirect symptom checker.

The pilot will initially allow people to check symptoms associated with fever and urinary problems and shortly be extended to include colds and flu, bites and stings, rashes, and other skin problems.

The Healthdirect chatbot can be accessed on the Healthdirect Australia Facebook page or directly in Facebook instant messenger.

https://about.healthdirect.gov.au/news/healthdirect-australia-launches-chatbot-pilot

Nibby – Nib health funds (nib) became the first Australian health insurer to introduce artificial intelligence technology to assist Australians with their health insurance enquiries. Known as nibby, the chatbot provides customers with access to simple responses regarding their health insurance. Unlike many other chatbots, nibby is integrated into nib's web platform, allowing it to intelligently move customers to the right sales or claims consultant as a customer's query becomes more complex and to offer assistance during key customer service moments [33].

Internet of Things and Consumer Empowerment in Health

In lay terms, the Internet of Things (IoT) is the network of physical devices, vehicles, home appliances, and other items embedded with electronics, software, sensors, actuators, and connectivity that enables these things to connect and exchange data, creating opportunities for more direct integration of the physical world into computer-based systems, resulting in efficiency improvements, economic benefits, and reduced human exertions. In healthcare, IoT offers a novel paradigm where objects with unique identities can be integrated into an information network to provide intelligent services for remote monitoring of health and wellbeing.

A report by Deloitte on IoT and patient-generated data (PGD) discusses how IoT technology provides the opportunity to bring to healthcare unprecedented levels of data generated by patients, making PGD an increasingly critical component of decision-making and delivery with significant potential to improve outcomes, lower costs, increase access to care, and improve the patient experience [34]. The areas highlighted by Deloitte for improving outcomes, lowering costs, and improving access to patient care and experience are short-term care planning, chronic-disease management and home care, and population-based evidence creation.

Wellness, prevention, and health promotion support provided via the use of mobile devices, particularly communication devices such as tablets, personal digital assistants (PDAs), and, most notably, mobile phones, have become pervasive in modern society. Consumer-facing technologies range from the most basic text messaging systems to highly interactive smartphone apps. Examples of text messaging services include appointment reminders, chronic disease management, laboratory results notifications, and lifestyle behavior modification tools.

Australian Case Studies

Springday is an Australian company that enables clients to embark on their wellbeing journey. Springday sources and collates wellbeing experts, learning modules, wearable technology integrations, and motivational and communication tools and connects them into a customizable and user-friendly experience, available via a web portal and iOS/android mobile apps. Users identify a starting point, set goals, and receive personalized guidance and lifestyle content. Users participate in company-wide and individual initiatives such as challenges, self-paced programs, face-to-face health services, and community events. Springday aggregates and reports on platform usage and behavior-change metrics in a real-time admin dashboard [35].

FoodSwitch is an initiative of the George Institute for Global Health and Bupa [36]. The FoodSwitch app enables consumers to get immediate, easy-to-understand nutritional information about packaged food products while they are at the supermarket, provides health star rating of food based on energy, saturated fat, sugar, and salt so users can see at a glance how healthy a given food item is, and then provides them with alternate healthier switches for their families based on their health and dietary preferences.

The New Horizon of Digital Health in Australia

Innovative approaches to care, enabled by digital health technology, can alleviate some of the most difficult problems in rural and remote healthcare in Australia. The establishment of the Australian Digital Health Agency in 2016 heralded a new era of policy development and strategic priorities in digital health in Australia. This was followed by the DHCRC, launched in 2018, which represents a major research, development, and translation program trying to facilitate governments, industry, and research to work together to realize the potential of data and digital technologies in supporting the health of all Australians.

Australian Digital Health Agency

Established in 2016, the Australian Digital Health Agency is leading the National Digital Health Strategy with a vision to provide better health for all Australians by enabling seamless, secure digital health services and technologies that provide a range of easy tools for both consumers and healthcare providers.

The strategy proposes seven priority outcomes that will enable

- health information to be available whenever and wherever it is needed through the implementation of a national My Health Record;
- secure health information exchange across authorized healthcare providers;
- the interoperability of clinical data across service settings supported by a standardized clinical terminology vocabulary;
- online medication management to reduce incidence of medication errors and adverse drug events,
- novel models of care that can drive improved accessibility, quality, and safety, especially in rural and remote areas;
- comprehensive workforce education so that healthcare professionals will have access to digital resources and be able to confidently maximize the benefits of digital health technologies; and
- a thriving innovative digital health industry that can create new services and apps to foster a sustainable and agile health system that supports the changing needs of both consumers and providers.

In the context of rural and remote care, the Australian Digital Health Agency works closely with the Northern Territory to provide increased telehealth services in remote areas to reduce significant amounts of travel time for both patients and health service providers [20].

Digital Health Cooperative Research Centre

The DHCRC, established in July 2018, is a 7-year national and international collaboration between 64 health and technology organizations and 16 Australian universities focused on enhancing the deployment and use of information technology, all forms of data, and computable knowledge to drive improvements in the wellness and healthcare of all citizens, efficiencies in the health system, and the growth of health and medical technology companies [37].

The DHCRC works closely with the Australian Digital Health Agency, with the goal of contributing to the achievement of its National Digital Health Strategy, particularly its goals of giving consumers more control over their healthcare decisions and promoting Australia's global leadership in digital health and innovation.

The DHCRC will also contribute to promoting a range of growth priorities of the medical technologies and pharmacy sector. The DHCRC's industry partner base covers public and private health organizations across all Australian jurisdictions. This coverage is indicative of the recognition of the transformational potential of digital health and their commitment to substantively contributing to unlocking this potential. Through this coverage, the DHCRC has the capacity to positively impact every Australian.

The DHCRC plans to achieve national impact through four interlocking research programs:

1. Information capture, storage, and flow.
2. Identifying and managing health risk.
3. Improving value, quality and safety through intelligent decision support.
4. Understanding clinical practice to support transparency and improve performance.

The plan is for research to focus on five diverse care settings:

- Home and work.
- Acute and primary care.
- Residential aged care.
- Rural and remote.
- Rehabilitation.

DHCRC Flagship Program for Rural and Remote Areas

The DHCRC plans to address the gaps in healthcare services in remote areas through a major flagship research program that focuses on the prevention and management of chronic diseases and improved access to care via digital technology.

At a more detailed level the research program may include the following features:

- Novel approaches to automated risk-based screening of consumers, automated triage, and treatment using solutions such as health-check booths or wearable devices (e.g., smart watches).
- Personalized wellness/support programs that integrate devices, apps, and virtual care/coaching.
- Integrated data and information flows to practitioners and consumers to support health and wellness programs.
- Integration with My Health Record and other shared records.
- Use of social determinants of health and other novel data points to identify high-risk consumers.
- Technological interventions modified by codesign processes for cultural safety and contextual factors.
- Use of telehealth technologies to improve access to care.

With industry partners from across the health ecosystem and across Australia, these research and development programs hold great promise to spur new ways of delivering care and supporting people in managing their health risks and making healthcare decisions.

Digital health and the use of data and digital technologies are at the beginning of an exciting journey of transforming health in Australia and offer the promise of improved health outcomes for rural and remote communities and, indeed, for all Australians.

References

1. National Strategic Framework for Rural and Remote Health 2016. Available from: http://health.gov.au/internet/main/publishing.nsf/Content/A76BD33A5D7A6897CA257F9B00095DA3/$File/NationalStrategicFrameworkforRuralandRemoteHealth.pdf. Accessed 10 July 2019.
2. Australia's Health. Australia: Australian Institute of Health and Welfare; 2018.
3. Glover B. The Australian health care system. Available from: https://international.commonwealthfund.org/countries/australia/. Accessed 10 July 2019.
4. Dobson A, Byles J, Dolja-Gore X, Fitzgerald D, Hockey R, Loxton D, et al. Rural, remote and regional differences in women's health: findings from the Australian longitudinal study on women's health. Newcastle: Women's Health Australia, University of Newcastle; 2011.
5. Health outside major cities: Australian Social Trends. Australia: ABS; 2011.
6. Kildea S, Tracy S, Sherwood J, Magick-Dennis F, Barclay L. Improving maternity services for Indignous women in Australia: moving from policy to practice. Med J Aust. 2016;205(8):375–9.
7. al. ADe. Australian Longitudinal study of Women's Health. Report. 2011.
8. Dobson AJ, Hockey R, Brown WJ, Byles JE, Loxton DJ, McLaughlin D, et al. Cohort profile update: Australian longitudinal study on women's health. Int J Epidemiol. 2015;44(5):1547–1547f.
9. Dobson A, McLaughlin D, Vagenas D, Wong KY. Why are death rates higher in rural areas? Evidence from the Australian Longitudinal Study on women's health. Aust N Z J Public Health. 2010;34(6):624–8. https://doi.org/10.1111/j1753-6405201000623x.

10. Commonwealth of Australia Department of Prime Minister and Cabinet. Closing the gap: Prime Minister's Report 2018. Canberra.; 2018.
11. Campo M, Tayton S. Domestic and family violence in regional, rural and remote communities. An overview of key issues. Melbourne: Commonwealth of Australia; 2015.
12. Wilson N, Couper I, De Vries E, Reid S, Fish T, Marais B. Inequitable distribution of health-care professionals to rural and remote areas. Rural Remote Health. 2009;9(1060).
13. The National Rural Health Alliance Fact Sheet May 2018. Available from: http://ruralhealth. org.au/sites/default/files/publications/nrha-factsheet-about-us-may-2018.pdf.Accessed   10 July 2019.
14. PHRN. Submission to the productivity commission data availability and use inquiry from the population health research network. July 2016 [Internet]. Pc.gov.au. 2018. Available from: http://www.phrn.org.au/media/80973/phrn-response-to-the-data-availability-and-use-inquiry_v10_29072016.pdf. Accessed 18 Aug 2018. 2019.
15. Srinivasan U, Ramachandran D, Quilty C, Rao S, Nolan M, Jonas D. Flying blind: Australian researchers and digital health, volume 2: health data series. Sydney: Digital Health Cooperative Research Centre; 2018.
16. Herrmann M, Boehme P, Mondritzki T, Ehlers JP, Kavadias S, Truebel H. Digital transformation and disruption of the health care sector: internet-based observational study. J Med Internet Res. 2018;20(3):e104. https://doi.org/10.2196/jmir9498.
17. My Health Record statistics 2018. Available from: https://www.myhealthrecord.gov.au/about/my-health-record-statistics. Accessed 10 July 2019.
18. Bradford NKC, Liam J, Smith AC. Telehealth services in rural and remote Australia: a systematic review of models of care and factors influencing success and sustainability. Rural Remote Health. 2016;16(4):4268.
19. Tomlinson J, Shaw T, Munro A, Johnson R, Madden DL, Phillips R, McGregor D. How does tele-learning compare with other forms of education delivery? A systematic review of tele-learning educational outcomes for health professionals. NSW Public Health Bull. 2013;24(2):70–5.
20. Northern Territory Telehealth Success 2016. Available from: http://www.amsant.org.au/nt-telehealth-success/. Accessed 10 July 2019.
21. Royal Far West – Telecare for Kids. Available from: http://www.amsant.org.au/nt-telehealth-success/. Accessed 10 July 2019.
22. NSW Paediatric Palliative Care Programme. Available from: https://www.caresearch.com.au/caresearch/tabid/2979/Default.aspx. Accessed 10 July 2019.
23. JASON. Artificial intelligence for health and health care. The MITRE Corporation 7515 Colshire Drive McLean, VA 22102-7508 2017.
24. F G. AI and Health. Sydney, Australia: Digital Health Cooperative Research Centre; 2018.
25. Moja L, Kwag KH, Lytras T, Bertizzolo L, Brandt L, Pecoraro V, et al. Effectiveness of computerized decision support systems linked to electronic health records: a systematic review and meta-analysis. Am J Public Health. 2014;104(12):e12–22.
26. Bright TJ, Wong A, Dhurjati R, Bristow E, Bastian L, Coeytaux RR, et al. Effect of clinical decision-support systems: a systematic review. Ann Intern Med. 2012;157(1):29–43.
27. Pinzari L, Mazumdar S, Girosi F. A framework for the identification and classification of homogeneous socioeconomic areas in the analysis of health care variation. Int J Health Geogr. 2018;17(1):42.
28. Khan A, Uddin S, Srinivasan U. Comorbidity network for chronic disease: a novel approach to understand type 2 diabetes progression. Int J Med Inform. 2018;115:1–9.
29. Road Safety in rural and remote Australia 2015. Available from: http://ruralhealth.org.au/media-release/road-safety-life-and-death-issue-rural-and-remote-australia.   Accessed   10 July 2019.
30. National Rural Health Alliance: Data issues relating to aspects of road safety in Australia 2015. Available from: http://ruralhealth.org.au/sites/default/files/documents/nrha-policy-doc-

ument/submissions/supplementary-supplementary-senate-data-and-road-traffic-accidents.pdf. Accessed 10 July 2019.

31. Esmaili N, Piccardi M, Kruger B, Girosi F. Analysis of healthcare service utilization after transport-related injuries by a mixture of hidden Markov models. PLoS One. 2018;13(11):e0206274.

32. Healthdirect Australia Chatbot 2017. Available from: https://about.healthdirect.gov.au/news/healthdirect-australia-launches-chatbot-pilot. Accessed 10 July 2019.

33. Nibby 2018. Available from: https://www.nib.com.au/nib-news/media/2017/12/nib-launches-australia-s-first-health-insurance-chatbot. Accessed 10 July 2019.

34. No appointment necessary. How the IoT and patient-generated data can unlock health care value.

35. Springday. Available from: https://corporate.myspringday.com.au/our-solution. Accessed 10 July 2019.

36. FoodSwitch [2018]. Available from: https://www.foodswitch.com.au/-/home. Accessed 10 July 2019.

37. Digital Health CRC. Available from: https://www.digitalhealthcrc.com/. Accessed 10 July 2019.

Chapter 11: Telehealth and Traumatic Brain Injury

Shana De Caro

Introduction

Traumatic brain injury (TBI) is a leading cause of disability in the United States.

It is estimated that 5.3 million U.S. residents are living with cognitive, psychological, and physical impairments caused by TBI. This alarming statistic equates to one out of every six Americans [1]. These multidimensional impairments affect all aspects of an individual's life, including day-to-day functioning, returning to work postinjury, and interpersonal relationships with both family and friends. Following a diagnosis of TBI in hospital emergency departments, many patients fail to receive follow-up care. In a recently reported study of patients with mild TBI, less than half self-reported receiving TBI educational material at discharge (353 patients [42%]) or seeing a physician or other healthcare practitioner within 3 months after injury (367 patients [44%]) [2]. Telemedicine, also called telehealth, has the potential to impact the quality of life and the delivery of medical, mental health, short-term, and long-term rehabilitative services to individuals suffering from the consequences of traumatic brain damage by improving access to care. The telemedicine modality has proven to be optimal for enhancing patient engagement and meeting the need for services.

The utilization of telemedicine, for both the diagnosis and treatment of the physical and mental health needs of individuals, is emerging as a beneficial tool, both medically and economically, and is a uniquely suitable modality for the remote diagnosis, care, and treatment of TBI. Telemedicine technologies can be especially effective for those suffering from these injuries by removing geographic barriers and providing access to institutions and providers capable of delivering quality care for those facing the lifelong consequences of brain damage.

S. De Caro (✉)
Esq. Attorney at Law, De Caro & Kaplen, LLP, Pleasantville, NY, USA
e-mail: shana@brainlaw.com

© Springer Nature Switzerland AG 2020
P. Murthy, A. Ansehl (eds.), *Technology and Global Public Health*,
https://doi.org/10.1007/978-3-030-46355-7_16

With the burgeoning problems associated with the shortage of doctors, and more particularly with specialists, it is necessary to address this unique healthcare crisis [3]. Compounded by the projected increase in the costs associated with addressing the physical, mental, and emotional needs of brain injury survivors, the U.S. medical system is currently unprepared to diagnose and treat those suffering from TBI [4].

Increasingly, federal agencies, including the Department of Defense (DOD), the Department of Veterans Affairs (VA), state Medicaid service providers, and medical facilities, have depended on telehealth to meet the needs of brain injury survivors and their family caregivers. Telepsychiatry allows those suffering the emotional and behavioral consequences of TBI who are too geographically remote to consult specialists in the required medical concentrations to gain access to qualified healthcare practitioners. Furthermore, access to telepsychiatry services provides patients suffering the emotional and behavioral ramifications of TBI an alternative to institutionalization by allowing them to receive care from the privacy and comfort of their homes and possibly live an otherwise independent life.

Telehealth and TBI

Telehealth is the remote delivery of healthcare services through many different telecommunication tools, including telephones, smartphones, computers, and videoconferencing [5]. Telehealth, in the context of delivery of services to victims of TBI, can ease access to care by identifying service providers, coordinating and providing access to care, and ultimately reducing costs. Additionally, telehealth methodology is beneficial in its utilization as a convenient educational tool for brain injury prevention programs; to provide background information about the signs and symptoms of brain injury; and for necessary screening of athletes following a concussion to determine when it is safe and appropriate to return to play.

TBI is an immensely misunderstood healthcare crisis among both the public and service providers alike. The use of webinars and other digital media is an efficient method to augment and supplement the awareness and knowledge of medical practitioners and other service providers of the signs and symptoms of TBI. This alternate educational material can also provide screening tools to ascertain whether someone has sustained a concussion or TBI.

Telemental health services, as a subcategory of telehealth, is defined as the "provision of mental health and substance abuse services from a distance" [6]. This is an intentionally all-encompassing characterization, allowing for flexible and wide-ranging applicability. Because psychiatry, by its nature, does not require physical interaction, the method of treatment lends itself to telecommunication technology. This type of intervention can be administered by many types of mental healthcare professionals and has broad application for individuals at a distance from healthcare professionals, including those who reside in rural areas and those with physical impairments that impede their ability to travel. The use of telemental health services ameliorates the pronounced "maldistribution of specialty care" [6]. These services and supports are exceptionally well suited for survivors of brain trauma who require an array of assistance to enable them to live within their community. Recognizing the utility of telemedicine services to provide care for TBI survivors, the U.S. Department of Health and Human Services Administration for Community Living awarded a statewide grant to the state of Arkansas for its inclusion of telehealth services to improve delivery of TBI-related healthcare [7].

Within the ambit of telemental health services is the specialty of telepsychiatry, which refers to psychiatric assessment and care through telecommunications technology, including videoconferencing [8]. The rationale and use of telepsychiatry allows clinicians to travel to patients rather than the reverse. No studies have been conducted on possible negative effects or impacts on patients who receive their mental healthcare services in this manner [6]. The prevalence of anxiety and depression in the traumatically brain injured population, including those suffering from postconcussion syndrome (PCS), and the lack of access to necessary treatment makes telepsychiatry particularly compatible for the delivery of services to those with emotional and behavioral impairments. Mental health support services are required to ameliorate problems with impaired self-image, inappropriate behavior, and interpersonal relationships among family and friends. Besides individual therapy sessions, support groups are often used to provide individuals increased information about their injury and to discuss the issues they face. These formal and informal support services can often be provided through telemental health and telepsychiatry programs.

Prevalence of TBI

Statistics released by the U.S. Centers for Disease Control and Prevention (CDC) in Atlanta, Georgia, reveal that TBI has become a national health epidemic. Using 2013 data, the CDC reported approximately 2.5 million emergency department (ED) visits, and 282,000 TBI-related hospitalizations. This represented approximately 1.9% of all hospital emergency room and hospital admissions during the year 2013 [9].

These staggering statistics fail to capture the full extent of the burgeoning public health crisis from TBI since many cases of brain trauma are unreported and therefore uncounted, especially in situations involving domestic violence and sports concussions. Many individuals are never seen in EDs, and when they receive treatment for concurrent injuries, criteria for brain assessment fail to include these patients [10]. This systemic breakdown has significant and widespread implications as it relates to adequate numbers of rehabilitation programs to manage the needs of this growing population, sufficient funding for both existing and new rehabilitation and long-term-care programs, and promulgation of injury prevention initiatives.

The populations most vulnerable to TBI are children aged 0–4 years, adolescents aged 15–19 years, and persons 75 years and older. These groups are most likely to have a TBI-related ED visit or hospitalization [11]. Generally, the leading cause of nonfatal TBI in the United States are falls (47%), blunt impacts to the head, either by being struck by a moving object or by the person's head striking a stationary object (15%), and motor vehicle–related injuries (14%) [12]. By population group, falls account for the largest proportion of TBI in children under age 4 and in the elderly, age 65 or older. Motor vehicle accidents and assaults are the primary causes of brain injury in teens and young adults aged 15 to 34 years [10]. The risk of TBI for males was determined to be twice that for females [10].

The annual financial and economic burdens associated with TBI are equally startling. In 2010, the CDC estimated annual economic costs associated with TBI to be $76.5 billion, including $11.5 billion in direct medical costs, and $64.8 billion in indirect costs, including lost wages, lost productivity, and nonmedical expenditures [10].

Notably absent from these financial estimates is the multidimensional toll taken on spouses, children, and the community because of TBI-associated disability. The CDC has recognized the significant noneconomic impact that brain injury has upon individuals and their families, stating, "For the estimated 5.3 million Americans who live with a TBI-related disability, the financial cost is only part of the burden. The long-term impairments and disabilities associated with TBI are grave and the full human cost is incalculable. Yet because these disabilities are not readily apparent to the public—unlike a broken leg—TBI is referred to as the "invisible epidemic." These disabilities, arising from cognitive, emotional, sensory, and motor impairments, often permanently alter a person's vocational aspirations and have profound effects on social and family relationships" [13].

Trauma and Brain Injury

Brain injury can occur absent any direct external trauma to the skull. The rapid acceleration and deceleration of the brain within the skull causes tearing, ripping, and stretching of nerve fibers. Damage also occurs when the brain strikes the interior of the skull due to the rapid head movement. The interior surface of the skull is composed of many sharp ridges and protrusions, which can cause damage to the soft tissue of the brain when it slides within the skull. When the brain is subjected to exterior forces causing it to move forward or backward or rotate within the closed skull cavity, it is forcefully propelled against the interior skull protrusions, causing bruising, bleeding, and destruction of nerve cells.

Most of the bony prominences are in the front and sides of the skull, injuring the frontal area of the brain (frontal lobe) and the side areas of the brain (temporal lobes) when the brain moves forcefully against these rough surfaces of the skull. The frontal and temporal lobes of the brain are responsible for cognitive skills, including memory and concentration, emotional functioning, including initiative, personality, and self-control.

Impairments and Disability Associated with TBI

Traditionally, the medical profession has classified brain injuries as mild, moderate, or severe, based solely on the patient's initial presenting signs and symptoms. The terms "mild traumatic brain injury (mTBI)," "concussion," and "mild closed head injury" are frequently used interchangeably and are often referred to collectively as PCS. While important to managing these injuries in the acute setting, these labels insufficiently reveal information on the long-term cognitive, emotional, and behavioral outcome. At least 75% of TBIs are classified as mild [14], and an estimated 15% of those who sustained a so-called mild TBI endured prolonged consequences [15].

Brain trauma can cause physical, cognitive, emotional, or behavioral impairments, and these impairments singularly or in combination affect an individual's ability to function day to day, at home, at school, or at work. Physical impairments following brain trauma include headaches, dizziness, visual disturbances, sensitivity to loud sound and bright light, and sleep disturbances. Cognitive impairments following injury to the brain include impaired memory, attention, and concentration. Frequently patients experience diminished ability to multitask or process and understand information. They have difficulties in planning, organizing, and assembling information and may experience difficulties in problem solving and decision-making. Emotional and behavioral impairments include anxiety, depression, and lack of self-control, including difficulty governing emotions and impulsivity.

Traditionally, both medical profession and insurance company evaluators have perceived brain injury as a singular event, rather than a long-term, chronic condition. Conventional analysis asserts that a broken brain is the equivalent of a broken bone. Once the brain is "fixed" or "healed," it will affect no other part of the body. A modern analysis of brain injury sees it as a persistent condition that must be approached and treated as a chronic disease with long-term consequences [16].

The consequences of a TBI are numerous and diverse. Brain damage may be the cause of neurological disorders, including epilepsy, sleep disorders, cognitive dysfunction, Alzheimer's disease, chronic traumatic encephalopathy, and Parkinson's disease. Neuroendocrine disorders, including thyroid and pituitary dysfunction, have been linked to brain trauma. Psychiatric disorders, including obsessive-compulsive disorder, anxiety, psychosis, mood disorders, and major depression, often develop following TBI. Victims of brain injury may also sustain sexual dysfunction, incontinence, and musculoskeletal dysfunction, including spasticity resulting from abnormal nerve transmission, associated with brain damage [16]. These conditions compound the cognitive, emotional, and behavioral consequences that frequently follow injury to the brain, referred to as PCS.

Necessary Services

Victims of brain trauma present a complex set of physical, emotional, and behavioral difficulties that differentiate them from individuals suffering from traditional disabilities. Recovery from a brain injury may be a long-term process persisting for many months or years with varying degrees of success. Brain injury survivors require continuing care following discharge from an acute-care setting. Individuals require home- and community-based services in many diverse areas such as cognitive, physical and occupational therapy, speech and language therapy, psychological support, mental health treatment, life care coaching, and vocational counseling. Because no two brain injuries are alike, the needs and services required to live within a community-based environment are many and varied. Community assistance includes independent living skills training and development services to assist in medication management, problem solving, household and money management; substance abuse program services to deal with alcohol and drug abuse; positive behavioral interventions and support services to provide guidance in the management of inappropriate behaviors; community integration counseling services to provide counseling and support for interpersonal relationships; and home and community support services to provide oversight and supervision in management of an individual's health and welfare [17]. A study comparing goal-oriented cognitive rehabilitation delivered in person with videoconferencing cautiously suggests cognitive rehabilitation can be adapted to telehealth videoconferencing for older adults with subjective and objective memory impairment [18]. Telemedicine services have also been found to be effective with the management of medications for dementia patients living in rural areas [19]. A review of studies reporting outcomes of structured telephone interventions following TBI found improvements in global functioning, posttraumatic symptoms, sleep quality, and depressive symptoms. Future controlled studies were recommended [20].

Impediments and Barriers to Care and Services for Persons with TBI

Despite efforts on the national and state levels since passage of the Traumatic Brain Injury Act of 1996 [21], there remains a paucity of postacute medical providers, rehabilitation centers, and therapists available and qualified to provide services to survivors of brain trauma. Telemedicine and the subcategory of telepsychiatry have the potential to address the needs of TBI survivors and provide necessary services and supports in both an accessible and cost-efficient manner.

As individuals recover from their brain trauma, their impairments and needs change. The transition of services from acute inpatient care to outpatient rehabilitation and the long-term assistance required presents difficulties in accessibility and the coordination of services among health and holistic support providers. Following discharge from the acute-care setting, most brain injury victims do not receive adequate and coordinated care. This is due to inadequate discharge planning arising from a lack of awareness by planners and patients of the types of care and assistance required, limited information regarding the categories and variety of programs and assistance available, the paucity of service providers, and geographic and transportation obstacles to accessing care, compounded by the limitations of insurance coverage.

In 2012, the State of New York examined the unmet needs of the brain-injured population. The analysis found that the most significant unmet needs were enhancing public knowledge of TBI treatment and prevention; improving availability/ access to community-based TBI services; enhancing TBI provider training, diagnosis, and treatment; and maximizing educational/vocational opportunities. Each of these can be addressed through carefully designed and implemented telehealth and telepsychiatric services.

The VA and DOD Experience with Telemedicine in Addressing the Needs of TBI Survivors

TBI, the signature injury of the Afghanistan (Operation Enduring Freedom [OEF]) and Iraq (Operation Iraqi Freedom, [OIF]) military conflicts, arises in a variety of situations. Acquired brain injury during military service occurs predominantly because of exposure to blasts, motor vehicle collisions, and gunshot wounds [22]. The Congressional Research Service, in analyzing data provided by the DOD, reported 233,425 TBI cases since 2000, with 178,961 reported as mild, 38,943 as moderate, and 6188 as severe or penetrating. An additional 9333 were incapable of classification [23]. It is difficult to ascertain the full extent of brain injury caused by blasts, because most available statistical information on TBI in the military is a compilation of all known causes. Accurate statistics are problematic because many traumatic brain injuries are not initially evident and may go unreported for long periods. These injuries may be overlapped by or confused with other service-related injuries, such as posttraumatic stress disorder. The consequences of brain trauma continue after termination of military service, with a persistent and substantial burden on the Veterans Health Administration, the agency responsible for medical and rehabilitative care of service members after discharge. Among service members separated from the military and enrolled with the VA, the estimated prevalence of history of TBI with persisting symptoms among those who presented was 7.1% [24].

The VA and the DOD are driving forces in implementing telemedicine for the diagnosis and treatment of TBI in active duty and returning service members. The military experience in using telemedicine and TBI can serve as a paradigm for the multitude of issues confronting brain injury survivors in the civilian population. In a 2014 report to Congress, the DOD stated that it "views telehealth as an important set of tools to improve access to PH/TBI (psychological health and traumatic brain injury care), as well as a range of other healthcare services, for beneficiaries in deployed and non-deployed settings. As telehealth services develop, they enhance the Department's readiness to deliver the right care, in the right place, at the right time" [25]. Patients who are "isolated by geography, poverty and disability" [26] are able to be supervised and treated by the Department of Veterans Affairs and the Veterans Health Administration utilizing telemedicine. "Veterans once at risk of being left untreated can now be monitored and cared for in their homes and communities" [26]. Over 690,000 veterans received remote care treatment in 2014. VA Secretary Robert A. McDonald commented that "a brick-and-mortar facility is not the only option for healthcare" [27].

In 2009, the U.S. Army's Medical Research and Material Command and the Telemedicine and Advanced Technology Research Center collaborated with the American Telemedicine Association to organize and conduct a symposium entitled "Innovative New Technologies to Identify and Treat Traumatic Brain Injuries: Crossover Technologies and Approaches Between Military and Civilian Applications" [28].

The symposium examined the role and use of telemedicine technology in the identification and treatment of service members with TBI for:

1. "Identification of concussion and mild TBI by using electronic cognitive assessment systems;
2. Provision of information so that clinical teams are able to collaborate on TBI care;
3. Provision of teletherapy and encouragement for patients with TBI receiving long-term rehabilitation services;
4. Provision of real-time video visits with family members or store-and-forward modalities;
5. Provision of video nursing supervision of patients with TBI in their home;
6. Management of medication and provision of an online response system;
7. Provision of cognitive therapy, speech and physical therapy in distance or rural areas; and
8. Provision of interactive video programs and Web courses to train medics, physician assistants (PAs), nurses and other providers in civilian and military settings" [28].

The symposium participants came to the following conclusion: "Whether the soldier is on the battlefield, in a military treatment facility, or at home, they need to have access to the appropriate clinical providers and telemedicine is one way that could enhance these connections" [28].

A website called TTWRL was created to support DOD and VA TBI case managers and care coordinators who advise and assist service members diagnosed with a TBI. This online tool is designed to provide rapid access to resources to support discharge planning and ongoing care required by service members, veterans, and their families dealing with a TBI [29].

Telemedicine and Brain Injury Diagnosis

Many injuries sustained by service members occur in remote areas where there is a dearth of trained medical professionals available and capable of diagnosing these conditions. It is critical to provide rapid screening and assessment for brain damage of service members exposed to blasts and other types of trauma. The Defense and Veterans Brain Injury Center (DVBIC) has utilized web-based programs that supply questionnaires and brief cognitive assessments that can be evaluated by clinicians in distant locations for diagnosis and to provide a baseline for follow-up when a combat soldier returns to base and even after his/her discharge [26].

Telehealth to Active Duty Service Members in Need of TBI Treatment

The DOD offers telepsychiatry clinics to active duty service members that connect these soldiers to psychiatric treatment at military facilities across the country by means of videoconferencing. In 2016, at a meeting of the American Telemedicine Association, David Shulkin, Under Secretary of Veterans Affairs for Health, announced the establishment of five VA Mental Telehealth Clinical Resource Centers, intended to provide enhanced mental health access and services to veterans in remote locations. The centers provide veterans with rapid access to services by eliminating barriers, such as remoteness from existing facilities. Among the services offered are clinical video telehealth (CVT), which uses real-time interactive videoconferencing to assess, treat, and provide care to patients remotely; home telehealth (HT), a program designed for veterans suffering from a chronic condition allowing coordination of care and case management, mobile monitoring, and two-way communication; and store-and-forward telehealth (SFT), which makes it possible to acquire, store, and access clinical information, including imaging studies [30].

Recognizing the need to remove existing barriers and allow the VA to provide treatment through physicians without regard to state licensing requirements, new regulations have been implemented by the VA to permit healthcare providers, including physicians and nurses, to administer care to veterans nationwide, without regard to state lines and outside of a federal facility [31]. Veterans are able to receive telemedicine treatment from any location under this recently enacted regulation, including in their homes or at a community center.

Telemedicine and Sports Concussions

The CDC estimates that about 325,000 children (age 19 or younger) are treated in EDs each year for sports- and recreation-related injuries whose diagnosis includes concussion or TBI [32]. From 2001 to 2009, the rate of ED visits for sports- and recreation-related injuries with a diagnosis of concussion or TBI, alone or combined with other injuries, rose 57% among children age 19 or younger [33]. A 2017 survey of students in grades 9 through 12 found that 15%, or 2.5 million youths, in the United States reported at least one concussion in the prior year [34].

Although there has been increased awareness of concussions within the context of sports over the last several years, there remains an urgent need for educating student athletes, parents, coaches, trainers, and other school personnel regarding concussion prevention, diagnosis, and management. Internet-based information systems provide an effective way of disseminating vital and functional information.

In May 2009, Washington State enacted the Zackery Lystedt Law, becoming the first state in the country to enact a comprehensive youth sports concussion safety law. Following enactment of this law, all 50 states now provide some form of protection for school-based athletic programs. Typically, these laws have an educational component, mandating training for school coaches in concussion recognition and how to make the important return-to-play decisions. These laws often require that students and parents receive information on the recognition of concussions, the importance of reporting symptoms, and the need to be symptom-free before returning to athletic participation.

In New York state, the Concussion Management and Awareness Act of 2011 requires school coaches, physical education teachers, nurses, and certified athletic trainers to complete a New York State Education Department–approved course on concussions and concussion management every 2 years. New York has approved Heads Up, Concussion in Youth Sports [35] for coaches and physical education teachers, which is a cost-free, web-based course developed by the CDC [36].

The use of telemedicine to assess athletes for sports-related concussions and medical determinations regarding return to play is an emerging area. Many schools and community teams lack access to trained professionals immediately available on the sidelines necessary to make timely decisions. Telemedicine through audio and visual links can provide quick and effective assessments of athletes by trained specialists at remote locations. The trained medical provider can interview patients, assess their complaints, and rapidly administer computer-based screening tests to determine whether a concussion was sustained. The University of Virginia's Center for Telehealth is developing audio-video conferencing capabilities to perform remote concussion assessment [37].

Following a concussion, a crucial decision must be made regarding when it is safe to allow athletes to return to play. Premature return to play can delay full recovery, lead to more serious injuries, and cause a life-threatening condition known as second-impact syndrome [38]. Neuropsychological testing is frequently relied upon in this decision-making process to ascertain when it is safe and appropriate to allow an athlete to return to play. The testing protocol often involves comparison of an athlete's preinjury neurocognitive status (baseline) with his postinjury condition. One such test, the Immediate Post-Concussion Assessment and Cognitive Testing (ImPACT) [39], is a computerized baseline neuropsychological test designed to be administered on a desktop or laptop computer. The test, which recently received

U.S. Food and Drug Administration (FDA) approval [40], can be administered remotely, with results stored and easily accessible for comparison by a trained professional after a player is diagnosed with a concussion. Similarly, in a telehealth setting, postinjury computerized neuropsychological test batteries can be administered easily to players after they have sustained a concussion. The Barrow Neurological Institute in Phoenix, Arizona, and A.T. Still University of Health Sciences in Mesa, Arizona, have developed a software-based telemedicine program using ImPACT for the evaluation and reevaluation of athletes. A concussion specialist remotely reviews the pre- and postinjury testing, which is uploaded, and then provides a written assessment that can be transmitted electronically. The protocols also permit a video consultation with an on-call physician when appropriate and necessary [41]. The remote comparison of pre- and postinjury testing is an effective and efficient way to assist in the evaluation of cognitive recovery following a sports-based concussion.

Telemedicine and Domestic Violence

Domestic violence is a common and often overlooked cause of TBI. The CDC estimates that within their lifetimes almost a quarter of women in the United States are victims of physical abuse at the hands of domestic partners. Extrapolating from these data, 20 million women could exhibit signs and symptoms of a TBI each year [42].

Repeated blows to the head, violent shaking, being thrown up against a wall, and strangulation are frequent causes of TBI. Recent research reveals that 60% of victims of domestic violence suffer a TBI [43].

Victims of domestic abuse face significant barriers to obtaining necessary services, including isolation, low self-esteem, and a lack of social support, insurance, and transportation [44]. One study found that offering telepsychiatric services to domestic abuse victims provided effective access to services and supports [45]. Domestic violence victims, however, are not routinely screened for a TBI even when examined in an ED or physician's office. Additionally, despite proper screening, the victim may be prevented from accessing medical care or rehabilitation services, scheduling or keeping appointments, or having necessary service providers in the home if she still resides with an abusive partner [46]. A study of the effectiveness and feasibility of providing evidence-based, trauma-focused treatment via videoconferencing to rural survivors of domestic violence and sexual assault determined that this modality of treatment was both beneficial and effective in providing psychological services to this fragile population [47]. Telehealth affords a means of educating and improving awareness of the signs and symptoms of brain trauma to victims of domestic violence and caregivers, expanding access to necessary screening tools, and removing barriers to support services following brain injury caused by domestic violence.

Telemedicine for Caregivers

Brain injury survivors frequently return home following discharge from acute and subacute rehabilitation facilities, placing inestimable burdens upon family members for continuing care, assistance, and support. These individuals frequently lack sufficient skills or training to provide care and also confront their own emotional turmoil resulting from the brain damage sustained by their loved ones. Caregivers often suffer from anxiety, depression, marital stress, and impaired life satisfaction because of the demands placed upon them.

Similar to those problems faced by brain injury survivors, caregivers also encounter obstacles to obtaining the training, assistance, and support they need. These barriers include limited availability of service providers, transportation issues, and time constraints. Telehealth holds the potential and promise to provide problem-solving interventional training, therapy, and emotional support to caregivers otherwise unable to access these benefits. Recent studies using a telephone-based model individualized to the unique needs of a caregiver have shown this category of intervention is associated with improved emotional outcomes for family members [48]. Telemedicine technology has proven effective at educating caregivers about the skills necessary to provide care and allowing feedback to improve outcomes for children living at home following a TBI [49].

Conclusion

Telemedicine and telepsychiatry have enormous potential benefits in addressing the prevention, diagnosis, and treatment of TBI. Telehealth can break through existing barriers preventing access to treatment for many victims of brain trauma and offers a practical solution to the existing uneven access to resources. The military experience provides a useful paradigm. The utilization of telehealth to address the needs and multifaceted problems associated with those suffering the lifelong consequences of brain injury can and should be replicated among the civilian population. Implementing telehealth services permits patients with TBI-related disabilities to access care from their own homes and possibly live independent lives, rather than be forced to remain institutionalized.

References

1. Corrigan JD, Selassi AW, Orman JA. The epidemiology of traumatic brain injury. J Head Trauma Rehabil. 2010;25(2):72–80. https://doi.org/10.1097/HTR.0b013e3181ccc8b4.
2. Seabury SA, Gaudette É, Goldman DP, et al. Assessment of follow-up care after emergency department presentation for mild traumatic brain injury and concussion: results from the TRACK-TBI study. JAMA Netw Open. 2018;1(1):e180210. https://doi.org/10.1001/jamanetworkopen.2018.0210.

3. Dall T, Chakrabarti R, Iacobucci W, Hansari A, West T. 2017 update: the complexities of physician supply and demand: projections from 2015 to 2030 final report. Washington DC: Association of Medical Colleges; 2017.. https://aamc-black.global.ssl.fastly.net/production/media/filer_public/a5/c3/a5c3d565-14ec-48fb-974b-99fafaeecb00/aamc_projections_update_2017.pdf. Accessed 18 Sept 2018

4. García-Lizana F, Muñoz-Mayorga I. What about telepsychiatry? A systematic review. Prim Care Companion J Clin Psychiatry. 2010;12(2):PCC.09m00831. https://doi.org/10.4088/PCC.09m00831whi.

5. Dorsey ER, Topol EJ. State of telehealth. N Engl J Med. 2016;375(2):154–61. https://doi.org/10.1056/NEJMra1601705.

6. Turvey C, Coleman M, Dennison O, et al. Practice guidelines for video-based online mental health services. American Telemedicine Association; 2013. https://www.integration.samhsa.gov/operations-administration/practice-guidelines-for-video-based-online-mental-health-services_ATA_5_29_13.pdf. Accessed 18 Sept 2018.

7. Talk Business & Politics staff. UAMS awarded $450,000 telemedicine grant to serve traumatic brain injury survivors. Talk Business & Politics Web site. https://talkbusiness.net/2018/07/uams-awarded-450000-telemedicine-grant-to-serve-traumatic-brain-injury-survivors/. Published July 19, 2018. Accessed 18 Sept 2018.

8. Crane, K. Telepsychiatry: the new frontier in mental health. U.S. News & World Report Web site. https://health.usnews.com/health-news/patient-advice/articles/2015/01/15/telepsychiatry-the-new-frontier-in-mental-health. Published January 15, 2018. Accessed 18 Sept 2018.

9. Taylor CA, Bell JM, Breiding MJ, Xu L. Traumatic brain injury–related emergency department visits, hospitalizations, and deaths — United States, 2007 and 2013. MMWR Surveill Summ. 2017;66(SS-9):1–16. https://doi.org/10.15585/mmwr.ss6609a1.

10. Centers for Disease Control and Prevention. CDC grand rounds: reducing severe traumatic brain injury in the united sates. MMWR. 2013;62(27):549–52.

11. Thurman DJ. National Center for Injury Prevention and Control (U.S.) [Accessed June 3, 2011]; Division of Acute Care Rehabilitation Research and Disability Prevention. Traumatic Brain Injury in the United States: A Report to Congress; 2018.

12. TBI: Get the Facts. Centers for disease control and prevention Website. https://www.cdc.gov/traumaticbraininjury/get_the_facts.html. Last updated April 27, 2017. Accessed 18 Sep 2018.

13. National Center for Injury Prevention and Control. Traumatic brain injury in the United States, a report to congress. Atlanta: Centers for Disease Control and Prevention; 1999.

14. National Center for Injury Prevention and Control. Report to congress on mild traumatic brain injury in the United States: steps to prevent a serious public health problem. Atlanta: Centers for Disease Control and Prevention; 2003.

15. Alexander MP. Mild traumatic brain injury: pathophysiology, natural history, and clinical management. Neurology. 1995;45(7):1253–60.; McMillan TM, Teasdale GM, Stewart E. Disability in young people and adults after head injury: 12–14 year follow-up of a prospective cohort. J Neurol Neurosurg Psychiatry. 2012;83(11):1086–91. doi: https://doi.org/10.1136/jnnp-2012-302746. Epub 2012 May 29.

16. Masel BE, DeWitt DS. Traumatic brain injury: a disease process, not an event. J Neurotrauma. 2010;27(8):1529–40. https://doi.org/10.1089/neu.2010.1358.

17. New York State Department of Health, Brain Association of New York State. New York state department of health traumatic brain injury Medicaid Waiver Program. https://www.health.ny.gov/publications/1111.pdf. Accessed 18 Sept 2018.

18. Burton RL, O'Connell ME. Telehealth Rehabilitation for Cognitive Impairment: Randomized Controlled Feasibility Trial. Eddens K, ed. JMIR Res Protoc. 2018;7(2):e43. https://doi.org/10.2196/resprot.9420.

19. Chang W, Homer M, Rossi MI. Use of clinical video telehealth as a tool for optimizing medications for rural older veterans with dementia. Geriatrics. 2018;3(3):44. https://doi.org/10.3390/geriatrics3030044.

20. Ownsworth T, Arnautovska U, Beadle E, Shum DHK, Moyle W. Efficacy of telerehabilitation for adults with traumatic brain injury: a systematic review. J Head Trauma Rehabil. 2018;33(4):E33–46. https://doi.org/10.1097/HTR.0000000000000350.
21. Public Law 104–166.
22. Office of Research & Development. VA research on traumatic brain injury (TBI). US Department of Veterans Affairs Web site. https://www.research.va.gov/topics/tbi.cfm. n.d. Accessed 17 Oct 2018.
23. Fischer H. U.S. Military Casualty Statistics: Operation New Dawn, Operation Iraqi Freedom, and Operation Enduring Freedom. Congressional Research Service; 2012. http://digital.library. unt.edu/ark:/67531/metadc98128/m1/1/high_res_d/RS22452_2012Jun12.pdf. Accessed 18 Sept 2018.
24. Silver JM, McAllister TW, Yudofsky SC. Textbook of traumatic brain injury. 2nd ed. Washington, DC: American Psychiatric Publishing; 2011. p. 18.
25. US Department of Defense. Report to congress: national defense authorization act for fiscal year 2014, section 702(b) use of telemedicine to improve the diagnosis and treatment of post-traumatic stress disorder, traumatic brain injuries and mental health conditions. Washington, DC: US Department of Defense; 2014.
26. Girad P. Military and VA telemedicine systems for patients with traumatic brain injury. J Rehabil Res Dev. 2007;44(7):1017–26.
27. United States Department of Veterans Affairs, Office of Public and Intergovernmental Affairs. VA Telehealth Services Served Over 690,000 Veterans In Fiscal Year 2014. http://www.va.gov/ opa/pressrel/pressrelease.cfm?id=2646. Published October 10, 2014. Accessed 18 Sept 2018.
28. Doarn CR, McVeigh F, Poropatich R. Innovative new technologies to identify and treat traumatic brain injuries: crossover technologies and approaches between military and civilian applications. Telemed J E Health. 2010 Apr;16(3):373–81. https://doi.org/10.1089/tmj.2010.0009.
29. Defense Centers of Excellence. For TBI case managers in support of service members, veterans and their families. Telehealth & Technology Website and Resource Locator Web site. https://ttwrl.dcoe.mil/. Updated April 14, 2016. Accessed 18 Sept 2018.
30. U.S. Department of Veterans Affairs, Office of Public and Intergovernmental Affairs. VA Announces Health Clinical Resources Centers During Telemedicine Association Gathering. http://www.va.gov/opa/pressrel/pressrelease.cfm?id=2789. Published May 16, 2016. Accessed 18 Sept 2018.
31. Unit 38 Code of Federal Regulations §17.417.
32. Coronado VG, Haileyesus T, Cheng TA, et al. Trends in sports- and recreation-related traumatic brain injuries treated in US emergency departments: the National Electronic Injury Surveillance System-all Injury Program (NEISS-AIP) 2001–2012. J Head Trauma Rehabil. 2015;30(3):185–97. https://doi.org/10.1097/HTR.0000000000000156.
33. TBI: Get the facts. Centers for disease control and prevention Web site. http://www.cdc.gov/ traumaticbraininjury/get_the_facts.html. Updated April 27, 2017. Accessed 18 Sept 2018.
34. DePadilla L, Miller GF, Jones SE, Peterson AB, Breiding MJ. Self-reported concussions from playing a sport or being physically active among high school students — United States, 2017. MMWR Morb Mortal Wkly Rep. 2018;67(24):682–5. https://doi.org/10.15585/mmwr. mm6724a3.
35. HEADS UP to youth sports: Online training. Centers for disease control and prevention Web site. https://www.cdc.gov/headsup/youthsports/training/index.html. Updated October 4, 2018. Accessed 17 Oct 2018.
36. The University of the State of New York, The State Education Department University. Guidelines for concussion Management in the School Setting. Albany: Office of Student Support Services; 2012.
37. Westerman AS. UVa. Center considers use of telemedicine to assess sports concussions. Capital News Service Web Site. http://cnsmaryland.org/2014/05/21/uva-center-considers-use-of-telemedicine-to-assess-sports-concussions/. Published May 21, 2014. Accessed 18 Sept 2018.

38. Cantu RC. Second-impact syndrome. Clin Sports Med. 1998;17(1):37–44.
39. Home page. ImPACT Applications, Inc. Web site. https://impacttest.com/. n.d., Accessed 18 Sept 2018.
40. FDA allows marketing of first-of-kind computerized cognitive tests to help assess cognitive skills after a head injury. U.S Food and Drug Administration Web site. https://www.fda.gov/newsevents/newsroom/pressannouncements/ucm517526.htm. Published August 22, 2016. Accessed 18 Sept 2018.
41. Cardenas JF, McLeon TV. ImPACT as a Component of Telemedicine Management for Concussion. Impact Research Report; 2016 Winter,4. https://www.impacttest.com/_admin/uploads/impact-researchreport-telemedicine-management-concussion.pdf. Accessed 18 Sept 2018.
42. Sojourner center launches first-of-its-kind effort to study link between domestic violence and traumatic brain injury. Sojourner Center Web site. https://www.sojournercenter.org/sojourner-center-launches-first-of-its-kind-effort-to-study-link-between-domestic-violence-and-traumatic-brain-injury/. Published June 2, 2015. Accessed 18 Sept 2018.
43. Monahan K, O'Leary KD. Head injury and battered women: an initial inquiry. Health Soc Work. 1999;24(4):269–78.
44. Gray MJ, Hassija CM, Jaconis M, et al. Provision of evidence-based therapies to rural survivors of domestic violence and sexual assault via telehealth: treatment outcomes and clinical training benefits. Train Educ Prof Psychol. 2015;9(3):235–41.
45. Thomas CR, Miller G, Hartshorn Jeanette C, et al. Telepsychiatry program for rural victims of domestic violence. Telemed J E Health. 2005;11(5):567–73. https://doi.org/10.1089/tmj.2005.11.567.
46. Langois J. Breaking the silence: violence as a cause and consequence of traumatic brain injury. BrainLine Web site. http://www.brainline.org/content/2008/07/breaking-silence-violence-cause-and-consequence-traumatic-brain-injury_pageall.html. Published July 25, 2008. Accessed 18 Sept 2018.
47. Hassija C, Gray MJ. The effectiveness and feasibility of videoconferencing technology to provide evidence-based treatment to rural domestic violence and sexual assault populations. Telemed J E Health. 2011;17(4):309–15. https://doi.org/10.1089/tmj.2010.0147.. Epub 2011 Apr 1
48. Powell JM, Fraser R, Brockway JA, Temkin N, Bell KR. A telehealth approach to caregiver self-management following traumatic brain injury: a randomized controlled trial. J Head Trauma Rehabil. 2016;31(3):180–90. https://doi.org/10.1097/HTR.0000000000000167.
49. Witt MR, Stokes TF, Parsonson BS, Dudding CC. Effect of distance caregiver coaching on functional skills of a child with traumatic brain injury. Brain Inj. 2018;32(7):894–9. https://doi.org/10.1080/02699052.2018.1466365.. Epub 2018 Apr 24

Chapter 12: Leveraging Technology for Attaining Sustainable Development Goal 3: The Road Ahead

Gopal Sankaran

Introduction - Challenges and Opportunities

Millennium Development Goals

The Millennium Summit, held in September 2000 at United Nations headquarters in New York City, brought together heads of state, government, and high-ranking officials representing 189 member nations [1]. They adopted the United Nations Millennium Declaration in recognition of their collective responsibility to uphold the principles of human dignity, equality, and equity at the global level [2]. The leaders committed their respective nations to a new global partnership for advancing a series of eight goals, referred to as the Millennium Development Goals (MDGs), with the deadline of 2015 for achieving them. The agreed upon MDGs were to: (1) eradicate extreme poverty and hunger; (2) achieve universal primary education; (3) promote gender equality and empower women; (4) reduce child mortality; (5) improve maternal health; (6) combat HIV/AIDS, malaria, and other diseases; (7) ensure environmental sustainability; and (8) develop a global partnership for development [1]. The final evaluation report of the MDGs in 2015 [3] showed several remarkable accomplishments. Successful efforts included lifting more than a billion people out of extreme poverty, enabling more girls to attend school than ever before, reducing hunger, and protecting planetary resources. The MDGs generated a wave of innovative partnerships and demonstrated that ambitious goals could be achieved. However, these accomplishments were tempered by the realization that progress was uneven among nations and even within nations. Specific challenges, such as maternal morbidity and mortality, rural-urban disparities, income inequality, and lack of progress among the disadvantaged, were sill prevalent [3].

G. Sankaran (✉)
West Chester University, West Chester, PA, USA
e-mail: gsankaran@wcupa.edu

© Springer Nature Switzerland AG 2020
P. Murthy, A. Ansehl (eds.), *Technology and Global Public Health*,
https://doi.org/10.1007/978-3-030-46355-7_17

Sustainable Development Goals

While progress was being made toward the attainment of MDGs, the United Nations embarked on an even more ambitious process of setting goals for the next 15 years. In October 2015, the United Nations General Assembly adopted a resolution (A/RES/70/1), Transforming our world: the 2030 Agenda for Sustainable Development [4], that paved the way to the 17 Sustainable Development Goals (SDGs) with 169 targets [5]. The SDGs sought to build on the MDGs and complete what had not yet been achieved. The 17 SDGs are to: (1) end poverty in all its forms everywhere; (2) end hunger, achieve food security and improved nutrition, and promote sustainable agriculture; (3) ensure healthy lives and promote well-being for all at all ages; (4) ensure inclusive and equitable quality education and promote lifelong learning opportunities for all; (5) achieve gender equality and empower all women and girls; (6) ensure availability and sustainable management of water and sanitation for all; (7) ensure access to affordable, reliable, sustainable, and modern energy for all; (8) promote sustained inclusive and sustainable economic growth, full and productive employment, and decent work for all; (9) build resilient infrastructure, promote inclusive and sustainable industrialization, and foster innovation; (10) reduce inequality within and among countries; (11) make cities and human settlements inclusive, safe, resilient, and sustainable; (12) ensure sustainable consumption and production patterns; (13) take urgent action to combat climate change and its impact; (14) conserve and sustainably use the oceans, seas, and marine resources for sustainable development; (15) protect, restore, and promote sustainable use of terrestrial ecosystems, sustainably manage forests, combat desertification, halt and reverse land degradation, and halt biodiversity loss; (16) promote peaceful and inclusive societies for sustainable development, provide access to justice for all, and build effective, accountable, and inclusive institutions at all levels; and (17) strengthen the means of implementation and revitalize the Global Partnership for Sustainable Development [5].

Transitioning from MDGs to SDGs – Ambition Meets Challenges

The report *Transitioning from MDGs to SDGs* [6], jointly published by the United Nations Development Programme and the International Bank for Reconstruction and Development/World Bank, details the key lessons learned from the MDG Acceleration Reviews undertaken under the auspices of the UN System Chief Executives Board for Coordination (CEB) during a period of 2+ years (April 2013–November 2015). This report identifies several challenges and offers possible solutions. For example, information gaps in household-level data were noted, making it difficult to know the direction of change for some measures such as poverty alleviation (whether are people rising out of poverty or falling back into it). A solution is to conduct household-level surveys in the poor populations every 3 years to see changes in key measures over time. Thus, lack of quality data and analysis was identified as a serious constraint on timely monitoring, policy development, and the ability to target interventions where most needed [6]. Such lessons need to be remembered because the SDGs are more ambitious than the MDGs in several ways. For example, SDGs 1 and 2 are stated in absolute terms (SDG 1 requires ending poverty in all its forms everywhere, while SDG 2 is focused on ending hunger). The 2018 UNDP report [7] *What Does It Mean to Leave No One Behind?*, noting the commitment of the 193 United Nations member states' pledge to ensure "no one will be left behind" and to "endeavour to reach the furthest behind first" offers a framework that governments and various stakeholders can use in their nations to act to leave no one behind. This would pave the way to enabling and accelerating national progress to achieve the SDGs. The framework identifies five key factors for who is being left behind and why: discrimination, geography, governance, socio-economic status, and shocks and fragility [7].

Achieving these goals globally will require innovation and a commitment of resources on a long-term basis that so far has not been seen in the development arena. The 2018 UNDP report [7] urges every nation to implement from early on three mutually reinforcing "levers." They are as follows: (1) examine: disaggregated and people-driven data and information; (2) empower: civic engagement and voice; and (3) enact: integrated, equity-focused SDG policies, interventions, and budgets. The report recommends that integrated approaches be employed to move all three "levers" at the same time to accrue the desired outcome [7].

Sustainable Development Goal 3

While all SDGs are interconnected, the focus here is on SDG 3: Ensure healthy lives and promote well-being for all at all ages [8]. The general information about targets 3.1 through 3.9 is as follows:

3.1 By 2030, reduce the global maternal mortality ratio to less than 70 per 100,000 live births.
3.2 By 2030, end preventable deaths of newborns and children under 5 years of age.
3.3 By 2030, end the epidemics of AIDS, tuberculosis, malaria, and neglected tropical diseases.
3.4 By 2030, reduce by one-third premature mortality from noncommunicable diseases through prevention and treatment.
3.5 Strengthen the prevention and treatment of substance abuse.
3.6 By 2020, halve the number of global deaths and injuries from road traffic accidents.
3.7 By 2030, ensure universal access to sexual and reproductive healthcare services.
3.8 Achieve universal health coverage.
3.9 By 2030, substantially reduce the number of deaths and illnesses from hazardous chemicals.

In addition to the nine targets presented (3.1 through 3.9), four additional means of implementing targets addressing overarching themes, such as application of World Health Organization Framework Convention on Tobacco Control, research and development, health financing and human capacity building, and risk surveillance and management, are also included and are labeled 3.a to 3.d [8, 9]. Each of the nine targets and an additional four means of implementing targets have a total of 26 indicators [8, 9] to be used for monitoring and evaluation of SDG 3 over time.

In the 2018 report *Towards a Global Action Plan For Healthy Lives and Well-being for All*, developed jointly by the World Health Organization and 10 other development-focused organizations, it is noted that the SDGs "represent an ambitious vision of the healthier, more prosperous, inclusive and resilient world we all want" [10](p. 1). The report notes that fragmentation, duplication, and inefficiency are pushing us off track in terms of achieving these ambitious goals by 2030, and underscores the need to "recalibrate and amplify our efforts now or else we will not even come close to reaching many of the health-related targets" [10](p.1).

Role of Technology in SDG 3 – Barriers and Opportunities

We live in a technological era marked by advances that a few years ago were unimaginable. As Klaus Schwab indicates, "The possibilities of billions of people connected by mobile devices, with unprecedented processing power, storage capacity, and access to knowledge, are unlimited" [11]. In his essay, Schwab posits that we are currently in the Fourth Industrial Revolution that has been happening since the 1950s. He outlines the earlier ones as follows: water and steam power to mechanize production constituted the First Industrial Revolution; electric power to create production on a mass scale marked the Second Industrial Revolution; the Third Industrial Revolution used electronics and information technology to automate production. The Fourth Industrial Revolution is blurring the lines between the physical, digital, and biological spheres because of the fusion of technologies [11].

The current revolution is evolving at an exponential pace, is disruptive, and has no historical precedents [11]. Technology comes with the twin features of high price (when it is newly introduced in the market) and a short shelf life, both less cumbersome to both providers and consumers in resource-rich nations. However, in developing nations, these two features could serve as potential barriers that are too difficult to overcome. *The Lancet* Commission's report *Technologies for Global Health* begins by stating that the "Availability of health technology is inversely related to health need" [12](p. 507). The report makes the case for focusing on technologies for health rather than on narrowly focused health technology. Their broader concept of technologies for health includes the traditional health technologies (medical devices, biological products, drugs, organizational systems, medical and surgical procedures, and support systems), along with information and communications technology (ICT), including the Internet, television, radio, and mobile phones, and collateral benefits accrued from the use of improvements in agricultural equipment, road safety technologies, bioengineered foods, and sanitation. The authors argue convincingly that such a broad understanding of the scope of technologies for health is particularly of value in low-income nations. They also emphasize the value of "frugal technology" – technology that is specifically developed to meet the needs of the world's poorest people; an example is Jaipur foot for those who have below-knee amputations – so that the needs of people in low-income situations could be best met through lower cost, better adaptability, and enhanced functionality [12]. The 2017 *Fast-forward for Progress* report highlights the use of ICTs in improving global health "by improving the ability to gather, analyze, manage, and exchange information in all areas of health" [13](p.25). ICTs are valuable in improving the timeliness and accuracy of public health reporting, in addition to facilitating disease monitoring and surveillance. The widespread global adoption of mobile technologies has certainly enhanced the opportunity for outreach to those who are separated by distance and difficult terrain. As demand to keep costs low and increase the efficiency of operations increases, eHealth will play a more important role both in low-income and middle-income nations [13]. It is notable that by 2015, over 120 countries had adopted national policies, including objectives on how ICTs, eHealth, or telehealth can support universal healthcare [14].

The use of social media by the public has been increasing, as has the widespread use of social media in health. Social media has been used by healthcare organizations to promote health messages as a part of health promotion campaigns, help manage patient appointments, seek feedback on services rendered, make general health announcements, and make emergency announcements. Similarly, social media has been utilized to a variable extent by individuals and communities to learn about health issues, help decide what health services to use, provide feedback to health facilities or health professionals, run community-based health campaigns, and participate in community-based health forums [14]. On the other hand, policies and strategies to use social media in the health domain by national governments are lagging and need strengthening.

The advent of artificial intelligence, robotics, machine learning, blockchain, big data processing, and other emerging technologies has been leveraged for relevant applications in resource-rich settings [15]. These technologies' widespread use in low- and middle-income nations with resource constraints along with an urgent need for enhancing the health status of communities and populations to achieve SDG 3 are not easily discernible. Novillo-Ortiz, Marin, and Saigí-Rubió [16] highlight how our daily lives have changed since the publication of the MDGs in 2000. They assert that the major changes in our day-to-day routine activities, such as how we access information or provide data, make purchases or sell goods, communicate with one another, and do our work, have been greatly influenced by one common factor – the growth and spread of ICTs. Thus, while in the MDG era, technology was an add-on, the progress toward achieving the SDGs is greatly influenced by the ever improving and expanding technology and its applications. The 2017 International Telecommunication Union's *Fast Forward Progress* report [13] indicates that science, technology, and innovation (STI), along with appropriate resources for development, were identified by the United Nations as two core means of making progress toward and achieving the SDGs by 2030. The report further shows that STI cuts across all SDGs and is valuable now and in future.

What needs emphasizing is that in the world of 2019, there is a technological divide between the "haves" and "have nots." While some forms of technology and their applications such as mobile technology, e-commerce, and ICTs have become common in resource-poor settings, there is still a yawning gap in the availability, accessibility, and affordability of technology between rich and poor nations. Widening income inequality between and within nations has also contributed to the reality of the "digital poor" being left behind. In addition, with automation, artificial intelligence, machine learning, and robotics, there is an inherent fear in resource-poor settings about the loss of jobs that are repetitive and are often the lifeline for families in many communities around the globe. Tran and Ravaud [17] point out that even with frugal innovations (i.e., a set of activities providing effective functional solutions to common problems encountered by "the many," with a minimal use of resources) issues related to safety and efficacy, acceptability and adaptability, and scaling up may thwart their wider application. It is important to note that these frugal innovations often arise out of necessity and often in resource-poor settings with the potential for wider adaptability. Some of the frugal innovations discussed by the authors [17] include the use of text messages through mobile phones to ensure adherence to prescribed medications, "kangaroo care" for preterm infants, and the use of Solarclave (a locally manufactured autoclave with locally available components). Such innovations and adaptations have great potential for scalability if safety, efficacy, and acceptability are thoughtfully considered and appropriate resources are made available.

The Lancet Commission's Technologies for Global Health [12] lays out well the challenges to poorer nations in the use of technology to enhance health. The report classifies the barriers to greater use of technology for global health into three categories: (1) necessary technology does not exist; (2) technology exists but is not accessible; and (3) accessible technology is not adopted. Each category is driven by a different set of factors, but the outcome is the uneven spread of the benefits of technology to promote global health. Another danger to consider is technology transfer without careful consideration of resource constraints among recipients. Providing earlier-generation technology to resource-poor settings, where repairs to donated machines are not available or too expensive for institutions to bear, comes with its own set of adverse consequences such as non-use and unmet needs.

Given the challenges outlined earlier, how do we then go about leveraging technology to make progress toward achieving the SDGs and particularly SDG 3? Dr. Margaret Chan, the past director-general of the World Health Organization, outlined several strategies in the 2017 International Telecommunication Union's Fast Forward Progress report [13]. These include the following: (1) sharing of knowledge of Research4Life (www.research4life.org), available to low- and middle-income nations on topics related to health, agriculture, the environment, and science and technology; (2) moving health interventions from expensive hospital settings and rechanneling them into people's homes through telemedicine, remote care, and mHealth with the ability to transform health services and systems; (3) aligning key stakeholders in eHealth around a national vision and strategy with sustained commitment, investment, and political will; (4) making eHealth the core of strategic health planning in nations aided by collaboration and partnership among sectors, building capacity, strengthening public ownership, and protecting privacy and confidentiality through an ethical and legal framework. Novillo-Ortiz, Marin, and Saigí-Rubió [16] advocate aligning digital health approaches and solutions with the specific needs of a country's health system and culture. They emphasize the need for technologically appropriate solutions that are within the limits of the social, cultural, environmental, and economic conditions of the area to which they are applied, promoting self-sufficiency. In addition, digital health interventions that arise from interdisciplinary and intersectoral collaboration, realistic public-private partnerships, and shared best ideas and key knowledge with proven evidence for efficacy and effectiveness are likely to prove sustainable. Furthermore, affordability and cost-effectiveness are other factors that are bound to facilitate the continued use of such digital interventions [16]. It is evident that there is no one path or one method that is applicable to all. The beauty of technological innovation is that it is flexible and lends itself to local adaptation.

Conclusion

The SDGs, including SDG 3, provide the most ambitious targets for the betterment of populations and our planet. The journey toward attaining these goals is neither linear nor easy. We have just over a decade to attain them. Several goals, such as SDGs 1 and 2, are absolute and no one anywhere can be left behind. Populations displaced by natural disasters, climate change, or other factors such as civil unrest or outright war could slow down the efforts. Technology is not a panacea. It is at best a tool, and a double-edged tool at that. Given its cost and barriers to access, the adoption of technology may be hampered in poor and remote areas, accentuating the digital divide. While these barriers are daunting, there is good news to share. The penetration of digital technology to remote areas of the globe and the widespread adoption of technology (e.g., mobile phones), particularly by those living in resource-poor settings, and innovations due to human ingenuity are occurring daily, providing rays of hope and reassurance. ICT has brought the world closer, and the newer generations across the globe are ready to test, use, and contribute to the new technology. Technology has become a part of everyday life, and very few people yearn for a life without technological devices, systems, and benefits. The recent World Health Organization draft report, *Global Strategy for Digital Health, 2020–2024* [17], incorporates the following vision: "Improve health for everyone, everywhere by accelerating the adoption of appropriate digital health" (p. 5). It is, then, our collective responsibility to harness the power of technology and leverage it to seek the best possible outcomes for all of us and our planet.

References

1. United Nations. Millennium Summit (6–8 September 2000). https://www.un.org/en/events/pastevents/millennium_summit.shtml. Accessed 28 Apr 2019.
2. United Nations. United Nations millennium declaration. A/RES/55/2. 2000. https://www.un.org/millennium/declaration/ares552e.pdf. Accessed 28 Apr 2019.
3. United Nations. The millennium development goals report. 2015. https://www.un.org/millenniumgoals/2015_MDG_Report/pdf/MDG%202015%20rev%20(July%201).pdf. Accessed 28 Apr 2019.
4. United Nations. Transforming our world: the 2030 agenda for sustainable development. A/RES/70/1. 2015. https://www.un.org/ga/search/view_doc.asp?symbol=A/RES/70/1&Lang=E. Accessed 28 Apr 2019.
5. United Nations. Transforming our world: the 2030 agenda for sustainable development. A/RES/70/1. 2015. https://sustainabledevelopment.un.org/content/documents/21252030%20Agenda%20for%20Sustainable%20Development%20web.pdf. Accessed 28 Apr 2019.
6. United Nations Development Programme and International Bank for Reconstruction and Development/The World Bank. Transitioning from the MDGs to the SDGs. https://www.undp.org/content/dam/undp/library/SDGs/English/Transitioning%20from%20the%20MDGs%20to%20the%20SDGs.pdf. Accessed 30 Apr 2019.
7. United Nations Development Programme. What does it mean not to leave no one behind? 2018. https://www.undp.org/content/undp/en/home/librarypage/poverty-reduction/what-does-it-mean-to-leave-no-one-behind-.html. Accessed 7 May 2019.
8. United Nations Sustainable Development Goals Knowledge Platform. Sustainable development goal 3. https://sustainabledevelopment.un.org/sdg3. Accessed 2 May 2019.
9. World Health Organization. Health in 2015: from MDGs, millennium development goals to SDGs, sustainable development goals. 2015. https://apps.who.int/iris/bitstream/handle/10665/200009/9789241565110_eng.pdf;jsessionid=040005918F4FD02FC604043B0EF88075?sequence=1. Accessed 2 May 2019.
10. World Health Organization. Towards a global action plan for healthy lives and well-being for all. 2018. https://www.who.int/sdg/global-action-plan/Global_Action_Plan_Phase_I.pdf. Accessed 4 May 2019.
11. Schwab K. The fourth industrial revolution: what it means, how to respond. World Economic Forum. https://www.weforum.org/agenda/2016/01/the-fourth-industrial-revolution-what-it-means-and-how-to-respond/. Published 14 Jan 2016. Accessed 29 Apr 2019.
12. Howitt P, Darzi A, Yang G-Z, et al. Technologies for global health. Lancet. 2012;380(9840):507–35.
13. International Telecommunication Union. Fast-forward progress. 2017. https://www.itu.int/en/sustainable-world/Pages/report-hlpf-2017.aspx. Accessed 5 May 2019.
14. Global Observatory for eHealth. Atlas of eHealth country profiles. 2016. World Health Organization. https://apps.who.int/iris/bitstream/handle/10665/204523/9789241565219_eng.pdf?sequence=1. Accessed on 5 May 2019.
15. Mohieldin M. Leveraging technology to achieve the sustainable development goals. World Bank Blogs. Published May 10, 2018. Accessed 11 May 2019.
16. Novillo-Ortiz D, Marin HDF, Saigí-Rubió F. The role of digital health in supporting the achievement of the sustainable development goals (SDGs). Int J Med Inform. 2018;114:106–7. https://doi.org/10.1016/j.ijmedinf.2018.03.011.
17. World Health Organization. Global strategy on digital health, 2020–2024. Draft. 2019. https://extranet.who.int/dataform/upload/surveys/183439/files/Draft%20Global%20Strategy%20on%20Digital%20Health.pdf. Accessed on 9 May 2019.

Part III
Types of Innovative Technology in Health Care

Chapter 13: Technology vs. Mercury: The Metal That Scars Civilization

Diane E. Heck, Laurie B. Joseph, Padmini Murthy, Amy Ansehl, Yi-Hua Jan, Gabriella Composto Wahler, and Hong-Duck Kim

Abbreviations

CH_3Hg^+	$MeHg^+$ methyl mercury
Hg (II)	mercury with $^{+2}$ valence
Hg	mercury
Hg^0	elemental mercury

Erethism and the Making of Hats

Mercury poisoning was one of the first occupational diseases to be associated with a specific industrial process rather than a company or an industry. The disorder, referred to as mad hatter disease, or erethism mercurialis, was an endemic disease among hat makers and felting industry workers resulting from chronic mercury poisoning. This disease was also a harbinger of a spectrum of widely disseminated disorders resulting from exposure to the metal [1–11]. Erethism mercurialis was first defined because it affected workers in the hat-making industry using a process where felting work involved prolonged exposure to gaseous mercury. Sufferers were recognized by their exhibition of a sequela of physiological and behavioral

D. E. Heck (✉) · P. Murthy · A. Ansehl · H.-D. Kim
Division of Environmental Health Sciences, SHSP, New York Medical College,
Valhalla, NY, USA
e-mail: diane_heck@nymc.edu

L. B. Joseph
Division of Environmental Health Sciences, SHSP, New York Medical College,
Valhalla, NY, USA

Ernest Mario School of Pharmacy, Rutgers University, Piscataway, NJ, USA

Y.-H. Jan
Department of Environmental and Occupational Medicine, Rutgers University-Robert Wood
Johnson Medical School, Piscataway, NJ, USA

G. C. Wahler
Ernest Mario School of Pharmacy, Rutgers University, Piscataway, NJ, USA

© Springer Nature Switzerland AG 2020
P. Murthy, A. Ansehl (eds.), *Technology and Global Public Health*,
https://doi.org/10.1007/978-3-030-46355-7_18

changes that include irritability, low self-confidence, timidity, depression, apathy, shyness, and, ultimately, social phobia [11]. These unique characteristics are best exemplified by the Mad Hatter Character found in Lewis Carrol's *Alice's Adventures in Wonderland* [12]. We now know that, along with the behavioral changes of delirium, physiological changes and memory loss can also occur, although these latter effects are primarily exhibited in extreme cases where individuals are subjected to high levels of or prolonged exposure to mercury. Although most of the effects of erethism are neurological, other physiological changes, including headaches, generalized pain, decreases in neuromuscular strength, irregular cardiac rhythms, and tremors, can also occur [1–5, 13–16]. In fact, as early as the nineteenth century, it was noted that "the tremor in the hands can be so severe that the victim is unable to hold a glass of water without spilling its contents" [11].

Erethism became widespread among eighteenth- and nineteenth-century hat makers after inorganic mercury in the form of mercuric nitrate was introduced for the production of felt for hats in a process called carroting. In this process, furs from small animals such as rabbits or beavers were separated from their skins and matted together, and an orange-colored solution containing mercuric nitrate was used to stabilize and smooth the scales of the fur shaft so they would lock together, forming a batt. Numerous batts were combined into a felt, which was then shaped into cone-shaped hat precursors, shrunk in boiling water, and dried. In this felting process, volatile free mercury was slowly released into the confined areas where the milliners typically worked [14, 16–18].

It is believed that the Huguenots in seventeenth-century France brought the use of mercury to hat making to England and eventually the U.S. This process was initially a trade secret in France, and at the end of the seventeenth century migrating Huguenots brought the process to England. During the Victorian era, hatter's disease became so widespread that it became known in the form of popular colloquial expressions like "mad as a hatter" and "hatter's shakes" [16, 18–21].

In the late nineteenth century, erethism became one of the first U.S. diseases clearly associated with occupational exposures as it specifically affected laborers in the hat-making industry using the mercuric process. In the U.S., the hat-making industry was largely geographically centered in New Jersey cities and towns, including Newark, Orange, and Bloomfield. Factory inspectors were appointed and recommendations for addressing the issue including the statement that "A proper regard for the health of this class of citizens demands that mercury should not be used so extensively in the manufacture of hats, and that if its use is essential, that the hat finishers' room should be large, with a high ceiling, and well ventilated." [22–25] Unfortunately, because the New Jersey hatters were primarily impoverished new immigrants, the condition became confounded by the prevalence of respiratory disease, tuberculosis, alcoholism, and unsanitary living conditions, as well as a pronounced bias against immigrants. Therefore, little was done to reduce mercury exposure. The use of mercury in hat making continued until the advent of World War II when limited supplies of mercury were needed for the U.S. war effort. In a meeting convened by the U.S. Public Health Service (USPHS) in 1941 on December 1, 1941, the USPHS banned the use of mercury. The felt manufacturers voluntarily agreed to adopt a readily available alternative process using hydrogen peroxide [23, 25–30].

More recently, the global impacts of mercury have been assessed for three potential future anthropogenic greenhouse gas (GHG) emission scenarios under the international Intergovernmental Panel on Climate Change Special Report on Emission Scenarios (IPCC SRES). It is important to note that, unlike with most other atmospheric pollutants, the environmental effects and health impacts of mercury are only indirectly related to ambient atmospheric concentrations of Hg (II) or Hg (Hg^0, elemental mercury, exists both as vapor or as nonatmospheric liquid metal). The effects and toxicity result from the net conversion of Hg (Hg^0 and HgII) to the more bioaccumulative organomercuries ethyl- and principally methylmercury [31–33]. Toxicity is mediated by the conversion to organic mercury through processes that generally occur in wetlands and sediments, watersheds and coastal zones, as well as in the upper ocean [31, 33]. Exposure of humans and wildlife to organic mercury overwhelmingly occurs by the consumption of methylmercury-contaminated ocean, freshwater, and terrestrial organisms. As a result, the impact of Hg on ecosystem health is related not only to the magnitude of regional and global emissions and deposition, but also the potential for microbes and biological entities in watersheds and the oceans to convert ionic Hg (II) to organomercuries, of food webs to biomagnify methylmercury concentrations, and ecosystem disturbances that alter net methylation and trophic transfer [32, 34, 35]. Due to its deposition in the atmosphere and accumulation in the planet's oceans, increasing levels of mercury pose a significant threat to human health worldwide [32–35]. Overall, total global Hg emissions to the atmosphere range from 6500 to 8200 Mg/year, of which natural environmental processes and secondary release generate 4600–5300 Mg/year. It is estimated that human-derived processes release 1900–2900 Mg/year, compared with primary natural (geogenic) inputs of 80–600 Mg/year [36–38]. Unfortunately, as developing nations make increasing use of fossil fuel sources (principally coal), Hg emissions are expected to continue to increase unless emission controls are widely implemented.

Human Mercury Toxicity

The organic mercury monomethylmercury (CH_3Hg) is a neurotoxin that can cause diminished intellectual capacity (measured by standard IQ evaluation) and long-term developmental delays in children and is associated with an array of conditions, including muscle weakness, poor coordination, numbness in the hands and feet, skin rashes, anxiety, memory problems, speech problems, hearing problems, vision problems, kidney disorders, and compromised cardiovascular health in adults [1–5, 39].

On a global scale, airborne emission levels are rising, and the bulk of increases in Hg emissions is generally attributed to the expansion of coal-fired electricity generation in the developing world. Evaluations of this hypothesis by Sundseth et al. confirmed the high socioeconomic cost of the projected increases in emissions. In these studies, it was estimated that by 2020, the annual cost of the associated decrease in human IQ would reach USD3.7 billion in 2005 dollars [40–43].

Molecular Mechanisms

On the molecular scale, mechanisms underlying mercury toxicity include irreversible inhibition of sulfhydro groups in enzymes and, in particular, selenoenzymes such as thioredoxin reductase. Thioredoxin reductase is critical for the maintenance of reduction/oxidation (redox) balance in mammalian cells [44–46]. Altered redox status can result in excessive levels of free radicals, resulting in oxidative damage to critical cellular macromolecules. Neurons are particularly sensitive to oxidative damage, and this effect has been attributed to the profound developmental effects that result from fetal exposure to mercury [1–5, 44–47]. Inhibition of other selenium-dependent enzymes by mercury also contributes to mercury toxicity (poisoning). For example, mercury inhibits the enzyme S-adenosyl-methionine. This alters vital cellular processes, including the synthesis of proteins required for development, wound healing, tissue repair, tRNA and rRNA methylation, immune responses, and nerve function. Through these mechanisms, exposure to mercury may result in profound neurological and neuromuscular deficits [1–5, 44–48].

Toxicity and Mercury Valency: Mercury Form and Differing Effects

In humans, elemental mercury (Hg^0) may be the least toxic form. Although mercury toxicity is primarily associated with ionic Hg^{+2} (HgII), the relatively nonreactive elemental state (Hg^0) of the metal is very poorly absorbed through the skin and gastrointestinal (GI) tract. While inhalation and, in particular, chronic inhalation of elemental mercury (Hg^0) can result in cognitive, sensory, emotional, and neuromuscular dysfunction, mercury salts/ionic mercury are water-soluble and can be absorbed from the GI tract. However, these charged ions only cross the blood-brain barrier following massive exposures. Mercuric (Hg^{+2}) salts are more toxic than mercurous (Hg^{+1}) salts. The primary site of injury resulting from exposure to these salts is the kidney, and in extreme cases the damage may be severe [1–5, 49–51].

Generation of Organic Mercuries

By far the most toxic forms of mercury are organic mercuries, primarily methyl- and ethyl- mercury. These forms of mercury cross the blood-brain barrier and are readily taken up by neurons and neuronal cells. Exposure to organic mercury has been found to result in intellectual and behavioral anomalies, with the most profound deficits arising following organic mercury exposure during fetal development [51, 52]. Organic mercury is formed within aquatic microbes exposed to high concentrations of airborne and waterborne inorganic mercury, once airborne metals largely derived from the burning of fossil fuels. Inorganic mercury vapor and ionic congeners in particulates released to the air, which can travel for months and across thousands of miles and are largely deposited in the aquatic ecosystems that comprise most of the Earth's surface. Following conversion, organic mercury bioaccumulates within food chains in these environments. Organic mercury production in inland and marine ecosystems has been primarily attributed to the activity of anaerobic bacteria in the sediment. In this process, aquatic microbes take up inorganic mercury and "methylmercury," a shorthand term for "methylmercury cation." The methylmercury (II) cation is created intracellularly through the formation of complexes composed of a methyl group (CH_3-) bonded to a mercury ion, resulting in a compound with the chemical formula of CH_3Hg + (MeHg+). In this process, the positively charged ion combines with anions such as chloride (Cl−), hydroxide (OH−), and nitrate (NO_3-) and has a particularly high affinity for sulfur-containing anions, particularly the thiol (−SH) groups on the amino acid cysteine in proteins containing cysteine, forming a covalent bond. Multiple cysteine moieties can coordinate with methylmercury, and methylmercury may migrate to other metal-binding sites in proteins. Alternatively, recent studies have revealed that peaks in methylmercury in the ocean water column and strong associations between methylmercury, nutrients, and organic matter remineralization suggest water column production of methylmercury during carbon remineralization [53–56]. In the past, in addition to nature-mediated conversion of ionic mercury, processes involved in purifying gold following extraction from mines also generated significant release of methylmercury into the air in industrialized nations [57]. Although in modern commercial gold mining, this process has been modified to protect the air, smaller releases of mercury resulting from the cottage industry's gold purification processes in developing nations have also been identified as a growing concern. Recent advances in the use of nanomaterials have significantly enhanced the detection of mercury poisoning. In this regard, gold nanoparticles (AuNPs) have been developed for rapid, cheap, and sensitive detection of organic mercury through identification of the thymine-bound mercury ions that result following human exposure to mercury. Silver nanoparticles are used as a sensitive detector of low-concentration Hg^{2+} ions in homogeneous aqueous solutions [79, 80].

Global Sources of Mercury Exposure

Overwhelming human exposure to inorganic mercury results from the burning of fossil fuels, principally coal. In the formation of coal, ionic mercury accumulated with organic waste results in mercury-contaminated coal. Burning mercury-contaminated coal releases both ionic mercury and mercury vapor into the air [1–5, 38, 42].

Industrial Emissions

In 2003, the Northeast States for Coordinated Air Use Management found that "Coal-burning power plants are the largest source of mercury emissions related to human activity in the U.S. In December 2003, the Environmental Protection Agency (EPA) issued regulations designed to control mercury emissions from these sources. Our ability to adequately protect the public from the adverse health effects associated with exposure to mercury is closely tied to the effectiveness and compliance to this rule." [58]

In one of our earliest industrial processes, gold amalgam was used to extract gold when it could not be extracted from crushed ore using hydromechanical methods. In this procedure, large amounts of mercury were used in placer mining, where deposits of granite slurry were washed in moving water, generally falling into streams, and separated in long runs of "riffle boxes" with mercury dumped in at the top of the run downstream; this generates a gray amalgam. The use of mercury in nineteenth-century placer mining in California is considered the source of ongoing extensive pollution in river and estuarine environments to this day [58–60]. Although this process and the use of mercury in industrial gold purification are banned, the use of the process by artisan gold miners in Peru, South America, and Africa remains a persistent problem [1–5, 61, 62].

Mercury is used in the production of an array of products, including barometers, manometers, float valves, mercury switches, mercury relays, fluorescent lamps, and other devices. Historically, mercury was used in medical equipment, including thermometers and sphygmomanometers; however, safety concerns have prompted the replacement of mercury with safer materials such as alcohol- or galinstan-filled glass thermometers and thermistor- or infrared-based electronic instruments. Likewise, mechanical pressure gauges and electronic strain gauge sensors have replaced mercury sphygmomanometers. Mercury is still used in scientific research applications and in amalgam for dental restoration; it is also used for fluorescent lighting where electricity passed through mercury vapor in a fluorescent lamp produces shortwave ultraviolet light that causes the phosphor in the tube to fluoresce [63].

Mercury in Waste (Emerging High-Tech Waste Issues)

Increasingly, electronic devices, including smartphones, tablets, laptops, LEDs, LCDs, DVD players, and portable music players, are made to be replaced. As a result of this largely planned obsolescence, it is estimated that 30–50 tons of e-waste are produced annually in the U.S. alone. Because only approximately 12% of e-waste is recycled, serious concerns arise about resulting air pollution, water pollution, and soil pollution. Air is contaminated when scavengers burn electronic waste to get the copper and other metals. If not stored or disposed of properly, toxins from electronic waste enter the soil and water supplies, potentially contaminating groundwater. Unfortunately, the bulk of e-waste contains gold, copper, and other valuable metals, as well as operational devices that could be reused or repurposed, which encourages scavenging of waste accumulation sites [64, 65]. The short lifespans of electronic devices, encouraged or designed by manufacturers, have led to consumers interpreting working electronics as insufficient or unusable. The appeal and value of discarded devices, their salable components, and the metals they contain have led to extensive scavenging by children from poor families in third-world countries. As a result, numerous children worldwide are being exposed to toxic chemicals including mercury, lead, and polycyclic aromatic hydrocarbons. These exposures can result in serious long-term neurological deficits in developing children as well as both chronic and acute maladies [65–69].

Protecting the Environment from Mercury Accumulation with Technology

The adage "the solution to pollution is dilution," as outdated as it seems, is indeed an accurate reflection of how we have concentrated naturally occurring metals to potentially toxic levels, and, as a result, contaminated the earth. This is notably exemplified in the case of mercury accumulation in food. Fish is a primary foodstuff and source of nutrients for populations worldwide. Most human exposures result from human consumption of mercury-contaminated fleshy, large fish, including mackerel, tilefish, bluefin tuna, swordfish, and other long-lived fish. This occurs because organic mercury bioaccumulates in the food chains of aquatic systems. Low levels of mercury are found in microbes and eventually residing in high concentrations in the flesh of long-lived large fish [1–5, 70–74]. Fortunately, this process has recently been interrupted by the advent of mercury scrubbers. In the scrubbing process, the exhaust gases of combustion that may contain mercury and other substances considered harmful to the environment are contained, and the scrubbing process removes or neutralizes the toxins. A wet scrubber is used for cleaning air of the noxious gases and particulates containing various pollutants and pollutant-contaminated dust particles. Wet scrubbing works through the physical contact of the noxious compounds or toxin-containing particulates with the scrubbing agent. Solutions may simply be water (for simple particulates) or solutions of reagents that chemically complex with noxious compounds. While wet scrubbers are effective for the removal of soluble mercury species, such as oxidized mercury, Hg^{2+}, mercury vapor and other contaminants in their elemental or uncharged forms that are insoluble are not removed. To remove other mercury requires an additional process, known as dry scrubbing, where mercury is converted to other ionic species, which is required for mercury capture. Usually halogens are added to the scrubber for this. The type of metal-contaminated coal or hydrocarbon burned and the presence of these selective catalytic reduction units both affect the degree to which mercury is removed [75, 76].

Regulations requiring mercury scrubbers in fossil fuel–burning power plants are yielding surprising successes in lowering organic mercury levels worldwide. For example, mercury emissions significantly dropped in North America between 1990 and 2007. According to peer-reviewed studies in 2010 and 2013, mercury emissions decreased 2.8% per year. Over a similar period, mercury levels in North Atlantic waters dropped 4.3% annually. And between 2001 and 2009, mercury in the air above the North Atlantic declined by 20%, approximately 2.5% a year. In related studies, researchers from Stony Brook University, the University of Massachusetts, and Harvard University analyzed Atlantic bluefin tuna captured between 2004 and 2012. Tests for mercury levels revealed that the mercury concentration in the fish was diminished by an average of 19%. These findings suggest that potential reductions in mercury emissions rapidly lead to reduced mercury concentrations in some marine fish [77, 78].

International Responses

Global concerns regarding widespread organic mercury contamination have led to international initiatives to evaluate current knowledge on atmospheric Hg emissions, transport, and its effects on terrestrial and aquatic ecosystems. These studies include ones spearheaded by the United Nations Environment Programme (UNEP) (www.unep.org/PDF/PressReleases/GlobalMercuryAssessment2013.Pdf) and that of the United Nations Economic Commission for Europe Convention on Longrange Transboundary Air Pollution (UNECE-LRTAP) Task Force on Hemispheric Transport of Air Pollution (TF HTAP). The UNEP initiative is focused on limiting human health and environmental risks from the release of Hg as well as improving information on international Hg emissions and their transport and fate. An international treaty, the Minimata Convention, signed in January 2013, was devised to control the global release of Hg to the environment. Additional programs are also being developed to monitor Hg in the atmosphere and marine and terrestrial ecosystems through partnerships among regional Hg-monitoring programs. There were ambitious expectations that these programs would yield information that would improve understanding of the global impacts of Hg pollution and help evaluate the effectiveness of national and international policies. Unfortunately, regulatory restriction rollbacks in the U.S. on airborne release of mercury have recently produced a threat to the global environment. Even worse, reduced pressure on coalburning industries is compromising the emerging industry centered on producing technologically advanced, cheaper, and more efficient scrubbing processes. Without strong leadership in limiting mercury emissions, fewer developing nations are likely to encourage their industries to employ emission-cleaning techniques. This is a significant problem, as coal burning by developing nations has become a significant contributor to global mercury emissions. The world's countries share the oceans and their abundant food supply; taken together, the unfortunate rollbacks of restrictions and increasing coal burning by developing nations are presenting an increasing threat to the global food supply.

Mercury is both a naturally occurring mineral and a major human toxicant. As inhabitants of the planet, emerging technologies have provided us with tools to detect and address this problem. However, we are faced with the dilemma of choosing between addressing the problem and the cost to society. Addressing the problem of mercury toxicity evolved through the modification of major pollution-generating technologies, including new and enhanced techniques for burning of various fossil fuels for the generation of electricity and through advances in the detection of mercury in humans and foodstuffs. Evolving techniques are significantly lowering the cost of addressing mercury toxicity; however, the cost to society of not attacking the problem is not universally valued. With the tools in hand, the answer to the problem depends largely on the focus and attention of the planet's policymakers. Their activities reflect the priorities of many nations and will ultimately have to answer to history.

Acknowledgements This work was supported by the National Institutes of Health CounterACT program through the National Institutes of Arthritis and Musculoskeletal and Skin Diseases U54AR055073, by ES005022 and by T32ES007148 (GCW).

References

1. Bernhoft RA. Mercury toxicity and treatment: a review of the literature. J Environ Public Health. 2012:460508.. PMCID: PMC3253456
2. Park J-D, Zheng W. Human exposure and health effects of inorganic and elemental mercury. J Prev Med Public Health. 2012;45(6):344–52., PMCID: PMC3514464.
3. Driscoll CT, Mason RP, Chan HM, Jacob DJ, Pirrone N. Mercury as a global pollutant: sources, pathways, and effects. J Prev Med Public Health. 2012;45(6):344–52., PMCID: PMC3514464.
4. Bjørklund G, Dadar M, Mutter J, Aaseth J. The toxicology of mercury: current research and emerging trends. Environ Res. 2017;159:545–54. https://doi.org/10.1016/j.envres.2017.08.051.. Epub 2017 Sep 8. PMID: 28889024.
5. Counter SA, Buchanan LH. Mercury exposure in children: a review. Toxicol Appl Pharmacol. 2004;198(2):209–30., PMID: 15236954.
6. Chang LW. The Neurotoxicology and pathology of Organomercury, Organolead, and organotin. J Toxicol Sci. 1990;15(Suppl 4):125–51., PMID: 2100318.
7. Sunderland EM, Krabbenhoft DP, Moreau JW, Strode SA, Landing WM. Mercury sources, distribution, and bioavailability in the North Pacific Ocean: insights from data and models. Glob Biogeochem Cycles. 2009;23(2):GB2010. ISSN 1944-9224. https://doi.org/10.1029/2008GB003425.
8. Griggs MB. Mercury Scrubbers On Power Plants Clean Up Other Pollutants, Too. Pop Sci. 2015.
9. Lafontaine S, Schrlau J, Butler J, Jia Y, Harper B, Harris S, Bramer LM, Waters KM, Harding A. Relative influence of trans-Pacific and regional atmospheric transport of PAHs in the Pacific Northwest, U.S. Environ Sci Technol. ISSN 0013-936X. 2015; https://doi.org/10.1021/acs.est.5b00800.

10. Lee C-S, Lutcavage ME, Chandler E, Madigan DJ, Cerrato RM, Fisher NS. Declining mercury concentrations in Bluefin tuna reflect reduced emissions to the North Atlantic Ocean. Environ Sci Technol. 2016; https://doi.org/10.1021/acs.est.6b04328.

11. Tchounwou PB, Ayensu WK, Ninashvili N, Sutton D. Environmental exposure to mercury and its toxicopathologic implications for public health. Environ Toxicol. 2003;18(3):149–75. https://doi.org/10.1002/tox.10116.

12. Waldron HA. Did the mad hatter have mercury poisoning? Br Med J. 1961. PMC 1550196 Freely accessible;287(6409) https://doi.org/10.1136/bmj.287.6409.

13. Medicine Health. Mercury poisoning. Emedicine Health. N.p., 23 Apr. 2010. Web. 23 Apr. 2012. <http://www.emedicinehealth.com/mercury_poisoning/article_em.htm>.

14. Mad Hatter syndrome. Stedman's Medical Dictionary. MediLexicon International Ltd. 2013.

15. Kitzmiller K. The Not-So-Mad Hatter: occupational hazards of mercury. Chemical Abstracts Service. American Chemical Society. 2013.

16. Lee WR. The history of the statutory control of mercury poisoning in Great Britain. Br J Ind Med. 1968;25(1):52–62. PMC 1008662 Freely accessible. https://doi.org/10.1136/oem.25.1.52.

17. Clarkson TW. The toxicology of mercury. Crit Rev Clin Lab Sci. 1997;34(4):369–403.. PMID: 9288445

18. Bateman T. Notes of a case of mercurial Erethism. Med Chir Trans. 1918;9(Pt 1):220–33.. PMCID: PMC2128877

19. Buckell M, Hunter D, Milton R, Perry KM. Chronic mercury poisoning. Br J Ind Med. 1993;50(2):97–106. PMCID: PMC1061245.

20. Waldron HA. Did the mad hatter have mercury poisoning? Br Med J (Clin Res Ed). 1983;287(6409):1961., PMCID: PMC1550196.

21. Devine ET, Kellogg PU eds. The Survey. 51; 1924. Survey Associates: 457. Retrieved 10 March 2013.

22. Wedeen RP. Were the hatters of New Jersey 'mad'? Am J Ind Med. 1989;16(2):225–33. https://doi.org/10.1002/ajim.4700160213.. What remains most remarkable about the hatters of New Jersey is that they expressed no anger about their working conditions. Minutes of the Hat Finisher's Association of the City of Newark from 1853 to 1870 make no reference to hatters' shakes. Neither the hatters nor the public nor the medical community was mad about the health costs of industrial progress

23. Freeman JA. Mercurial disease among hatters. Trans Med Soc New Jersey: 61–64. During the winter of 1858–59 and following spring, there prevailed quite extensively among the hatters of Orange, Newark, Bloomfield, and Milburn a disease showing all the medical characteristics of Mercurial Salivation and Stomatitis. More than a hundred cases occurred in Orange alone. The usual symptoms were ulceration of the gums, loosening of the teeth, foeter of the breath, abnormal saliva, tremors of the upper extremities, or a shaking palsy, the result of inhaling air impregnated with mercury vapor. (Cited in Wedeen, 1989). 1860.

24. Wedeen RP. Were the hatters of new Jersey "mad"? Am J Ind Med. 1989;16(2):225–33.

25. Neal PA, Jones RR, Bloomfield JJ, Dallavalle JM, Edwards TI. A study of chronic mereurialism in the hatter's fur-cutting industry. <http://www.cabdirect.org/abstracts/19382700038.html;jsessionid=A3145BBE9D19C0C4CDAE4F82B9FF9883, 1937.

26. Merler E, Boffetta P, Masala G, Monechi V, Bani F. A cohort study of workers compensated for mercury intoxication following employment in the fur hat industry. J Occupat Med. 1994;36(11):1260–4. https://doi.org/10.1097/00043764-199411000-00016.

27. Dennis, L. Hatting: as effecting the health of operatives. Rep New Jersey State Board Health. 1878; 2: 67–85..

28. Stickler JW. Hatters' consumption. New York Med J. 1896; 43: 598–602. (Cited in Wedeen, 1989).

29. Stickler JW. The hygiene of occupations. II. Diseases of hatters. Tenth Annual Report of the Board of Health of New Jersey and Report of the Bureau of Vital Statistics 1886. Trenton: John L. Murphy Publishing Co; 1887. pp. 166–188. (Cited in Wedeen, 1989).

30. Stainsby, W. Diseases and disease tendencies of occupations: the glass industry and the hatting industry. Twenty-Fourth Annual Report of the Bureau of Statistics of New Jersey. Trenton; 1901. (Cited in Wedeen, 1989).
31. Sundseth K, Pacyna JM, Pacyna EG, Pirrone N, Thorne RJ. Global sources and pathways of mercury in the context of human health. Int J Environ Res Public Health. 2017;14(1):105. https://doi.org/10.3390/ijerph14010105.
32. Kim M-K, Zoh K-D. Fate and transport of mercury in environmental media and human exposure. J Prev Med Public Health. 2012; 45(6): 335–343. Published online 2012 Nov 29. https://doi.org/10.3961/jpmph.2012.45.6.335, PMCID: PMC3514463.
33. Driscoll CT, Mason RP, Chan HM, Jacob DJ, Pirrone N. Mercury as a global pollutant: sources, pathways, and effects. Environ Sci Technol. 2013; 47(10): 4967–4983. Published online 2013 Apr 16. https://doi.org/10.1021/es305071v PMCID: PMC3701261.
34. Sheehan MC, Burke TA, Navas-Acien A, Breysse PN, McGready J, Fox MA. Global methylmercury exposure from seafood consumption and risk of developmental neurotoxicity: a systematic review, Bull World Health Organ. 2014; 92(4): 254–269F. Published online https://doi.org/10.2471/BLT.12.116152, PMCID: PMC3967569.
35. Schartup AT, Mason RP, Balcom PH, Hollweg TA, Chen CY, Methylmercury production in estuarine sediments: role of organic matter. Environ Sci Technol. Author manuscript; available in PMC, Published in final edited form as: Environ Sci Technol. 2013; 47(2): 695–700. Published online 2012 Dec 21. https://doi.org/10.1021/es302566w, PMCID: PMC4066882.
36. Gworek B, Dmuchowski W, Baczewska AH, Brągoszewska P, Bemowska-Kałabun O, Wrzosek-Jakubowska J. Air Contamination by Mercury, Emissions and Transformations—a Review. Water Air Soil Pollut. 2017; 228(4): 123. Published online 2017 Mar 3. https://doi.org/10.1007/s11270-017-3311-y, PMCID: PMC5336545.
37. Zhang Y, Jacob DJ, Horowitz HM, Chen L, Amos HM, Krabbenhoft DP, Slemr F, Vincent LS Louis, Sunderland EM. Observed decrease in atmospheric mercury explained by global decline in anthropogenic emissions. Proc Natl Acad Sci U S A. 2016; 113(3): 526–531. Published online 2016 Jan 4. https://doi.org/10.1073/pnas.1516312113, PMCID: PMC4725498.
38. Chen CY, Driscoll CT, Lambert KF, Mason RP, Rardin LR, Serrell N, Sunderland EM. Marine mercury fate: from sources to seafood consumers. Environ Res 2012; 119:1–2. https://doi.org/10.1016/j.envres.2012.10.001. Epub 2012 Oct 31. PMID: 23121885.
39. Sheehan MC, Burke TA, Navas-Acien A, Breysse PN, McGready J, Fox MA. Global methylmercury exposure from seafood consumption and risk of developmental neurotoxicity: a systematic review. Bull World Health Organ. 2014; 92(4): 254–269F. Published online 2014 Jan 10. https://doi.org/10.2471/BLT.12.116152, PMCID: PMC3967569.
40. Gworek B, Dmuchowski W, Baczewska AH, Brągoszewska P, Bemowska-Kałabun O, Wrzosek-Jakubowska J. Air contamination by mercury, emissions and transformations—a Review. Water Air Soil Pollut. 2017; 228(4): 123. Published online 2017 Mar 3. doi: https://doi.org/10.1007/s11270-017-3311-y, PMCID: PMC5336545.
41. Burger J, Gochfeld M. Mercury and selenium levels in 19 species of saltwater fish from New Jersey as a function of species, size, and season. Sci Total Environ. Author manuscript; available in PMC 2015 Jan 20, Published in final edited form as: Sci Total Environ. 2011; 409(8): 1418–1429. Published online 2011 Feb 2. https://doi.org/10.1016/j.scitotenv.2010.12.034, PMCID: PMC4300121.
42. Sundseth K, Pacyna JM, Pacyna EG, Pirrone N, Thorne RJ. Global sources and pathways of mercury in the context of human health. Int J Environ Res Public Health. 2017;14(1):pii: E105. https://doi.org/10.3390/ijerph14010105., PMID: 28117743.
43. Pacyna JM, Sundseth K, Pacyna EG, Jozewicz W, Munthe J, Belhaj M, Aström S. An assessment of costs and benefits associated with mercury emission reductions from major anthropogenic sources. J Air Waste Manag Assoc. 2010;60(3):302–15., PMID: 20397560.
44. Fields CA, Borak J, Louis ED. Mercury-induced motor and sensory neurotoxicity: systematic review of workers currently exposed to mercury vapor. Crit Rev Toxicol. 2017; 47(10):811–844. https://doi.org/10.1080/10408444.2017.1342598. Epub 2017 Jul 18, PMID: 28718354.

45. Holmgren A, Lu J. Thioredoxin and thioredoxin reductase: current research with special reference to human disease. Biochem Biophys Res Commun. 2010;396(1):120–4. https://doi.org/10.1016/j.bbrc.2010.03.083., PMID: 20494123.

46. Farina M, Aschner M. Methylmercury-induced neurotoxicity: focus on pro-oxidative events and related consequences. Adv Neurobiol. 2017;18:267–86. https://doi.org/10.1007/978-3-319-60189-2_13., PMID: 28889272.

47. Farina M, Aschner M. Methylmercury-induced neurotoxicity: focus on pro-oxidative events and related consequences. Adv Neurobiol. 2017;18:267–86. https://doi.org/10.1007/978-3-319-60189-2_13., PMID: 28889272.

48. Karita K, Sakamoto M, Yoshida M, Tatsuta N, Nakai K, Iwai-Shimada M, Iwata T, Maeda E, Yaginuma-Sakurai K, Satoh H, Murata K. Recent epidemiological studies on methylmercury, mercury and selenium. Nihon Eiseigaku Zasshi. 2016;71(3):236–51. Japanese.

49. Yokel RA, Lasley SM, Dorman DC. The speciation of metals in mammals influences their toxicokinetics and toxicodynamics and therefore human health risk assessment. J Toxicol Environ Health B Crit Rev. 2006;9(1):63–85., PMID: 16393870.

50. Kim KH, Kabir E, Jahan SA. A review on the distribution of hg in the environment and its human health impacts. J Hazard Mater. 2016;306:376–85. https://doi.org/10.1016/j.jhazmat.2015.11.031. Epub 2015 Nov 21, PMID: 26826963.

51. Bjørklund G, Dadar M, Mutter J, Aaseth J. The toxicology of mercury: current research and emerging trends. Environ Res. 2017;159:545–54. https://doi.org/10.1016/j.envres.2017.08.051.. Epub 2017 Sep 8, PMID: 28889024.

52. Li WC, Tse HF. Health risk and significance of mercury in the environment. Environ Sci Pollut Res Int. 1:192, 2015–201. https://doi.org/10.1007/s11356-014-3544-x.. Epub 2014 Sep 16, PMID: 25220768.

53. Kim MK, Zoh KD. Fate and transport of mercury in environmental media and human exposure. J Prev Med Public Health. 45(6):335–43. https://doi.org/10.3961/jpmph.2012.45.6.335. Epub 2012 Nov 29. Review. Erratum in: J Prev Med Public Health. 2013 Jul. 2012;46(4):211. PMID: 23230463.

54. Ullrich S, Tanton T, Abdrashitova S. Mercury in the aquatic environment: a review of factors affecting methylation. Crit Rev Environ Sci Technol. 2001;31(3):241–93. https://doi.org/10.1080/20016491089226.

55. Govindaswamy N, Moy J, Millar M, Koch SA. A distorted mercury [hg(SR)4]2− complex with alkanethiolate ligands: the fictile coordination sphere of monomeric [hg(SR)x] complexes. Inorg Chem. 1992;26(26):5343–4. https://doi.org/10.1021/ic00052a001.

56. Erni I, Geier G. Kinetics of extremely fast ligand exchange reactions with methylmercury(II)-complexes of 1-Methylpyridine-2-thione and 1-methyl-quinaldine-4-thione: rate-equilibria correlations. Helv Chim Acta. 1979;62(4):1007–15. https://doi.org/10.1002/hlca.19790620411.

57. Mining Technology in the Nineteenth Century | ONE www.onlinenevada.org/articles/mining-technology.

58. EPA mercury. Retrieved 2018, https://www.epa.gov/mercury/what-epa-doing-reduce-mercury-pollution-and-exposures-mercury.

59. Slowey AJ, Rytuba JJ, Brown GE Jr. Speciation of mercury and mode of transport from placer gold mine tailings. Environ Sci Technol. 39(6):1547–54.. PMID: 15819208

60. Domagalski JL, Alpers CN, Slotton DG, Suchanek TH, Ayers SM. Mercury and methylmercury concentrations and loads in the Cache Creek watershed, California. Sci Total Environ. 2004;327(1–3):215–37.. PMID: 15172583

61. Gworek B, Dmuchowski W, Baczewska AH, Bragoszewska P, Bemowska-Kałabun O, Wrzosek-Jakubowska J. Air contamination by mercury, emissions and transformations-a review. Water Air Soil Pollut. 2017;228(4):123. https://doi.org/10.1007/s11270-017-3311-y.. Epub 2017 Mar 3, PMID: 28316351.

62. Basu N, Clarke E, Green A, Calys-Tagoe B, Chan L, Dzodzomenyo M, Fobil J, Long RN, Neitzel RL, Obiri S, Odei E, Ovadje L, Quansah R, Rajaee M, Wilson ML. Integrated assessment of artisanal and small-scale gold mining in Ghana—Part 1: human health review. Int J

Environ Res Public Health. 2015; 12(5): 5143–5176. Published online 2015 May 13. https://doi.org/10.3390/ijerph120505143. PMCID: PMC4454960.

63. US EPA: Consumer and Commercial Products [containing mercury]. http://www.speciation.net/Database/Links/US-EPA-Consumer-and-Commercial-Products-containing-mercury-;i2582. Retrieved 2018.

64. Heacock M, Kelly CB, Suk WA. E-waste: the growing global problem and next steps. Rev Environ Health. 2016;31(1):131–5. https://doi.org/10.1515/reveh-2015-0045. PMID: 26820178.

65. Xu X, Zeng X, Boezen HM, Huo X. E-waste environmental contamination and harm to public health in China. Front Med. 2015;9(2):220–8. https://doi.org/10.1007/s11684-015-0391-1. Epub 2015 Mar 25, PMID: 25808646.

66. Lau WK, Liang P, Man YB, Chung SS, Wong MH. Human health risk assessment based on trace metals in suspended air particulates, surface dust, and floor dust from e-waste recycling workshops in Hong Kong, China. Environ Sci Pollut Res Int. 2014;21(5):3813–25. https://doi.org/10.1007/s11356-013-2372-8.. Epub 2013 Nov 28, PMID: 24288065.

67. Xu X, Zeng X, Boezen HM, Huo X. E-waste environmental contamination and harm to public health in China. Front Med. 2015;9(2):220–8. https://doi.org/10.1007/s11684-015-0391-1.. Epub 2015 Mar 25. PMID: 25808646

68. Julander A, Lundgren L, Skare L, Grandér M, Palm B, Vahter M, Lidén C. Formal recycling of e-waste leads to increased exposure to toxic metals: an occupational exposure study from Sweden. Environ Int. 2014;73:243–51. https://doi.org/10.1016/j.envint.2014.07.006. Epub 2014 Aug 27, PMID: 25300751.

69. Hussain M, Mumtaz S. E-waste: impacts, issues and management strategies. Rev Environ Health. 2014;29(1–2):53–8. https://doi.org/10.1515/reveh-2014-0016., PMID: 24695030.

70. Gworek B, Bemowska-Kałabun O, Kijeńska M, Wrzosek-Jakubowska J. Mercury in marine and oceanic waters-a review. Water Air Soil Pollut. 2016;227(10):371.. Epub 2016 Sep 7, PMID: 27656005.

71. Vilizzi L, Tarkan AS. Bioaccumulation of metals in common carp (Cyprinus carpio L.) from water bodies of Anatolia (Turkey): a review with implications for fisheries and human food consumption. Environ Monit Assess. 2016;188(4):243. https://doi.org/10.1007/s10661-016-5248-9.. Epub 2016 Mar 23, PMID: 27007291.

72. Chételat J, Braune B, Stow J, Tomlinson S. Special issue on mercury in Canada's north: summary and recommendations for future research. Sci Total Environ. 2015;509–510:260–2. https://doi.org/10.1016/j.scitotenv.2014.06.063., PMID: 25669603.

73. Rowe CL. Bioaccumulation and effects of metals and trace elements from aquatic disposal of coal combustion residues: recent advances and recommendations for further study. Sci Total Environ. 2014;485–486:490–6. https://doi.org/10.1016/j.scitotenv.2014.03.119. Epub 2014 Apr 16, PMID: 24742559.

74. Praveena SM, de Burbure C, Aris AZ, Hashim Z. Mini review of mercury contamination in environment and human with an emphasis on Malaysia: status and needs. Rev Environ Health. 2013;28(4):195–202. https://doi.org/10.1515/reveh-2013-0011. PMID: 24317783.

75. Griggs MB. Mercury scrubbers on power plants clean up other pollutants, too. Popular Science. 2015.

76. Lafontaine S, Schrlau J, Butler J, Jia Y, Harper B, Harris S, Bramer LM, Waters KM, Harding, A. Relative Influence of Trans-Pacific and Regional Atmospheric Transport of PAHs in the Pacific Northwest, U.S. Environ Sci Technol. 2015. ISSN 0013-936X. https://doi.org/10.1021/acs.est.5b00800.

77. Lee C-S, Lutcavage ME, Chandler E, Madigan DJ, Cerrato RM, Fisher NS. Declining mercury concentrations in Bluefin Tuna reflect reduced emissions to the North Atlantic Ocean. Environ Sci Technol. https://doi.org/10.1021/acs.est.6b04328, 2016.

78. Gworek B, Bemowska-Kałabun O, Kijeńska M, Wrzosek-Jakubowska J. Mercury in marine and oceanic waters-a review. Water Air Soil Pollut. 2016;227(10):371.. Epub 2016 Sep 7, PMID: 27656005.

79. Roller M. In vitro genotoxicity data of nanomaterials compared to carcinogenic potency of inorganic substances after inhalational exposure. Mutat Res. 2011;727(3):72–85. https://doi.org/10.1016/j.mrrev.2011.03.002. Epub 2011 Mar 30.
80. Rafati-Rahimzadeh M, Rafati-Rahimzadeh M, Kazemi S, Moghadamnia AA. Daru. Current approaches of the management of mercury poisoning: need of the hour. 2(22):46. https://doi.org/10.1186/2008-2231-22-46. 2014.

Chapter 14: Trafficking, Technology, and Public Health: The Malignant Malady of Modern Slavery

Melissa Jane Kronfeld

Introduction

Human trafficking and modern slavery (HTMS), as a matter of concern to healthcare professionals, is a critical, pressing, and frequently overlooked medical matter and one of the many unprecedented health challenges confronting the global community today. Touching upon a range of physical and psychological issues over the short and long term, HTMS is a complex and multidimensional threat in dire need of attention from the public healthcare space. And as HTMS rapidly shifts into the digital age, the crime is transforming, providing a broader range of target-rich environments as well as recruitment and conditioning tactics. As a result, the diversity of victims affected by the unrestricted reach of HTMS on communities around the world demonstrates that the problem requires solutions beyond those offered by a government's judicial, legislative, and social service agencies, as well as well-intentioned industry and civil society leaders or nonprofit organizations (NPOs) [1].

It is important to note that HTMS is, first and foremost, a crime; therefore, a law enforcement response is, and will always be, necessary. As Nick Grono, CEO of the Freedom Fund and the former chief of staff to the attorney general of Australia, points out, slavery is illegal everywhere; all countries have laws banning its practice, but yet it continues to exist in every corner of the Earth [1]. This implies that law enforcement is not enough to combat HTMS. Furthermore, the success of law enforcement – as well as the aforementioned antitrafficking actors and their associated offerings – depends entirely upon the health and well-being of victims and survivors of human trafficking. From participating in legal proceedings, sharing testimonies in open court, or participating in educational awareness and training

M. J. Kronfeld (✉)
Passion For A Purpose, Tel Aviv, Israel
e-mail: mj@pfapnyc.com

© Springer Nature Switzerland AG 2020
P. Murthy, A. Ansehl (eds.), *Technology and Global Public Health*,
https://doi.org/10.1007/978-3-030-46355-7_19

events, providing critical and necessary care for the trafficked (including men, women, children, and transgender persons) is the first step on their long road to recovery, rehabilitation, reentry, and reintegration back into society.

Mark Latonero writes, "As human trafficking, and many of today's most pressing social issues, become increasingly mediated by technologies, the negative and positive dimensions of technology's impact on social change and human rights must become vital considerations." [2]. Admittedly, by the time this is published and thereafter, the technologies described herein, whether employed by traffickers or by those who seek to disrupt their activities, may very well be irrelevant. In fact, during the course of researching and writing this chapter, Backpage.com – the most flagrant and widely used open-source platform for commercial sexual exploitation – was shut down by the U.S. Justice Department [3]. Its owners were swiftly charged with facilitating human trafficking and money laundering, among other associated crimes, ending over a decade of the platform's being used for the sale of human beings for sex [4]. In addition, Craigslist.com (alongside Reddit.com) took down its personal advertising pages (the former of which was described by Illinois Sheriff Thomas J. Dart in a 2009 lawsuit against the website as "the single largest source of prostitution in the nation") following the passage of the Fight Online Sex Trafficking Act (FOSTA) by the U.S. Congress and the Stop Enabling Sex Trafficking Act (SESTA) by the U.S. Senate in 2018 [5].

Just as slavery laid the foundations for the Industrial Revolution to thrive, today the technological revolution is working to strengthen the foundation upon which modern slavery survives. But the narrow focus of HTMS and technology featured herein does not discount the many additional forms of HTMS untouched by a digital footprint [6]. Every day and everywhere, individuals are trafficked into forced labor, domestic servitude, commercial sexual exploitation, child marriage or soldiering, and organ "donations" in their own homes, villages, towns, and cities by individuals who did not recruit them through the Internet or sell or exploit them over the Internet. But what does remain true is that the Internet, and its many associated platforms and applications, is rapidly redefining HTMS by lowering the bar for exploitation. And those fighting HTMS are failing to effectively wield technology in their favor. As a result, the capacity to respond to the immediate-, short-, and long-term "population health" of the survivor community, as well as ensure general population health management (PHM) for those who may be at risk of HTMS – in addition to those perceived as being unlikely targets (despite the lack of any specific trafficking victim profile) – is essential to deter, diminish, and eventually defeat the modern slave trade [4].

As Dr. Kevin Bales, founder of the Walk Free Foundation, notes, healthcare – in tandem with education and training in particular, and the reduction of corruption, poverty, and conflict more generally – is necessary to tackle HTMS [7]. And the role of healthcare professionals, in expanding their knowledge of and engagement in the anti-HTMS movement, is vital. To that end, research in the field remains both important and interesting because it adds incrementally to the literature addressing the topic [7].

Understanding Human Trafficking and Modern Slavery

To situate the role of public health in the context of HTMS, it is necessary to establish an understanding of exactly what HTMS is. At its most basic level, journalist and activist E. Benjamin Skinner defines a slave as an individual who is "forced to work, under threat of violence, for no pay beyond subsistence." [8]. In theory, slavery has been declared illegal by the international community as enshrined in a range of international treaties as well as a variety of regional and transregional, transnational, supranational, and domestic legal arrangements or legislation. For example, Article 4 of the 1949 Universal Declaration of Human Rights guarantees that "no one shall be held in slavery or servitude; slavery and the slave trade shall be prohibited in all their forms." [8]. But the document also recognizes that "slavery is not dead. It continues to be reported in a wide range of forms: traditional chattel slavery, bonded labour, serfdom, child labour, migrant labour, domestic labour, forced labour and slavery for ritual or religious purposes." [9].

The United Nations (UN) further defines human trafficking as "the recruitment, transportation, transfer, harbouring or receipt of persons, by means of threat or use of force or other forms of coercion, of abduction, of fraud, of deception, of the abuse of power or of a position of vulnerability or of the giving or receiving of payments or benefits to achieve the consent of a person having control over another person, for the purpose of exploitation." [9]. Importantly, the defining UN protocol goes on to note that "exploitation shall include, at a minimum, the exploitation of the prostitution of others or other forms of sexual exploitation, forced labour or services, slavery or practices similar to slavery, servitude or the removal of organs." [10]. The United States similarly defines human trafficking as "the recruitment, harboring, transportation, provision, or obtaining of a person for labor or services, through the use of force, fraud, or coercion for the purpose of subjection to involuntary servitude, peonage, debt bondage, or slavery." [11]. Human trafficking has three constituent elements: the act (what is done), the means (how it is done), and the purpose (why it is done), or the causal factors behind an individual's exploitation. It is furtherly important to point out that trafficking can occur within and across borders; it victimizes men, women, and children of all ages and backgrounds and frequently takes place without any involvement of any organized crime groups or transnational criminal organizations. Still, the definition of HTMS remains contentious. Cultural norms, religious practices, and general ignorance and disbelief persist in preventing the emergence of a universal anti-HTMS movement truly unified in opposition to this heinous crime. This is further compounded by the range of HTMS categories that exist under the current definition (including forced labor; bonded labor or debt bondage; domestic servitude; commercial sexual exploitation; organ trafficking; and an array of child exploitation including child labor, marriage, soldiering, and sex trafficking considered separate and distinct from adult exploitation) [12]. As a result, there exists a diverse array of context-specific approaches to combating HTMS and a range of distinct needs from different types of victims and survivors over the short and long term, which further silos the modern abolitionist community.

Human Trafficking and Modern Slavery in the Digital Age

Twenty-first century technology, as Pedro Szekely et al. write, is both "facilitating and disrupting trafficking" across the world [13]. This sentiment was prevalent across the survey and interview data acquired for this research. That being said, technology is neither inherently good nor bad, but rather who uses it and how, why, and to what end it is used determine the moral value of its utility. As the current modality of humanity, technology is at the forefront of HTMS for those who deal in it and those who fight against it. As John Temple, former assistant district attorney in the Manhattan District Attorney's Office in New York City and chief of its Human Trafficking Response Unit, noted in an interview for the purposes of this research, "Technology is moving so quickly that law enforcement and their ability to access that is [sic] going dark" (J. Temple, phone communication, April 4, 2018). Moreover, the rate at which technology is moving undermines efforts "to better understand how controllers and survivors utilize technology," as Vanessa Bouche writes in a report issued by the technology-based, anti-HTMS organization Thorn, because "this knowledge will inform our approach to disrupt extant methods used by controllers and create new and innovative interventions." [14].

In researching this chapter, a self-selecting, online survey was conducted from March 15 to April 1, 2018, and distributed to a range of individuals in the anti-HTMS movement, in conjunction with the NEXUS Working Group on Human Trafficking & Modern Slavery, the Global Modern Slavery Directory, and the Freedom Collaborative (written communication with anonymous subjects).

The 100 respondents included nonprofit professionals (62); human trafficking survivors (12); academic and think-tank researchers (9); representatives from companies, corporations, businesses, corporate social responsibility (CSR) offices or social enterprises whose business model or philanthropy prioritizes anti-HTMS efforts in some form (6); representatives from foundations, family offices, and grant-making organizations or philanthropists who fund antitrafficking initiatives (5); elected or appointed government officials and civil servants (2); members of the media who actively report on HTMS (2); retired or active-duty military and law enforcement officials (1); and medical professionals (1). Of the respondents, 68 were female and 32 were male, with ages ranging from 15 to 69 years old. Respondents represented 28 different countries including the United States (62), Canada (5), South Africa and Mexico (3 each), the Philippines, the United Kingdom, and Australia (2 each), and one respondent each from Austria, France, Ghana, India, Ireland, Italy, Jamaica, Jordan, Kosovo, the Netherlands, Nigeria, Macedonia, Malawi, Moldova, Nepal, New Zealand, Peru, Romania, Spain, Sweden, and Uganda.

Respondents were required to answer only one question: "Is technology more harmful or helpful in the context of human trafficking and modern slavery?" (anonymous subjects, written communication). A third option, that technology is equally harmful and helpful, was also included (Fig. 1).

The majority of survey respondents indicated they believe technology is equally harmful and helpful (66%). As one survey respondent noted, "Slavery is a product

Is technology more harmful or helpful in the context of human trafficking & modern slavery?

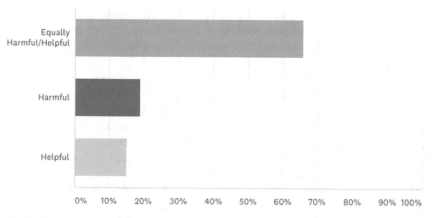

Fig. 1 The relationship between Technology and Trafficking

of power imbalances combined with coercion. Whether a technology increases or decreases a power imbalance is highly context-specific" (Subject 70, personal communication, n.d.). The subject added, "The Internet can help connect anonymous consumers to coerced supply of sexual services. But it can also connect and empower a community of survivors. Similarly, advancement in blockchain may be useful for distributed ledger technologies that help improve supply chain transparency. And it may assist criminal trafficking organizations to launder the proceeds of crime free from effective Anti-Money Laundering (AML) regulation" (Subject 70, personal communication, n.d.).

Interestingly, more survey respondents believed technology was harmful rather than helpful as a secondary choice (19% and 15%, respectively). Although this further reflects the majority view, that technology is equally harmful and helpful, it also implies a concern that the use of technology, in the context of HTMS, favors vice over virtue.

For the purpose of the research, a series of interviews were also conducted with a range of individuals in the anti-HTMS movement, including government officials, survivors, industry leaders, and NPO professionals. In general, interviewees conveyed five key points regarding HTMS in the context of technology. (Communication from U.S. Ambassador Susan Coppedge; Justin Dillon of Made In A Free World; Nathaniel Erb of Erb & Associates; Patrick Gage of the Scalibrini International Migration Network; Nick Grono of the Freedom Fund; Laura Hackney of AnnieCannons; Duncan Jepson of Liberty Asia; Siddharth Kara of Harvard University; U.S. Ambassador Mark Lagon; Bradley Myles of the Polaris Project; Rebecca Sadwick of the Luskin Center For Innovation; John Temple, formerly of the Manhattan District Attorney's Office; and Ehb Teng of ATHack).

First, interviewees emphasized that technology is not itself a solution to the problem, but rather a tool, and at times a limited one at best. Ambassador Mark Lagon, who served as Ambassador-at-Large and Director of the Department of State's Office to Monitor and Combat Trafficking in Persons (TIP), noted in his interview, "I think it's a classic American reaction that information technology will be the solution to things we've learned. But information technology is not necessarily the universal solvent in washing away the oppression and trafficking of others" (Mark Lagon, phone interview, March 23, 2018).

Bradley Myles, CEO of the Polaris Project, concurred, noting in his interview that technology provides "real efficiency gains" and is "a very critical tool, especially data analytics and reaching more victims and operating in scale." But he added that "there is still a very human element of the field that can't be replaced by technology, like sitting with a survivor and talking to them about the traumas that they've been through and endured. These are things technology can't really replace (Bradley Myles, phone interview, April 3, 2018).

Nathaniel Erb, founder of Erb & Associates, expanded on this in his interview, pointing out that "ignoring the impact of technology in our society is wrong; I think it would be a mistake to do so. But at the same time, I think it is not the Achilles heel to the mission…It comes down to the social science of humans and why people traffic other humans"(Nathaniel Erb, phone interview, March 22, 2018). He added, "Technology could be a great tool in addressing that, and providing a really good solution as well as helping bring to scale solutions in a way that we couldn't have done years ago, [but] it's not going to be the thing that fixes it because there's more that pertains to the issue that we can get away from: why people treat other people like slaves, why we traffic others." Erb further noted, "Technology is a great way for others to stay connected, but it does not cover the human aspect of why people traffic others in the first place, which is the most effective way to take on human trafficking" (Nathaniel Erb, phone interview, March 22, 2018).

And the use of technology, interviewees pointed out, is only relevant if the underlying issues sustaining HTMS are also addressed. As Grono noted in his interview, "Technology is a tool, not a solution in and of itself. Technology can be an amplifier, a multiplier of impact if used widely where there's a genuine attention to tackle the fundamental issues behind the exploitation of workers. Technology is really important, but only where there's a willingness to get to grips with real challenges" (Nick Grono, phone interview, March 29, 2018). He added that "tech is a tool that can be useful where it can be applied to support solutions that genuinely understand the model of exploitation and the power relationships" (Nick Grono, phone interview, March 29, 2018). Duncan Jepson, founder of Liberty Asia, concurred in his interview: "It is a matter of identifying what tools you need, and how you're going to use them. What people are trying to do is use technology to force a change, to create something that humans don't want to do. Technology won't change the behavior on its own" (Duncan Jepson, phone interview, March 20, 2018).

Indeed, as Ehb Teng, founder of ATHack!, pointed out in his interview, "The correct question to ask is what is happening at a human condition level that causes these things? Technology is completely up to us...Technology will only follow if we exploit each other" (Ehb Teng, phone interview, March 23, 2018).

Temple concurred: "Technology doesn't do anything unless we have human interaction; [it] doesn't do anything unless we can connect it to other meaningful data sets, and it doesn't mean anything if we don't enable ourselves to take action." [15]. He added that technology "helps increase the tools in your toolbox, but nothing will ever be a silver bullet for this, which makes it such a challenging problem" (J. Temple, private communication, n.d.).

Second, interviewees emphasized the distinction between so-called high and low forms of technology. As Justin Dillon, founder of Made In A Free World, noted in his interview, it is the simplest forms of technology that are most dangerous (J. Dillon, phone interview, March 21, 2018).

Laura Hackney, founder of AnnieCannons, concurred, noting in her interview that when working with survivors, it is the "everyday technologies" – such as social media and peer-to-peer messaging platforms – that are the most likely entry point for exploitation by traffickers, calling concerns over bitcoin and the "dark web" mostly hype (L. Hackney, phone interview, March 23, 2018).

Third, interviewees emphasized the importance of data collection and analysis. For example, Dillon pointed out that "it is really hard to use technology unless you have data...[but] what's important to understand when you're talking about technology and slavery is that we're tracking a behavior – we're not tracking zeros and ones, and we're not tracking a chemical emission. Behavior changes at will – it's actually more powerful than data" (J. Dillon, private communication, n.d.). He added, "We can never track down someone's motivation for why they do this, but what we can do is start to change the context around individuals who choose to harm another person for their own gain. So when we can make that activity less invisible, and we can change the context in which the marketplace affects government and vice versa – these things start to work together and not only makes this less invisible, it makes slavery just harder to pull off" (J. Dillon, private communication, n.d.).

Fourth, interviewees emphasized the critical importance of partnerships in building and employing technology to combat HTMS. As Rebecca Sadwick of the Luskin Center of Innovation emphasized, "It's important to stay one step ahead of the rapid evolution of the technological exploitation methods, and that's really why the partnerships between private providers and nonprofit agencies need to be as organized and aligned as possible" because, as she added, "traffickers are working together to stay against and ahead of law enforcement" (R. Sadwick, phone interview, March 26, 2018).

Siddharth Kara of Harvard University expanded on this point, noting that "it's also very important to switch the mindset away from playing catch-up, more towards being predictive. Meaning, let's convene a technology trust...some of the brightest minds in the tech world to think about how might our tools be used in the future, things that we haven't seen yet or thought about." He added it is critical that partnerships be employed to "think proactively about how [technology] might be used in the future, and then start solving for that today" (S. Kara, phone interview, April 17, 2018).

The role of partnerships as conveyed by interviewees was depicted in a variety of forms, including using technology to raise awareness, to track HTMS patterns and manage data to make more informed decisions, and to empower victims and survivors to access critical resources to end and recover from their various forms of exploitation. As Ambassador Susan Coppedge, who also served as ambassador-at-large in the Department of State's TIP Office, noted in her interview, "Getting technology into the hands of workers so that they can report labor abuses that can lead to trafficking is really important. That can be done with cell phones or through GPS, and then just equipping law enforcement." But, she added, "Just arresting and prosecuting successfully is only one component…in the fight against trafficking and certainly that needs to be supported to send a deterrent message. But I think to really end it we're going to have to engage businesses and technology to put companies on the alert" (S. Coppedge, phone interview, March 30, 2018).

Finally, significant emphasis was placed on empowering survivors through technology. One such means of empowerment, often unconsidered in the context of HTMS and technology, as Hackney pointed out, is providing technology-based education and employment opportunities for survivors of trafficking, in order to ensure financial stability and independence over the long term. Additionally, Hackney noted that empowering survivors through technology also includes employing survivors when building technology (L. Hackney, private communication, n.d.).

Much like the modern HTMS community, which endorses a survivor-led movement, Hackney perceives the same as being necessary in the context of the digital revolution. She noted that "we have a lot of people who are really well intentioned who want to build something to fight trafficking, but they don't have the perspective," adding that "we're not just hoping to build more technology, but help more people understand the problem, and that the technology being built will reflect the living experience of the people" (L. Hackney, oral communication, n.d.).

Patrick Gage, Director of Development at the Scalabrini International Migration Network, concurred in his interview: "Technological solutions need to be better informed, for survivors, and consider what would've helped them at the time," adding that "when informing technological solutions to be better, we have to not only ask for survivors' feedback, but to actually give them the tools and say that they can build what it is that they want if they were in that situation" (P. Gage, phone interview, n.d.).

As survey respondents pointed out, those very technologies used by government authorities to disrupt HTMS tend to be the same as those being used to facilitate it. But, unlike government authorities, traffickers are not limited by any laws or jurisdictions, ensuring that the government remains strategically and perpetually disadvantaged relative to traffickers. It is also important to note that although some generalizations can be made in the context of HTMS, different types of or uses for technology are employed for different forms of exploitation. For example, a victim of commercial sexual exploitation is more likely to be recruited by a trafficker through a social networking site or peer-to-peer messaging mobile application, while a victim of labor trafficking is more likely to be recruited through an ad-hosting site featuring employment opportunities. Furthermore, the Internet's perceived anonymity, the ease of deception, the swiftness of international communication, and the legitimate public-private security concerns regarding information online all contribute to advancing the capabilities of traffickers relative to those who seek to disrupt their activities. As Coppedge noted, "Technology is a tool for the trafficker to avoid detection" (S. Coppedge, private communication, n.d.).

In an extensive 2-year study published by the European Union in 2015, the Trafficking as a Criminal Enterprise (TRACE) project compiled a full review of the applications, software, and hardware that facilitate trafficking. The report included applications and software such as adult entertainment websites, advertising and classifieds, applications (web-based), computer games, the dark web, email, online dating sites, online forums, peer-to-peer networks, and social networking sites, while hardware included camera and video technologies; desktops, laptops, tablets, printers, scanners, telephones/cellphones, and television [16]. Survey respondents voluntarily listed most of the aforementioned technologies, in addition to blockchain technologies; cryptocurrencies; GPS-enabled devices or online platforms; employment, marriage, and tourism websites and recruitment services; encryption software or services; online marketplaces; wireless pagers; Tor and virtual private network (VPN) software; as well as a range of popular online platforms. Survey respondents conveyed a general belief that trafficking can be facilitated by any open-source forum that allows communication between two users, with each being target-rich environments for vulnerable persons, particularly youth.

The TRACE project also reviewed the applications, software, and hardware that are employed to combat HTMS. Notable are the similarities between the two lists, which, in the context of anti-HTMS efforts, include applications and software such as adult entertainment websites, (web-based) applications, case management tools, computer games, crowdsourcing, the dark web, e-learning training programs, email, facial reconstruction, financial tracking, geographic information systems, i2 software, online collaboration platforms, online forums, online petitions, peer-to-peer networks, podcasts, police database systems, social networking sites, supply chain management toolkits, and (generic) websites, while hardware included closed-circuit television, routers and backup devices, telephones/cellphones, and television [16]. In addition to many of the aforementioned technologies and tools, survey respondents added artificial intelligence (AI), advancements in biomedics for organ transplants, blockchain technologies, crisis hotlines (via phone of web-based peer-to-peer platforms), cybercrime tracking software, data management tools, ethical hacking, experimental algorithms, unmanned aerial vehicles, online awareness and educational campaigns, online law enforcement sting operations, and geospatial imagery and satellite mapping.

In essence, what these lists reveal is the extent to which technology is employed to either support or combat HTMS efforts and how, as Laura Hackney noted in her interview, common technologies used daily worldwide – for communicating with friends and family, conducting business, or engaging in leisure activities – are also the most common tools for the recruitment, conditioning, and enslaving of its users (L. Hackney, personal communication, n.d.).

For example, commonplace technologies such as mobile phones are used to facilitate commercial sexual exploitation by providing a direct link between trafficker and victim (for the purposes of recruitment and conditioning) as well as the trafficker, victim, and client to arrange the provision of services for the client from the victim and payment for services rendered by the client to the trafficker (V. Bouche and M. Latonero, private communication, n.d.). And with at least 75% of the world's population being connected or having access to mobile phones, vulnerable communities can be as likely to exist in a rural community as they are in a large urban setting (M. Latonero, private communication, n.d.). But according to research conducted by Siddhartha Sarkar on sex trafficking in India, Nepal, Thailand, and Hungary, survivors revealed that traffickers not only use mobile phones, but also sophisticated or advanced encryption software (alongside less sophisticated software) to preserve anonymity, including employing hosting services and online storage platforms to counteract digital forensic investigation conducted by law enforcement [17]. And so where there is a distinction between high and low technology, it is important to also recognize how the two are not mutually exclusive. As Teng noted, "There's [sic] pros and cons to every cent piece of technology out there, and traffickers have been kind of ahead of the game for a long time. The anti-trafficking efforts are only now catching up." He added that "for everything that we stop, something else pops up. You can't stop progress"(E. Teng, private communication, n.d.).

Finally, these lists illustrate how the diffusion of common technologies – specifically their availability and their accessibility – is vastly increasing the capability of criminals to engage in HTMS. Indeed, as one survey respondent noted, "Technology is not an either/or, good/bad proposition. The intent of the user matters most. I have not run across any technologies that were made specifically for human trafficking, only technologies that were created and have been creatively used by traffickers" (Communication, Subject 44, March 19, 2018). This emphasizes Dillon's view, who noted in his interview that the general approach to combatting HTMS through technology "should be about taking what we have and using it better" (J. Dillon, private communication, n.d.).

Fighting Human Trafficking and Modern Slavery in the Digital Age

Increasingly, government authorities and civil society actors are doing just that: employing technologies and analytical methodologies in equally creative ways to keep pace with the diffusion of, access to, and ease with which traffickers obtain and exploit technology for nefarious purposes. Although a relatively new approach to anti-HTMS – what Jepson labels nascent – the application of new technologies and innovative analytical methodologies has begun to emerge and be established as critical tools for government, law enforcement, and civil society to combat HTMS and provide services to victims and survivors.

As a result of a growing body of HTMS databases collected by transnational organizations, governments, local authorities, and civil society groups across the world, in addition to information gleaned from the use of open-source platforms used by traffickers, the true breadth and nature of HTMS have only just begun to be revealed. Longitudinal data acquired, for example, by the UN Office of Drugs and Crime, INTERPOL, the U.S. National and International Center for Missing and Exploited Children, the U.S. Department of Justice, the International Offices of Migration and Labor, the United Kingdom Internet Watch Foundation, and the Walk Free Foundation, among others, have finally grown to such an extent that their utility to modern methodological practice is just now being realized. Analytical tools, such as knowledge graphs, tailored search engines, and network analysis (which has been used to fight terrorist organizations, crime syndicates, and other illicit nonstate actors around the world), have also become more important [16]. So too have anti-HTMS-specific tools such as the Virtual Global Taskforce's Operation Pin (a collaborative effort between American, Australian, Canadian, and European law enforcement); Microsoft's Child Exploitation Tracking system and chatbot program Project Intercept; Polaris and Palantir's database management software as well as Polaris' SMS-based BeFree program (in collaboration with Thorn, Twilio, and the Salesforce Foundation); the National Center for Missing and Exploited Children's CyberTipline; the Federal Bureau of Investigation's FANTOM software; the Defense Advanced Research Projects Agency's Memex Program; Southern California's Annenberg School for Communication and Journalism's DIG tool; Marinus Analytics' Traffic Jam software; the Exchange Initiative's TraffickCam mobile application; the Wynyard Groups Advanced Crime and Analytics software; IBM's STOP APP; LexisNexis' Social Media Monitor [18]; and Thorn's Spotlight program have, in the last decade, begun to establish the necessary foundation for an innovative, digital-centric, big data approach to the threat posed by HTMS [19] (Godoy, Sadwick, and Baca; D.D. Suthers and M. Ibanez, private communications, op. cit.; P. Szekley, private communication, n.d.; H. Watson, private communication, n.d.).

And a range of transformative technologies, not specifically created for the purpose of antitrafficking but that have nonetheless been adopted by the movement (and those affected by the crime of HTMS), have also been exponentially scaled. For example, anti-money-laundering (AML) software employed by financial institutions to track terrorism and organized crime following the 2001 terrorist attacks on the United States has also proven instrumental in uncovering illicit financial flows from human trafficking operations [20]. Even awareness and education tools, such as Made In A Free World's SlaveryFootprint.com or the University of Nottingham's Slavery From Space project, have a critical role to play in utilizing big data to inform the public of its role in perpetuating HTMS in the most simple, accessible, and impactful way possible.

Despite the rise of modern techniques to combat HTMS and support survivors, big data in the context of HTMS remain limited in scope. And most NPOs lack the access or skills to utilize technological advancements that would increase their capacity to provide resources and services to victims and survivors or to advance their knowledge through analysis of the data they have acquired on this specific population [21]. As one survey respondent noted, "Information silos are continuing to occur when technology should allow us to communicate and collaborate to better prevent and respond to vulnerabilities and exploitation." [17]. Another subject expanded on this, pointing out that "there's a big disconnect between the individuals who understand emerging technologies and those who understand human trafficking. And I think there needs to be more opportunities for them to get into the same space, and just start understanding each other's work" (Subject 53, private communication, n.d.). A third subject added that "tech companies need to do a better job of engaging with anti-trafficking orgs and letting them know what internal initiatives they have put in place to combat online trafficking. NGOs need to take a more open-minded approach to the tech sector and break away from the 'all tech is evil' narrative that is being perpetuated" (Subject 44, private communication, n.d.). The respondent concluded by noting, "It's only together that we will be able to learn how to best leverage technology to combat trafficking issues" (Subject 44, private communication, n.d.).

However, it is also important to note that victims do not raise their hand to be counted (and often neither do survivors), and therefore insights into a community that frequently lacks a meaningful population sample size continues to frustrate efforts to better understand victims and survivors in order to serve their direct needs [22].

Human Trafficking, Modern Slavery, and Healthcare

For medical professionals, there are two primary opportunities for interacting with and providing services for slaves or trafficked individuals. This includes the treatment of victims while being trafficked or during the course of providing short- or long-term physical and psychological treatment and care of survivors. Each form of care, although showing some significant overlap, still presents unique and distinct challenges.

The primary barrier to entry for healthcare professionals in terms of serving victims and survivors of HTMS is a dearth of research and literature on the topic [22]. However, some primary insights can be gleaned from the existing survivor-centric research studies and data sets published over the last decade. A preliminary review of the data finds a concentrated focus on victims of commercial sexual exploitation in Europe (particularly eastern European survivors) as well as Southeast Asia, with an occasional study focused on Latin America or the Middle East, ranging in population sample size from as many as 4500 to as few 20 survivors [17, 23, 24]. In 2012, for example, Sian Oram et al. counted just 19 reports on survivors, specifically women and girls who had been commercially sexually exploited, illustrating methodological weakness and sample size bias in its lack of focus on men and boys [23]. There is a significant lack of research in the context of the United States, where locally focused studies tend toward diminutive population sample sizes of 100 or less [24, 25]. And studies focused on survivors of alternative forms of HTMS (including bonded labor, domestic labor, organ trafficking, and all forms of child exploitation) are in even lower supply [1, 3, 26].

The available data sets and general insights regarding victims of commercial sexual exploitation reveal a critical medical need both during and following exploitation. Common health problems found among victims and survivors include addiction to and complications from drug or alcohol abuse; unwanted pregnancies and unsafe abortions; physical abuse and fractures; sexually transmitted diseases; chronic back, vaginal, pelvic, or gastrointestinal pain; oral health problems and headaches; a range of skin conditions; fatigue and dizziness; post-traumatic stress disorder (PTSD); and anywhere between 10 and 20 or more concurrent symptoms [1, 23]. Victims and survivors of HTMS also tended to have a higher rate of HIV/AIDS than the general population and are exposed to a higher risk of workplace violence, with one study finding that those recruited and exploited before the age of 18 tend to suffer even higher rates of violence [23].

But perhaps the most interesting insight found consistently across many of these studies was the revelation that victims tend to interact with healthcare professionals while being exploited. One report revealed that more than 80% of victims of commercial sexual exploitation had received a consultation or treatment from a medical practitioner while being trafficked [24]. This is critical because it implies that there are integral opportunities for intervention during the cycle of exploitation that are being overlooked or ignored. This may be the result of a lack of awareness regarding the visible signs of HTMS, fear of reporting HTMS in the presence of a trafficker, or failure to adequately categorize HTMS as such, thereby preventing the due course of action for survivors (which includes judicial, legal, educational, and social services in addition to other forms of public and private anti-HTMS services).

A secondary barrier to collecting data stems from the nature of the subject. As a black market economy of scale, collecting data on HTMS – whether the focus is on victims or survivors – is often dangerous and raises methodological and ethical issues requiring a multidimensional approach across multiple disciplines, both internal and external to direct medical practice [22]. This is compounded by controversies regarding the definition of HTMS and, as result, those who are victims and survivors and qualify for any associated services or assistance [22].

Victims and survivors are, as previously mentioned, a unique population with unique needs that require healthcare professionals as a means of prevention, intervention, and recovery over the short and long term [22, 27].

Prevention

Models of prevention relevant to healthcare professionals include ensuring potential victims and the concentric communities in which they exist at the micro-, meso- and macro-level (including families, houses of worship, educational institutions, the general community and municipalities broadly defined) are informed of how individuals are recruited and conditioned to be trafficked. Promoting conversations on self-esteem and positive body image, providing healthy relationship and sexual education, as well as attention to mental wellness, family stability, or community cohesiveness is critical.

Intervention

Given the likelihood of encountering certain forms of trafficking in professional medical settings, intervening in the cycle of exploitation is another critical role public health practitioners can assume responsibility for. Understanding the signs of trafficking, creating culturally sensitive forms of engagement, and developing the capacity to report incidents of trafficking encountered in professional medical settings – without further endangering the victim or the practitioner – are essential.

Recovery

The process of recovering from HTMS is different for each survivor. Pathways to recovery, rehabilitation, reentry, and reintegration back into society require that healthcare professionals address survivors' physical and mental well-being, respond to each individual's unique needs (as defined by their specific forms of exploitation and trauma), commit to continued engagement over the lifetime of the survivors.

It is important to note that to effectively achieve the aforementioned goals, it is most critical to employ a trauma-informed and culturally sensitive approach to the physical and psychological well-being of each victim or survivor [28]. Furthermore, each of these three stages holds great potential for the use of technological solutions. It is therefore necessary for those in the public health space to be more creative, engage in more partnerships, and advocate for more funding to build and deploy technological tools in order to assist in achieving these ends.

Finally, it is essential to point out that working with victims and survivors of HTMS can have a significant effect on the psychological and physical well-being of service providers, including medical professionals. This unintended consequence is often discussed among service providers in the NPO space, where long, grueling hours and remote or dangerous locations are the norm when tending to a traumatized client population and dealing with its associated issues, including addiction, abuse, and other diseases. And with many providing these services pro bono or on a voluntary basis, self-care for those who work with victims and survivors, whether they be medical professionals or otherwise, is as necessary as the care they provide victims and survivors.

Solutions, Strategies, and Sustainable Impact to End Slavery Now

As this research has attempted to illustrate, the nature of the HTMS problem today implies that it cannot go ignored by healthcare professionals. As Tordes writes, "There are strong arguments in favor of deeming human trafficking a public health issue: its health implications are severe, and the scale of human trafficking, with possibly millions of victims annually, suggests population-level implications. Moreover, there is growing consensus that violence is a public health issue, and trafficking is clearly a severe form of violence." [1]. But, given the extent of the problem, developing strategic, effective, and successful methodologies and practices can seem daunting. However, there are four primary means through which medical professionals can position themselves as critical leaders and have a significant impact on the fight against HTMS. These include practice, profiling, partnerships, and philanthropy [1].

Practice

As Mitali Thakor and Danah Boyd write, "By creating new mechanisms to share information and connect, technology has the potential to increase exploitative transactions; but it also has the potential to create new opportunities to intervene." [21]. Increasing the level of education among medical professionals and providing safe and effective tools for reporting trafficking while protecting victims in their care, regardless of the presence of a trafficker in a medical facility, is most critical and pressing. As Tiffany Dovydaitis writes, "Human trafficking is a major global health problem, one that all healthcare providers cannot ignore. Although trafficking victims are unlikely to have adequate and timely access to health care, some victims will be seen in women's health care practices." As a result, the author writes, "They should be prepared to identify, treat, and assist victims of trafficking as part of their regular clinical practice." [22].

In addition, technological platforms and tools are critical in this regard. Whether through online training modules, HTMS victim assessment programs, peer-to-peer information sharing platforms, or discreet methods for reporting incidents of trafficking to authorities in real time, there is significant capacity to use technology to further education, intervention, and care. Furthermore, as Sadwick noted in her interview, over 60% of victims are able to access technology while being exploited, providing an underutilized pathway for intervention or the provision of telemedicine services (Godoy and Burke, oral presentation, n.d.).

As Lagon noted, "The fact that [victims] now have ways that they can use their handheld devices to get help, that's impressive for those who are invisible." [29]. And those in public heath, given their likelihood of interacting with survivors, can be the point of revelation, shining a light on this dark crime.

Profiling

As noted, the deficit of authoritative, longitudinal, and meaningful data continues to thwart efforts to create a comprehensive understanding of the healthcare needs of victims and survivors of all forms of HTMS. As Hackney noted, "The conversation is generally that the other person can receive services, but the question is never what services. They never asked about the duration and the quality of the services." And although a clearer picture of the health effects of commercial sexual exploitation is beginning to emerge, alternative forms of HTMS lack methodological or analytical understanding. Healthcare professionals are best situated to address this issue. By collecting, sharing, and analyzing data on victims and survivors, as well as compiling sociopsychological profiles of perpetrators, medical professionals will play an integral role in detecting and preventing HTMS.

The public health space must begin advocating for increased funding for anti-HTMS research in the context of public health by seeking out new types of innovative partnerships with governments, universities, philanthropists, and civil society groups to advance the use of data management and analysis tools. As Grono noted in his interview, fighting HTMS is about "understanding your audience, your target, and how your tech can best suit them." [2].

But collecting data can only assist in combatting HTMS to a certain extent. As this research has illustrated, the "human element" – in this specific case, interactions between victims, survivors, and medical professionals – will always be key. As Temple, noted, "We get so enamored with technology that when we leave out the human element, we always come up short on it" (J. Temple, oral communication, n.d.).

But as Jennifer Lynne Musto and Danah Boyd write, "As technologies grow more sophisticated, so too will the possibilities grow for staging innovative socio-technical interventions, yet capitalizing on this knowledge requires far more low-tech solutions, specifically, political will and agitation for redistributive justice, the hardest assets to find." By lending its voice to the anti-HTMS movement, the public heath space can begin to lay the foundation for the vital will and necessary agitation required to achieve justice for all victims and survivors [30].

Partnerships

As Hackney noted, "The more we can use technology to collaborate between organizations, the more we can head in the right direction." And partnerships between the public health space and technologists, civil society, businesses, governments, and law enforcement are necessary. As Jonathan Tordes writes, "Although a public health approach alone is not sufficient, public health methodologies can advance antitrafficking efforts in ways currently underutilized or not contemplated by a criminal law model and reveal deep-seated structural challenges impeding the success of current legislative and policy initiatives designed to combat human trafficking." [1].

Although slavery is illegal in every nation, until the passage of SESTA and FOSTA in the United States, few nations had had legislation directly addressing the role of technology in facilitating HTMS [3]. As Latonero writes, the "challenge for legislatures is finding a uniform way to define the technologies used to facilitate trafficking in an era of rapid change." [3]. Even in developed nations, it is often the case that the legal system has not caught up with the complexity of the crime. This stems in large measure from a lack of understanding of the issue as a result of the paucity of data. As Jepson commented, "There's not much point in gathering [data] if you're not using it; we're not doing it for research purposes. That's what's important. You're doing it for, ostensibly, to inform people, so they can make better decisions about what they do every day in relation to this problem," adding that "you want people to make better decisions" (D. Jepson, oral communication, September 2018). Teng agrees, noting in his interview that data collection and the use of AI in the anti-HTMS space will go a long way toward predicting local patterns and influence local legislative initiatives by better understanding the prevalence of the crime and the needs, particularly healthcare needs, of the survivor population [31] (E. Teng, personal communication, n.d.).

Lagon concurs, commenting that "technology might be helpful to count what the extent of the problem is and which policy can actually make a difference." [29]. The public health space, therefore, has a unique opportunity to lend its expertise to legislative efforts advocating for the passage of laws funding critical telemedicine initiatives for victims and survivors as well as funding the long-term care of survivors, some of whom will struggle their entire lives to remain gainfully employed due to a lack of necessary training, social stigma, psychological trauma, or chronic physical ailments.

Philanthropy

As was evident in the responses of interviewees, technology itself does not provide a simple solution to the problem of HTMS. What will always be necessary, as previously mentioned, is the human element. In this regard, medical professionals are uniquely situated to be leaders in the fight against HTMS.

Pro bono medical support for organizations, shelters or centers, and other groups offering critical services to survivors, as well as telemedicine platforms, is an immediate solution for the most pressing demands of the anti-HTMS movement. The provision of medical services – unlike general education, vocational training, shelter and child care provisions, security, and, to a lesser degree, legal support – requires a higher degree of specialized training, particularly in light of the client population and its unique physical and psychological conditions. Whether approaching an organization as an individual practitioner or through the creation of a public healthcare network connecting doctors and nurses to organizations in need (similar to those which exist in among lawyers and legal aid providers), the public health space must actively engage civil society leadership in direct contact with victims and survivors. By using preexisting platforms and networks already established by the anti-HTMS movement, direct and meaningful connections between those in need of medical services and those best suited to provide these services represent a readily available pathway for public health to lead the fight [32–37].

Conclusion

Throughout history, and when humanity has been confronted with its greatest and gravest threats, necessity has always driven innovation. This is perhaps most true when it comes to medicine, wherein our will to not only survive but live and thrive has thrust science, industry, governments, and its citizens hurtling toward radical and revolutionary solutions to ensure health, wellness, longevity, and capability over the longest term possible. The same can and should be true in the context of the role of public health practitioners in the fight against modern slavery.

But, as one survey respondent noted, it "is important that technology not be treated like a silver bullet. The more tools to fight trafficking, the better. But in the end, it's a complex human problem, and even if we suddenly had no technology at all, we'd still have trafficking. So the solutions must always be human-centered" [18] (Subject 53, private communication, n.d.). Indeed, just as HTMS has been affected by the rise of technology, there are as many victims of exploitation whose servitude remains untouched by any digital footprint. As a result, one survey respondent commented, "Technology cannot solve the problem of human trafficking, but the people who use it can" (Subject 6, oral communication, March 15, 2018).

This cursory review of HTMS in the context of healthcare and the digital age has implications for further research. How can public health professionals, and the industry as a whole, work to increase preventive measures to stem the tide of trafficking by diminishing the supply of vulnerable targets? What measures can be put in place to ensure that the use of specific technological tools and platforms (or their prohibition) will not contribute to exploiting or re-exploiting victims and survivors? How can the capacity to provide telemedicine be vastly scaled up to reach the growing survivor population that exists in diverse geographies including large cities, remote and rural villages, impoverished urban slums, and regions lacking significant digital penetration and connectivity? Finally, how can technology and medicine be better integrated and diffused to the range of actors in need across the anti-HTMS movement?

Musto and Boyd note, "Human trafficking is increasingly understood as a technological problem that invites collaborative, anti-trafficking solutions," with the result that "a growing cohort of state, non-governmental, and corporate actors in the United States have come together around the shared contention that technology functions as both a facilitator and disrupting force of trafficking." [30]. But the authors add that "despite increased attention to the trafficking-technology nexus, scant research to date has critically unpacked these shifts nor mapped how technology reconfigures anti-trafficking collaborations." [30]. Therefore, "widespread anxieties and overzealous optimism" might be misplaced and further efforts must be made to better understand the tangible and realized impact, or lack thereof, technology has had on furthering anti-HTMS efforts [21, 30].

As Dillon noted, "No-one is going to create an app that will end slavery. It's never going to happen. It has been around since the dawn of humankind. But for the first time ever, we have a way; we have this thing called technology and the Internet that wraps around the whole world" [19] (J. Dillon, oral communication n.d.). He adds that "the key right now is to remain curious…if you really want to see change happen, you have got to be willing to stay curious, and when a good idea comes along, to get behind it" (J. Dillon, oral communication n.d.). Perpetually on the forefront of innovation and life-saving technologies, those in the medical space – inherently curious as a result of their profession – are fully prepared and adequately equipped to be the source of this next "good idea" as well as to "get behind it."

Thakor and Boyd note, "Technology has a powerful role in everyday life" and has the capacity to "destabilize existing infrastructures of power in a networked society." [21]. This does not imply that technology will exclusively serve the greater good or those who wish to subvert it. Rather, it implies that the potential exists for leveraging technology for either. But the authors also note that "by using technology to build their own powerful networks, the anti-trafficking movement may have benefited as much, if not more, than the traffickers they seek to challenge." [21]. And it is the responsibility of those in public health to now do the same.

Acknowledgments This work could not have been completed without the unending commitment of research assistants Matthew Pinna and Joanna Lepuri of the University of Chicago. Additional gratitude is extended to Ambassador Susan Coppedge, Justin Dillon, Nathaniel Erb, Patrick Gage, Nick Grono, Rachel Cohen Gerrol, Laura Hackney, Duncan Jepson, Siddharth Kara, Ambassador Mark Lagon, Margo LaZaro, Diana Mao, Padmini Murthy, Bradley Myles, Yvonne O'Neal, Rebecca Sadwick, John Temple, Ehb Teng, Jonah Wittkamper, and the many members, supporters, and partners of the NEXUS Working Group on Human Trafficking & Modern Slavery and the NEXUS Youth Summit around the world.

References

1. Tordes J. Moving upstream: the merits of a public health law approach to human trafficking. N C Law Rev. 2011;89:147.
2. Grono N. Why does modern slavery persist? Huffington Post. 2015 Mar 30. https://www.huffingtonpost.com/nick-grono/why-does-modern-slavery-p_b_6960174.html. Accessed May 1, 2018
3. Latonero M. The rise of mobile and the diffusion of technology-facilitated trafficking. Los Angeles: University of Southern California Annenberg Center on Communication, Leadership & Policy; 2012. p. vi.
4. Selyukh A. Backpage founders indicted on charges of facilitating prostitution. NPR. 2018 Apr 9. https://www.npr.org/sections/thetwo-way/2018/04/09/600360618/backpage-founders-indicted-on-charges-of-facilitating-prostitution. Accessed 11 May 2018.
5. Selyukh A. Congress passes legislation to curb online sex trafficking of children. NPR. 2018 Feb 27. https://www.npr.org/2018/02/27/589279439/house-to-vote-on-online-sex-trafficking-bill. Accessed 17 Aug 2019.
6. CNN. Lawsuit accuses craigslist of promoting prostitution. CNN. 2009 Mar 5. http://www.cnn.com/2009/CRIME/03/05/craigs.list.prostitution/index.html. Accessed 17 Aug 2019.
7. Bales K. What predicts human trafficking. Int J Comp Appl Crim Just. 2007;31:269–79.
8. Skinner EB. A world enslaved. Foreign Policy. 2009 Oct 8.
9. United Nations. Universal declaration of human rights. 1949. https://www.un.org/en/universal-declaration-human-rights/. Accessed 17 Aug 2019.
10. United Nations. Protocol to Prevent, Suppress and Punish Trafficking in Persons, Especially Women and Children, supplementing the United Nations Convention against Transnational Organized Crime. 2000. https://www.unodc.org/unodc/en/organized-crime/intro/UNTOC.html
11. United Nations. 12. A. Protocol to Prevent Suppress and Punish Trafficking in Persons Especially Women and Children, supplementing the United Nations Convention against Transnational Organized Crime. 2000.
12. United States Congress. Victims of trafficking and violence protection Act of 2000. Washington, DC: United States Congress; 2000.
13. United Nations Vienna. Office on Drugs and Crime. For an overview of child exploitation in the digital age, see Study on the Effects of Information Technologies on the Abuse and Exploitation of Children. 2015.
14. Szekley P et al. The Semantic Web – ISWC 2015. Building and using a knowledge graph to combat human trafficking. 2015; p 205.
15. Bouchle V. A report on the use of technology to recruit, groom and sell domestic minor sex trafficking victims. Los Angeles: Thorn; 2015.
16. Watson H. Report on the role of current and emerging technologies in human trafficking. Brussels: European Union; 2015.
17. Sarkar S. Use of technology in human trafficking networks and sexual exploitation: a cross-sectional multi-country study. Trans Soc Rev. 2015;5:55–68.
18. Quinn K. Trajectory magazine. 2016. http://trajectorymagazinecom/modern-slavery/. Accessed 17 Aug 2019.
19. Sadwick R. Using AI to fight crime: the terrorism, trafficking and money laundering links. Forbes. 2018.
20. Sadwick R. Your money helps fight crime: using AI to fight terrorism, trafficking and money laundering. Forbes. 2018.
21. Thakor MD, Boyd BD. Networked trafficking: reflections on technology and the anti-trafficking movement. Dialect Anthropol. 2013;37(2):287.
22. Dovydaitis T. Human trafficking: the role of the health care provider. J Midwifery Women's Health. 2010;55:462–7.
23. Oram S, et al. Prevalence and risk of violence and the physical, mental and sexual health problems associated with human trafficking: systemic review. PLOS Med. 2012;9:1–13.

24. Lederer LJ, Wetzel CA. The health consequences of sex trafficking and their implications for identifying victims in healthcare facilities. Ann Health Law. 2014;23:61–91.
25. For example, see Lederer, op. cit. Family violence protection fund. Turning pain into power: trafficking survivors' perspectives on early intervention strategies. 2005.
26. Godoy S, Sadwick R, Baca K. Shedding light on sex trafficking: research, data and technologies with the greatest impact Los Angeles: Luskin Center for Innovation; 2010. Checked and cross checked till here.
27. Crane AP, Moreno M. Human trafficking: what is the role of the health care provider? J Appl Res. 2001;2(1)
28. https://digitalcommons.library.tmc.edu/childrenatrisk/vol2/iss1/7/. Accessed 18 Aug 2019.
29. Hemmings S, et al. Responding to the health needs of survivors of human trafficking: a systematic review. BMC Health Serv Res. 2016;16:320.
30. Lagon PM. The global abololition of human trafficking: the indispensible role of the United States. Georgetown J Int Aff. 2011;12(1 (Winter/Spring)):89–98.
31. Suthers DD, Ibanez M. Detection of domestic human trafficking indicators and movement trends using content available on open internet sources. Honolulu: The 47th Hawaii International Conference on System Science; 2014.. https://scholar.google.com/scholar?q=Detection+of+Domestic+Human+Trafficking+Indicators+and+Movement+Trends+Using+Content+Available+on+Open+Internet+Sources.&hl=en&as_sdt=0&as_vis=1&oi=scholart. Accessed 17 Aug 2019
32. Musto LJ, Danah B. The trafficking-technology nexus. Soc Polit Int Stud Gend State Soc. 2014, Fall;21(3):461–83. https://doi.org/10.1093/sp/jxu018.
33. United Nations Global Compact. Human trafficking: the facts. 2008.
34. https://www.unglobalcompact.org/library/88. Accessed 18 Aug 2019.
35. Heal Trafficking. Global modern slavery directory. 2019
36. https://healtrafficking.org/resources/global-modern-slavery-directory/. Accessed 18 Aug 2019.
37. NEXUS. Human trafficking and modern slavery. 2018. https://nexusglobal.org/human-trafficking-and-modern-slavery/ Accessed 18 Aug 2019

Chapter 15: The Worldwide Digital Divide and Access to Healthcare Technology

Irene M. Wohlman

Population Health Tools

Providing virtual healthcare depends upon the use of population health tools. Examples of population health tools include Doctor on Demand–type apps, electronic personal healthcare records available to both physicians and patients, computerized clinical decision support systems, and fitness/nutrition apps. Population health is "the health outcomes of specific groups of people, including the distribution of these outcomes within the group" [1]. Groups can be stratified by geographic region, city, town, or ethnicity, for example. Population health management (PHM) also encourages positive behavioral changes and healthy lifestyles by providing a variety of healthcare services [1]. Improvements in the quality of care and providing better access to and increasing the use of preventive care are three ways PHM strives to improve the health outcomes of groups of people. The model uses caregiver teams, which include care managers, physicians, specialists, and patients' family members [1].

PHM systems comprise several platforms. One is a population health intelligence platform (PHIP), which allows secure, cloud-based access to financial and clinical information for plan administrators and care teams. PHIP systems access patient and clinical data from a variety of sources and provide access to everything from hospital admissions to predictive analysis and population risk stratification information. Another type of PHM system is a medical management system (MMS). A MMS uses both people and data to create effective, personalized services for acute and chronic care and for the management of wellness. By identifying patients at risk, tracking results, analyzing care, and supporting wellness management, a MMS can reduce hospital and emergency room visits [1].

I. M. Wohlman (✉)
New York Medical College, Valhalla, NY, USA
e-mail: irene61@gmail.com

© Springer Nature Switzerland AG 2020
P. Murthy, A. Ansehl (eds.), *Technology and Global Public Health*,
https://doi.org/10.1007/978-3-030-46355-7_20

Risk stratification tools allow providers to establish the correct level of care and services to specific categories of patients [2]. Patterns of care, medical conditions, demographics, and utilization of resources are used to group patients into categories, including episode of care, high-risk and chronically ill patients, healthy patients with conditions or healthy patients [1]. An example is NextGen Software, which facilitates the sorting of patients into groups by chronic disease, condition severity, or demographics. Once the system identifies the at-risk patients, their level of risk is flagged as low, medium, or high, allowing physicians to decide how to best proceed with treatment [3]. High-risk patients can be identified early in a disease process using predictive or prescriptive analysis tools [1]. The goal of this approach is to use historical patient data to improve health outcomes for current patients. Once a health problem area is identified, existing data are gathered and used to evaluate different algorithms. The best algorithm is tested and validated with a separate data set, then is used in a real-world application [4].

Electronic Health Records

The combination of PHM with information technology (IT) and telecommunications allows physicians to provide a wide variety of healthcare tools to the public. Electronic health records (EHRs) or electronic medical records (EMRs) provided through patient portals allow sharing of information between providers and patients and encourage patients to take more personal responsibility in the management of their care. Improved control over chronic conditions such as diabetes can be maintained through remote patient monitoring. Patients can visit physicians remotely using audio and video conferencing, reducing the need for in-office visits and saving time and transportation costs. Referral tracking is facilitated using referral management tools, allowing physicians to track referrals to other providers while ensuring receipt of consultation results. Automated outreach systems send messages to patients receiving preventive care or care for chronic conditions; pharmacies use them for reminders to fill prescriptions [5].

EHRs make computerized clinical decision support systems (CCDSS) possible. CCDSSs improve clinical decision-making by matching individual patient characteristics to a computerized knowledge base, with patient-specific treatment recommendations generated by software algorithms [6]. Access to EHRs is necessary to create treatment algorithms. As these systems capture more data over time, the recommendations become more statistically accurate. They will not replace the human element of medical treatment, but they are a reliable tool for doctors and medical personnel to help with their decision-making.

Healthcare Applications

A variety of healthcare applications, or apps, are available for smartphone users. While there are many to choose from, the two most popular categories include those that people use to monitor their health and fitness, while others target medical information.

Digital fitness wearables allow consumers to track a variety of health-based metrics through apps downloaded to a smartphone or computer. Many fitness apps are free or very inexpensive to download and are easy to use. They allow users to keep track of data such as the foods they eat, how far they walk, calories burned, amount of sleep, heart rate, and pulse [7].

With the advent of personal monitoring systems, such as Fit Bit, individuals can receive constant updates on their vital signs and physical activity [7]. In the future, technology will continue to upgrade and provide users with even more information. These apps and devices provide a consistent way to monitor basic health parameters and, for regular users, a way to set a baseline of physical activity and health. If they notice a change, they can seek out medical attention before a problem becomes too big.

Other apps are available that match symptoms with a possible underlying cause. WebMD was one of the leading pioneer websites providing comprehensive information of this type with its WebMD Symptom Checker. It effortlessly migrated to a mobile platform when smartphones became part of our lives [8]. Even health insurance providers have apps that their members can utilize. One example is Kaiser Permanente, a large integrated hospital and health insurance system. In 2017, its digital patient interactions exceeded office visits. Over 140,000 video and 8.4 million member visits *via* telephone were logged with its nearly 12 million patients. Oscar Health, a New York start-up insurance company, reported that almost two-thirds of its patient interactions in 2017 were virtual, from telemedicine consultations to appointment scheduling with in-network physicians [9].

Disease Reporting and Epidemiology

Epidemiology is the science determining the reasons for disease and how a disease can spread through a geographic area or population. It is the foundation for public health practices and shapes the methods for preventive healthcare to slow down or prevent the spread of disease [10].

E-epidemiology utilizes epidemiological information to further refine knowledge on conditions using such digital media as the Internet, smartphones, and other communication technology. E-epidemiology speeds up the traditional method of epidemiology that once relied only on paper questionnaires to gather information on a particular condition, disease incident, or outbreak. Once the information gathered using paper questionnaires was sorted, it would take time to process and analyze before finally deciding on a course of action [11].

Using modern communication tools allows e-epidemiologists to not only gather similar data quickly, but in a more cost-effective manner. Information can be downloaded immediately onto a computer to do the number crunching. The result is more data assembled and efficiently analyzed for more accurate statistical information. The method also enables the efficient capture of data from patients, doctors, medical centers, hospitals, or health departments [11].

Good data are at the crux of any preventive strategy against a disease or illness. The 2017–2018 flu season is an example. Information gathered through e-epidemiology tracked the progress of flu activity throughout the country, and the numbers showed that particular flu season to be worse than most based on past data [12]. This information helped health professionals formulate a plan to prevent the flu from infecting more people. In a state like New Jersey, the department of health can give a week-by-week report of, for example, the number of cases of influenza in each county or the severity and effects on the population [13]. Having an almost real-time snapshot of how a disease is progressing through a population helps in planning treatment and ensuring there are enough doctors, facilities, and medicines to meet the demand.

Data Mining

The ability to access current information in large quantities helps health experts to perform data mining on a disease. Data mining involves sorting through large amounts of data in a particular category to identify patterns and establish connections [14]. In health-related matters, it helps with preventing further spread of disease. After a health crisis passes, data mining enables medical specialists to look back and carefully build a model considering how the condition began, how it spread, and what steps slowed down or eradicated the threat. By doing this, health professionals can put in place a plan to deal with a similar crisis in the future.

Health Information and News Reporting

Communication technology allows information on diseases to be broadcast quickly through various news outlets on the Internet. Not that many years ago, health crisis notification meant waiting for information to come out in the newspaper or on one of the few newscasts available on radio or TV. In our world of 24/7 media, if a message needs to go out about a health crisis, it is immediately sent out over the airwaves. Furthermore, every media outlet is well-represented on the Internet. While the evening news broadcasts a story on a severe outbreak of influenza, for example, an alert on a cell phone allows a user to read the story at 2:00 in the afternoon.

The Internet also provides a forum for doctors or health experts to share their expertise and immediately make the information accessible to anyone who needs it. Writing blogs or recording the video equivalent ("vlogs") makes a great deal of information available for other healthcare professionals to study [15]. Healthcare is a constant process of researching and finding out what works and what doesn't against a given illness or disease. Solutions to health problems are usually a collaborative effort where doctors and scientists build on the information of others. There was a time when such information could be found only in printed journals or books, but now the choices are much broader and readily available.

Social Media

An extension of reporting diseases and helping to prevent them on the Internet is through the use of social media. There are social media sites geared toward healthcare professionals; an example is a site called Sermo. With over a half-million users, the site allows doctors to connect with each other and offers the opportunity for doctors to elicit their peers' opinion on a current medical problem [16]. Many of these sites allow instant communication among medical professionals regarding general medical issues or those dealt with in a specialist's practice.

General social media sites are also an important source of information. The Pew Research Center determined that, in general, Facebook and other social media sites played an important role in providing news information to the public. The combined figure reported for Facebook and YouTube was 64% [17]. Throw in all other forms of social media, and one can grasp the impact on the population. Therefore, if there is news on an epidemic or if information needs to be gathered from the general population, social media can be utilized as another outlet.

Online Teaching

Online education is prevalent across every subject on many different levels, including health and medicine. Many colleges have an online presence for classes, as do specialty schools that concentrate on one discipline. For medical professionals, this helps them keep up with the latest medical information and enables them to work on their formal continuing medical education credits to maintain their certification or to earn other degrees in health and medicine.

There are several advantages to online education. It is usually easier to work online courses into a person's schedule. Most people in the health field are so busy doing their job that it can be almost impossible to find the time to drive to a school and go to class on a set schedule. At least with online learning, they don't need to commute, and many online courses contain video lectures, so a doctor or health professional can fit them into their schedule, even at 11:00 p.m.

As with most things on the Internet, online courses can make immediate use of the latest information. As we have seen, current information is critical in the health and medical field. Also, professionals in rural areas or developing countries can receive the same up-to-date material that students are receiving at Harvard Medical School. Online teaching has been a significant factor in breaking down the barriers of distance and the lack of local teaching facilities for health professionals. Finally, online courses are usually much less expensive than ones held on-campus, and students can avoid transportation, housing, and parking costs as an added benefit [18].

It isn't only professionals that benefit from the boom in online learning. The Internet has given anyone with a computer and the means to connect the opportunity to learn anything about the health field. Organizations like UNICEF and Doctors Without Borders use digital technology to help educate people on essential issues like basic clean water, sanitation, and hygiene [19]. People from all over the world can become connected and obtain information on health issues and solutions.

Barriers to Access

The biggest obstacle to the use of digital healthcare options is that people first need to have the Internet and then have a device to access it.

Connectivity

First, let us look at hooking up to the Internet. In the early years of Internet connectivity, a computer was hooked up to a telephone line and dialed into an Internet service provider, but dial-up speeds were too slow for downloading large files or streaming sound clips or videos, and access meant tying up telephone lines. By the late 1990s, the fastest dial-up connection available to most users was only 56 Kbps. Then in the early 2000s, broadband technology was developed and the Internet became a high-speed network. Not only could users connect without the use of a telephone line, but connections were much faster [20]. By 2001, broadband subscriptions had increased by 50% and, by 2010, it was used by over 65% of households in the United States [21]. Since then, developments such as 4G mobile broadband and fiber optic cable have allowed faster and more reliable Internet access. Most of the eHealth technology developments discussed in this chapter would not be viable without broadband technology.

However, even today, not everyone has access to high-speed Internet, including within the United States. According to Federal Communications Commission (FCC) reports, although 21 million Americans gained access to broadband by 2016, 34 million residents remained without broadband providers in their community [22]. For example, most areas in the state of Connecticut have high-speed Internet access, while in Mississippi, the number is closer to one-third of residents. At the local level, residents in more than 200 counties have no broadband access [22].

This scenario plays itself out across the world. Many regions in developing countries, such as in Africa or Asia, as well as those in more technologically advanced countries, cannot make use of the software, apps, and online tools discussed here because they cannot connect to the high-speed Internet. Most Internet companies are private, and if they are looking at a specific geographical area and decide that installing broadband service will be unprofitable, they will move on to an area that will. In developing countries, often the necessary infrastructure is lacking to establish a network. In these areas people rely on dial-up or satellite if either is available.

Affordability

Having broadband service in an area is only one part of the equation. Another is the issue of affordability. In the United States, many households cannot afford to contract with a local service provider. Ninety-two percent of U.S. households with incomes greater than USD75,000 have broadband subscriptions, while less than half with incomes of less than USD20,000 per year can afford one [22]. In Canada, income plays the greatest role in determining Internet access, more than level of education, location, age, or gender [23]. In addition, service providers may decide against installing expensive equipment and infrastructure if they don't believe there is demand for it on the part of consumers. Rural, lower-income, or aging communities may be left out since they are less likely to subscribe [22]. A related issue involves people who cannot afford to buy a laptop, phone, or tablet to access the Internet. Even finding a doctor becomes a formidable challenge when a prospective patient cannot go online.

Digital and Health Literacy

In addition to technological and financial access barriers to online health services, there is also the issue of so-called health literacy, or the ability to obtain, process, and understand basic healthcare information and how the healthcare system works and then use this information to make the proper healthcare -related choices [1]. A closely related concept is that of digital literacy, or the ability to find and use digital content, create digital content, and communicate or share it [24].

Some of the same factors behind the digital divide and digital literacy also drive health literacy, issues of access and communication, physical or mental limitations, and social factors, such as level of education, language, culture, or age. In the United States, the National Institutes of Health (NIH) reported that more than 90 million people had low health literacy [25]. Individuals with low health literacy tend to be more skeptical of health technologies and find themselves overwhelmed by the vast amount of available information. They are less likely to spend time online reading about health and new treatment options or creating online accounts for medical records access.

Demographics Issues – Age, Ethnicity, and Race

Many individuals with low health literacy are older or elderly. Internet usage by people over the age of 65 drops off noticeably, and while cost can certainly be a factor for a retired person on a fixed income, often individuals at this stage in life without Internet never learned how to use a computer and see no reason to use one or to become connected to cyberspace. Approximately one-third of Americans over 65 do not use broadband, compared to the less than one-fifth of Americans below 65 who do [22].

There is also evidence that race and ethnicity affect a person's ability to access the Internet. The U.S. Census Bureau's 2017 statistics on the digital divide indicated 36.4% of black non-Hispanics had no broadband or computer, followed by 30.3% Hispanics, 21.2% whites, and 11.9% Asians [26]. Learning online is one indicator of this effect. In a survey of online education, the racial identification of such students in the United States was white 46.6%, black 24.8%, Hispanic 20.8%, 3.2% Asian, and 4.6% all other groups [27].

Cultural Barriers

The interplay between cultural norms, lack of Internet access, and low health literacy creates barriers to eHealth service access, especially in developing countries. The most severely affected groups are often women and children. In some countries, women may face sociocultural norms that discourage independence and prevent them from making financial decisions, including purchasing and using a cell phone or computer. According to a 2014 Telecom Regulatory Authority of India report, out of 900 million-plus cell phone subscribers, only 30% were female [28]. Fears of mobile phone use leading to adultery and distraction from studies led to a ban on cell phone use in villages in three Indian states, while in Morocco a woman was stoned to death for owning a cell phone. In sub-Saharan Africa, women are 43% less likely to be online [29]. While in the developing world 25% fewer women than men can access the Internet, in regions like sub-Saharan Africa the gender gap approaches 45% [30]. In contrast, Internet use by all is highly encouraged in some Asian countries, such as South Korea, where it is viewed as an educational tool with the potential to improve one's status or future [31].

English proficiency plays a crucial role, given that much of online content is in the English language. In countries like Singapore or in Hong Kong, where English is one of the official languages, Internet use is much higher [32]. In countries where

English language education is not readily available, obtaining, using, and sharing information via the Internet is more difficult. Although social media and mobile phones in native languages allow more opportunities for access and information, English proficiency remains a significant barrier of access to online education, eHealth applications, and information [32].

Efforts to Reduce the Digital Healthcare Divide

The digital divide exists primarily because of cost and accessibility. However, electricity was once looked upon as a luxury and not a necessity; now the Internet is experiencing the same transformation around the world. Most countries realize that it is a vital tool to bind nations together and to provide valuable services to the world's citizens, including healthcare. The United Nations has identified Internet access as a basic human right [33].

Telemedicine and other Internet-based platforms are becoming more and more popular in the United States. Many of the web-based health services discussed earlier in the chapter are available to and utilized by a growing number of people. As many as 15 million people in the U.S. utilized telemedicine services in 2015, an increase of 50% over previous years [34]. However, even in a developed country like the U.S., more effort is needed to bridge the digital divide. The FCC's Universal Service Fund and the Department of Agriculture's Rural Utility Service program are making efforts to bring broadband to all parts of the country, much like it did with electrifying the entire country in the 1930s [35]. The cost is not cheap. The 2010 National Broadband Initiative estimated that a USD24 billion federal investment is necessary to bring rural America up to an adequate level of broadband service [36]. In 2015, President Obama announced a broadband initiative, ConnectHome, to assist low-income and rural students in connecting to the Internet at home. A joint venture between the Department of Housing and Urban Development (HUD), private companies, and nonprofits was put together to overcome the "homework gap" caused by lower-income/rural students' inability to access the Internet to complete homework assignments. The goal was to connect 20 million people to high-speed Internet by 2020. Since 2015, 37% of HUD-assisted homes with children have gained Internet access through the ConnectHome program [37].

In Europe, the European Union (EU) has taken on a bold initiative to ensure universal access to broadband across the continent by 2020. The EU recognizes the many advantages of the high-speed Internet and is working at erasing the digital divide. Europe's lack of monopoly providers ensures that there is more competition, resulting in better technology, higher-quality service, and cheaper Internet access [38]. However, as in the United States, the biggest issue is connecting rural communities. The EU has launched initiatives using monetary incentives to encourage Internet providers to move into geographical areas they normally would not consider [39]. Recognizing the power of the Internet as an epidemiology tool, the EU began programs like MEDISYS, a "media monitoring system providing event-based surveillance to rapidly identify potential public health threats using information from media reports" [40]. The system displays only those articles with interest to public health (e.g., diseases, plant pests, and psychoactive substances), analyzes news reports, and warns users via automatically generated alerts [40]. European interest in new digital health options is also reflected in the popularity of two health and fitness apps, in the UK (Your.MD) and in Sweden (KRY) [41]. Europe lags behind the U.S. in use of telemedicine, and as of 2015, Europe was without regulatory guidance regarding reimbursement by the public healthcare sector. The demand for Internet healthcare services is there, but the market conditions need to improve, and further innovation in healthcare apps is necessary for the market to grow [42].

In India, Telemedicine is the country's ambitious program of examining, treating, and monitoring patients through wireless broadband facilities. As with most countries, the problem is delivering broadband access to the many rural communities in India. According to the World Bank, "Over the past five years, there has been a veritable explosion of technology and consumerism in India, but this has occurred largely in urban and middle-class communities" [43]. However, rural India has 600,000 villages scattered throughout rural areas of the country, with over 500 million inhabitants who remain behind technologically. These communities have remained unchanged through the centuries, a multitude of villages encircled by small farms, the laborers low-income and landless with little opportunity to improve their standard of living. Knowledge of best agricultural practices, larger-scale markets, or information about earnings opportunities is beyond reach [43].

For both its Telemedicine program and broadband access, India still has a long way to go. However, the government's goal is a digital economy, and broadband Internet is an excellent foundation to build on. Like the EU, when the government takes high-speed Internet access seriously, it can cause implementation to move faster than without government support.

According to June 2019 statistics, about 39.8% of the African population has Internet access [44]. The challenge in Africa is the vast expanse of rural areas that can comprise anything from impenetrable jungles to endless deserts. In these regions, the growth of broadband Internet is not the only problem; many homes throughout Africa are not even connected to the electric grid [45]. The big cities are better connected as government institutions, businesses, banking, and health services require high-speed service. South Africa is an enthusiastic utilizer of online education, and the country is establishing broadband service as quickly as it can [46], with 33.7% of the country's residents 15 years or older using the Internet [45]. For the very remote areas, satellite companies are establishing service to reduce the need to expand broadband infrastructure into those towns [47].

The technical body of the African Union, the New Partnership for Africa's Development (NEPAD), provides support for infrastructure development in part through its Programme for Infrastructure Development (PIDA). PIDA supports the promotion of a favorable policy environment for information and communications technology (ICT) growth in Africa by mobilizing financial capital and providing open markets with free and fair competition [48]. The related Community of

Practice on Regional Integration and Trade focuses on the improvement of infrastructure, market development, and trade across Africa. Its goal is for the African continent to establish a reliable, modern infrastructure to help support its businesses and population [49].

For those with connectivity, groups like Telemedicine Africa and eHealth Africa (eHA) are striving to provide virtual health services to underserved and distant populations. Telemedicine Africa, founded by female African physician Moretlo Molefi, is a network of physicians and other healthcare professionals that provide interactive healthcare solutions in South Africa. The Telemedicine Center of Excellence facility is staffed with a general practitioner and medical specialists who monitor and diagnose cases reported from referral sites. Once a referral site has the proper equipment, it can connect to the Virtual Telehealth Centre network and take advantage of the service. The network provides community care, clinical basic healthcare, and services to local hospitals, along with wellness management and corporate health solutions [50].

eHA is based in Nigeria but provides public health emergency systems, disease surveillance systems, laboratory and diagnostic centers, and nutrition and food security systems to communities in Guinea, Sierra Leone, and Liberia. Working with the Sierra Leone Ministry of Health and Sanitation, eHA established a 117-call center as part of a health reporting system during the recent Ebola outbreak and set up a field epidemiologists training program (FETP) to build a local public health workforce to monitor disease. In Nigeria, eHA expanded the health system's capacity to provide services to populations in hard-to-reach areas using a central tracking system on a weekly basis to gather data on immunization rates and services provided by local healthcare facilities. Currently, solutions include Aether, a secure and reliable information-sharing platform, Electronic Integrated Disease Surveillance and Response (eIDSR), which tracks epidemiologically relevant data on challenging health conditions and diseases, the LOMIS logistics organization and tracking system, and VaxTrac, a vaccination registry used in the field to track immunization records [51].

Like Africa, Asia is an expansive continent, and there is a significant disparity of broadband availability. The UN Economic and Social Commission for Asia and the Pacific (ESCAP) has found that broadband capabilities and access are highly concentrated in East and Northeast Asia, at 74% of total fixed broadband subscriptions. South and Southwest Asia follow at 9.77%, North and Central Asia at 7.68%, Southeast Asia at 5.74%, and the Pacific at just 1.93%, according to a 2015 study conducted by ESCAP [52]. This means that in Asian countries, developed areas like South Korea and the highly developed regions of China have a more established broadband infrastructure and services. As observed throughout the rest of the world, bringing broadband into undeveloped areas takes a long time because of infrastructure issues and cost.

Conclusion

The digital divide is very real for much of the world, but hard to comprehend if you live in an area with easy and immediate access to anything digital. The good news is that many governments and economic bodies realize the advantages of high-speed Internet access. Studies show that it increases prosperity, lowers unemployment, facilitates commerce and healthcare, and leads to a better-informed society. When government bodies or individual nations take these advantages to heart, they make broadband access a policy priority. For larger countries with a great deal of rural territory, the prospect of bringing the country together with high-speed Internet can be daunting. As with many national issues, the problems revolve around cost. Countries that align their policies with financial support stand a better chance of achieving their goals than countries that do not.

Necessity also drives the need for expanded broadband coverage. As discussed here, many healthcare programs and apps utilizing the Internet are ineffective or completely useless without high-speed Internet access. When you factor in banking, other financial venues, commerce, logistics, and other aspects, countries will find it easy to justify wiring up their citizens.

While cost and connectivity are the most significant barriers, the constant turnover of communications technologies can reduce those constraints. Most technology becomes less expensive over time. Its efficiency increases, better production methods lower costs, and competition drives prices down. One need only look at the price of consumer items like flat-screen televisions and computers over the past 10 years to see how dramatically prices can fall.

Technology is also an unknown in the sense that we don't know what is around the corner. Smartphones are now a staple in our lives, yet the first iPhone celebrated its tenth anniversary just recently in 2017 [53]. We can predict what the near future might bring, but we don't know what lies beyond that. Some corporation or even just two people tinkering in a garage might invent a device to connect more people to broadband more cheaply than ever before.

There is a digital divide, but nations, companies, and individuals are working hard at overcoming it. Overcoming that divide will improve the life of every man, woman, and child with respect to healthcare, education, economic prospects, and general quality.

Case Study: Rural Village Clinic

You have been working as an internal medicine physician along with a nurse practitioner in a small rural African village, located approximately 121 kilometers outside a metropolitan area. Although you initially encounter some resistance, you set up a small clinic to care for the basic health needs of the villagers. In most cases, they have been able to provide care using folk medicine, and the primary role of the clinic has been to monitor the villagers' general health and document the effectiveness of their traditional treatment methods. Thus far, recordkeeping has consisted of handwritten notes and files on laptops. There is some Internet connectivity – Wi-Fi is very unreliable, so most of the connectivity is provided via satellite.

The village lies along a well-traveled road, and members of other villages often pass through to trade goods and visit friends and relatives. Recently visitors have been describing a strange illness, resistant to all traditional remedies, affecting the old and very young in a neighboring village. From their description, it sounds like the flu, but you can't be sure. You realize you and the villagers could be in danger of contracting this illness, and you need to come up with a plan to handle what could turn out to be an epidemic.

1. Problem statement: Identify the problems involved with your situation.
2. Decision criteria: Develop appropriate decision criteria to use in addressing the problems.
3. Planning and priority setting: Describe your short- and long-term goals based on the foregoing information and in the chapter.
4. Operational issues: Identify a minimum of three key operational issues you will need to address, and discuss what strategies you will employ.
5. Evaluation: Identify three organizational outcomes you will use to evaluate your success. Include how and how frequently they will be measured and tracked.

References

1. McInnis M. Population health management 101: new strategies and tools to care for high-risk patients. Healthcare IT News. https://www.healthcareitnews.com/news/population-health-management-101-new-strategies-and-tools-care-high-risk-patients. Published February 3, 2016. Accessed 26 July 2019.
2. Population Health Management – nachc.org. http://www.nachc.org/wp-content/uploads/2018/02/Action-Guide_Pop-Health_Risk-Stratification-Sept-2017.pdf. Accessed 25 July 2019.
3. Loria G. Population health tools for small practices. Software Advice. https://www.softwareadvice.com/resources/population-health-tools/. Published January 18, 2019. Accessed 26 July 2019.
4. Predictive Analytics Solutions in Healthcare. Health Catalyst. https://www.healthcatalyst.com/predictive-analytics. Accessed 26 July 2019.
5. Pennic F. 10 Recommended health IT tools to achieve population health management. Healthcare IT News. http://hitconsultant.net/2013/10/18/10-recommended-health-tools-achieve-population-health-management/. Published October 18, 2013. Accessed 26 July 2019.
6. Garg AX, Adhikari NK, McDonald H, et al. Effects of computerized clinical decision support systems on practitioner performance and patient outcomes: a systematic review. JAMA. 2005;293:1223–38.
7. Duffy J. The best fitness apps for 2019. PCMAG. https://www.pcmag.com/article2/0,2817,2485287,00.asp. Published December 28, 2018. Accessed 26 July 2019.
8. In-Depth: How WebMD navigated the rise of digital health. MobiHealthNews. https://www.mobihealthnews.com/content/depth-how-webmd-navigated-rise-digital-health. Published January 29, 2016. Accessed 26 July 2019.
9. Coombs B. Health-care insurers are beefing up their apps to make you like them more. CNBC. https://www.cnbc.com/2018/01/26/health-care-insurers-are-beefing-up-their-apps-to-make-you-like-them-more.html. Published January 27, 2018. Accessed 26 July 2019.

10. What is Epidemiology? | Teacher Roadmap | Career Paths to Public Health | CDC. Centers for Disease Control and Prevention. https://www.cdc.gov/careerpaths/k12teacherroadmap/epidemiology.html. Accessed 26 July 2019.
11. van Gelder MMHJ, Pijpe A. E-epidemiology: a comprehensive update. OA Epidemiol. 2013;1(1):5.
12. Estimated Influenza Illnesses, Medical visits, Hospitalizations, and Deaths in the United States – 2017–2018 influenza season | CDC. Centers for Disease Control and Prevention. https://www.cdc.gov/flu/about/burden/2017-2018.htm. Accessed 26 July 2019.
13. Patel J. Communicable Disease Service. Department of Health | Communicable Disease Service | Seasonal Influenza. https://www.state.nj.us/health/cd/topics/flu.shtml. Accessed 26 July 2019.
14. Joshi S, Nair MK. Prediction of Heart Disease Using Classification Based Data Mining Techniques. SpringerLink. https://link.springer.com/chapter/10.1007/978-81-322-2208-8_46. Published January 1, 1970. Accessed 26 July 2019.
15. Indiana University. Online video blogs (a.k.a. vlogs) as tools for patient engagement: Is seeing engaging? ScienceDaily. https://www.sciencedaily.com/releases/2017/02/170202123037.htm. Published February 2, 2017. Accessed 26 July 2019.
16. Wertens L. Top 20 social networks for Doctors and Healthcare professionals. UpCity. https://upcity.com/blog/top-20-social-networks-for-doctors/. Published June 4, 2019. Accessed 26 July 2019.
17. Kozlowska H. Facebook is still a hugely popular news source in the US, though users expect the news to be fake. Quartz. https://qz.com/1386624/americans-are-still-getting-a-lot-of-their-news-from-facebook/. Published September 11, 2018. Accessed 26 July 2019.
18. Rapp A. Why Online Medical Education Is Here To Stay: Part I. Electronic Medical Certification. https://emedcert.com/blog/online-medical-education-part1. Published September 22, 2015. Accessed 26 July 2019.
19. UNICEF. https://www.unicef.org/. Accessed 26 July 2019.
20. Warner D. The history of broadband from the '80s to today. uSwitch. https://www.uswitch.com/broadband/guides/broadband_history/. Published April 1, 2019. Accessed 26 July 2019.
21. Eha BP. An accelerated history of internet speed (Infographic). Entrepreneur. https://www.entrepreneur.com/article/228489. Published September 25, 2013. Accessed 26 July 2019.
22. Heinrich M. America's digital divide. Democratic Staff of the U.S. Congress Joint Economic Committee. September 2017.
23. Reddick A, Boucher C, Groseilliers M. The dual digital divide, the information highway in Canada. Ottowa: Public Interest Advocacy Center; 2000.
24. Heitin L. What is digital literacy? Education Week. https://www.edweek.org/ew/articles/2016/11/09/what-is-digital-literacy.html. Published February 20, 2019. Accessed 26 July 2019.
25. Health Literacy. MedlinePlus. https://medlineplus.gov/healthliteracy.html. Published May 1, 2019. Accessed 26 July 2019.
26. The Digital Divide. Percentage of Households by Broadband Internet Subscription, Computer Type, Race and Hispanic Origin. US Department of Commerce, Economics and Statistics Administration https://www.census.gov/content/dam/Census/library/visualizations/2017/comm/digital-divide-percent.jpg. Accessed 26 July 2019.
27. Education and Careers. https://blog.classesandcareers.com/education/infographics/student-demographics-infographic/. Accessed 26 July 2019.
28. Potnis D. 8 Economic Barriers Responsible for India's Gender Digital Divide. ICTworks. https://www.ictworks.org/8-economic-barriers-responsible-for-indias-gender-digital-divide/. Published January 2, 2018. Accessed 26 July 2019.
29. Edwards S. Cultural barriers need to be challenged to close the gender digital divide. Devex. https://www.devex.com/news/cultural-barriers-need-to-be-challenged-to-close-the-gender-digital-divide-90213. Published May 8, 2017. Accessed 26 July 2019.

30. Sow R. Women and ICT in Africa: A new digital gap. Africa | Al Jazeera. http://www.aljazeera.com/indepth/opinion/2014/05/women-ict-africa-new-digital-ga-201452210244121558.html. Published May 23, 2014. Accessed 26 July 2019.

31. Sang-hun C. In South Korea, all of life is mobile. The New York Times. https://www.nytimes.com/2009/05/25/technology/25iht-mobile.html. Published May 24, 2009. Accessed 26 July 2019.

32. Pearce KE, Rice RE. The language divide – the persistence of English proficiency as a gateway to the internet: the cases of Armenia, Azerbaijan, and Georgia. Intl J of Comm. 2014;8:2834–59.

33. Sandle T. UN thinks internet access is a human right. Business Insider. Digital Journal. http://www.businessinsider.com/un-says-internet-access-is-a-human-right-2016-7. Published July 22, 2016. Accessed 26 July 2019.

34. InDemand Interpreting. Telehealth. https://www.indemandinterpreting.com/wp-content/uploads/2017/03/InDemand-Interpreting-Trends-patient-telehealth.pdf. Accessed 26 July 2019.

35. Universal Service. Federal Communications Commission. https://www.fcc.gov/general/universal-service. Published July 25, 2019. Accessed 26 July 2019.

36. Kruger LG, Gilroy AA, Goldfarb CB. The National Broadband Plan. CRS Report for Congress. Congressional Research Service. July 9, 2010.

37. ConnectHomeUSA. https://connecthomeusa.org/. Accessed 26 July 2019.

38. Miller CC. Why the U.S. Has Fallen Behind in Internet Speed and Affordability. The New York Times. https://www.nytimes.com/2014/10/31/upshot/why-the-us-has-fallen-behind-in-internet-speed-and-affordability.html. Published October 30, 2014. Accessed 26 July 2019.

39. Stupp C. Rural areas have bad internet access in most member states. euractiv.com. https://www.euractiv.com/section/broadband/interview/rural-areas-have-bad-internet-access-in-most-member-states/. Published August 4, 2017. Accessed 26 July 2019.

40. FPFIS Team. Medical Information System – MEDISYS. EU Science Hub – European Commission. https://ec.europa.eu/jrc/en/scientific-tool/medical-information-system. Published July 26, 2017. Accessed 26 July 2019.

41. Annicelli C. Investors Place Bets on European Healthcare Apps. eMarketer. https://www.emarketer.com/Article/Investors-Place-Bets-on-European-Healthcare-Apps/1016110. Published June 30, 2017. Accessed 26 July 2019.

42. Jahns R-G. European countries are behind the USA in regards to telemedicine maturity, but they're beginning to catch up. research2guidance. https://research2guidance.com/european-countries-are-behind-the-usa-in-regards-to-telemedicine-maturity-but-theyre-beginning-to-catch-up/. Published February 28, 2019. Accessed 26 July 2019.

43. Hay KAJ. Expanding broadband access in rural India: the role of alternative telecommunications networks (English) | The World Bank. http://documents.worldbank.org/curated/en/918041468258540682/Expanding-broadband-access-in-rural-India-the-role-of-alternative-telecommunications-networks. Published July 1, 2010. Accessed 26 July 2019.

44. Africa Internet Users, 2019 Population and Facebook Statistics. Internet World Stats Usage and Population Statistics. http://www.internetworldstats.com/stats1.htm. Accessed 26 July 2019.

45. Stork C, Calandro E, Gamage R. The future of Broadband in Africa. Research ICT Africa – policy brief. Published July 2013. Accessed 26 July 2019.

46. Sidler V. Online learning – the future of education in South Africa. MyBroadband.. https://mybroadband.co.za/news/industrynews/265149-online-learning-the-future-of-education-in-south-africa.html. Accessed 26 July 2019.

47. 10 Positive Roles of Satellite Internet Providers in Africa. Answers Africa. https://answersafrica.com/satellite-internet-africa.html. Published May 3, 2018. Accessed 26 July 2019.

48. Navuri A. African Governments urged to rethink ICT as a prime and primary sector. Virtual PIDA Information Centre. http://www.au-pida.org/news/african-governments-urged-to-rethink-ict-as-a-prime-and-primary-sector/. Published July 18, 2019. Accessed 26 July 2019.

49. Integration R. Infrastructure and trade: AUDA. NEPAD. . https://www.nepad.org/cop/regional-integration-infrastructure-and-trade. Accessed 26 July 2019

50. Telemedicine Africa – About Us. http://www.telemedafrica.co.za/about-us. Accessed 26 July 2019.
51. Health Delivery Systems. eHealth Africa – Building stronger health systems in Africa. https://www.ehealthafrica.org/health-delivery/. Accessed 26 July 2019.
52. Okuda A, Vakataki 'Ofa S, Dukda S, Kravchenko A. State of ICT in Asia and the Pacific 2016: Uncovering the Widening Broadband Divide. Information and Communications Technology and Disaster Risk Reduction Division. ReliefWeb. https://reliefweb.int/report/world/state-ict-asia-and-pacific-2016-uncovering-widening-broadband-divide. Accessed 26 July 2019.
53. Berak D. iPhone 10 year anniversary – how smartphones changed our lives. Chinavasion. https://blog.chinavasion.com/45582/iphone-10-year-anniversary-how-smartphones-changed-our-lives/. Published June 29, 2017. Accessed 26 July 2019.

Chapter 16: Technology for Creating Better Professional Teams to Strengthen Healthcare Systems

Elvira Beracochea and Aaron Pied

The Importance of Teams and a Strong Workforce

Healthcare providers, including doctors, nurses, and other health professionals, are the foundation of any health system. Health systems need competent people to follow and implement programs and to deliver healthcare services in an effective, efficient, and organized fashion. Healthcare has become complex, and thus the days of a solo practitioner are past. Healthcare today requires teams of primary healthcare providers, specialists, and laboratory, radiology, information, and pharmacy technicians, as well as many other workers, to deliver quality healthcare according to accepted evidence-based standards. An effective and competent health team is essential to deliver healthcare efficiently and consistently. In addition to sound clinical skills, a health team also needs the skills and tools of public health, healthcare management, human resource management, and financial knowledge. The challenge of pre-service education is to provide future healthcare providers with the knowledge, skills, and tools required to meet the health needs of a country's people. The challenge of continuous education is to continue improving the performance of healthcare providers throughout their career to meet the changing needs of a population.

Before we go further, let us step back and look at a health system as we define it, to provide a perspective on the impact of technology in preparing current and future healthcare providers to implement new, improved public health policies and programs and to deliver quality services. Healthcare providers from donor countries come to help their colleagues in host countries to find ways to solve the many health

E. Beracochea (✉)
Realizing Global Health, Fairfax, VA, USA
e-mail: elvira@realizingglobalhealth.com

A. Pied
Abt Associates, Boston, MA, USA

system problems. Then, the healthcare providers in the host country system must ultimately ensure whether disease control and healthcare delivery programs succeed or fail in saving lives.

A Healthcare System Defined

A healthcare system is the organization of a country to deliver a continuum of care to its people, from promotion and prevention to diagnostic, treatment, and rehabilitation services. Every country has an organized system to deliver a continuum of services through public and private health facilities. These facilities are responsible for implementing health programs developed and usually led by the host country governments; health programs are the means through which health systems function. Every country designs its health programs to better conform to the epidemiological profile of their people to meet the needs of all, or at least those that need the most help and are most vulnerable. For that reason, there are child health programs, programs for safe motherhood, for the elderly, and to control diseases such as acquired immunodeficiency syndrome (AIDS), diabetes, cancer, and malaria. The goal is to have health programs that guide the services the facilities provide. A health program defines who does what and how and sets standards of care. For example, a maternal health program sets that at minimum a pregnant mother needs to have four antenatal care visits and to be delivered by a trained healthcare provider.

Health systems are the vehicle through which health programs are implemented and healthcare services are delivered. Without a system, quality and access to healthcare for all cannot be ensured or sustained consistently across an entire nation. Without quality health systems, we cannot ensure that people can be tested and treated for human immunodeficiency virus (HIV), that every infant is protected against vaccine-preventable conditions, or that a complicated pregnancy undergoes the timely care that saves a woman's life. Donor-funded projects help improve how health programs are implemented and how health facilities work. However, although a project funded by a donor may, for example, train healthcare providers and provide supplies to ensure all pregnant women are tested for HIV, if the health system teams are not strengthened, all these improvements will end when the project ends, with a return to earlier conditions. In short, if the results achieved by the donor-funded intervention are not integrated as part of the health system, these changes are not sustainable.

Therefore, after decades of trying to improve only the programs, such as HIV or malaria programs, or to improve provision of services, through such interventions as antenatal, delivery, or postpartum care, global health leaders now realize they must invest in strengthening the country's health system to sustain these programs and services and maintain the benefit of donor investments. Now, strengthening the health systems is finally receiving deserved attention, particularly to achieve universal health coverage as part of Sustainable Development Goal 3 (SDG3).

Health system strengthening has three main goals:

1. **Better programs.** Here, strengthening focuses on improving the country's public health programs, not the donor's projects such as PEPFAR or Feed the Future, but to improve the organization and management of the country's programs.
2. **Better services.** Here, strengthening focuses on improving the operational procedures for health facilities, that is, community-based posts, clinics, health centers, and hospitals, to deliver quality health services efficiently and consistently to every person, everywhere, every day. Effective standard operating procedures based on evidence-based standards help ensure the quality of care delivered in every facility by every healthcare provider.
3. **Better teams.** Here, strengthening focuses on improving the knowledge and skills of health professionals and the management support they receive to function as more effective teams. To have better teams of healthcare providers, the country must improve its pre-service and continuous education programs, human resource management, and support of professional associations to ensure health professionals can meet professional accreditation and certification standards and continue to do so consistently.

The Right to Health, Country Ownership, and Sustainable Development Goal 3 (SDG3)

You may be wondering about the purpose of all these statements and why a country's government must be involved. The answer is that the main purpose of a health system is to protect and fulfill the right to health of every citizen in the country. Under international human rights law, the government of each country is responsible for protecting and fulfilling that right, among all other human rights. The law does not state the government must provide healthcare for all, although some countries choose to do so, but seeks to ensure vulnerable citizens are protected and everyone has access to quality healthcare. Because the right to health has not been fulfilled in every country, the progressive realization of this right remains a global health goal: hence, SDG3.

With today's technology and the knowledge to treat, even cure, most of the diseases that kill millions, we now are much closer to fulfilling this right for most of the world's populations. Thus, this chapter is important. Using technology we can reach every healthcare provider and ensure their access to up-to-date knowledge, their opportunities to improve and reinforce their healthcare delivery skills, and the support they need to address challenges and solve problems in their work.

The implementation of solutions to strengthen the health system of a country, to realize the right to health, requires strengthening the leadership of the country. Health system strengthening must empower its leaders who must have full country ownership of its health system and its development. Technology also helps support a country's leaders to make the right decisions with the right knowledge, evidence-based information, skills, and tools. Leadership empowerment and sustainability can also be developed using technology, and this will be accomplished by empowering them to develop the workforce that will implement improved programs and deliver better services.

Given the thousands of healthcare providers who are involved in a health system, an affordable and effective strategy and the means to continue to develop their knowledge and skills, and which provides the tools to deliver quality healthcare that meets the changing needs of the people they serve, are essential. This is where internet-based education comes in.

What Does Effective Internet-Based Education Look Like?

When talking about using technology to educate healthcare providers and a country's health leadership, many different terms are used: eLearning, mLearning, online education, digital learning, social learning, distance learning, computer learning, mobile education, and blended learning. All these terms overlap, and many are used interchangeably, but there are differences in their application. This chapter does not explore all these terms but is concerned specifically with internet-based education, which is a component of the commonly used term eLearning (electronic learning). eLearning includes learning via all types of electronic media, to improve how healthcare leaders and providers perform in developing countries.

Internet-based education is material delivered via the internet, such as accessing a learning management platform via the web or downloading a syllabus and materials to learn about a specific topic. The main distinction here is that all learning is done remotely, without physical presence (classroom). Many of the terms already mentioned are a component, or an offshoot, of internet-based education, and we touch upon them; however, it should be noted that much research on the efficacy of internet-based education is limited to wealthy and middle-income countries and universities. Therefore, as we discuss the potential and current application of internet-based education for health professionals in developing countries, we are largely extrapolating strategies based on current data and our own experience of internet-based training in the field of global health.

Why Internet-Based Training for Global Health?

Despite the obvious challenges with infrastructure, in developing countries events are developing rapidly. For example, "many African countries are upgrading their internal digital infrastructure, and international internet connectivity is rapidly moving from satellites to high bandwidth undersea cables" [1]. Therefore, although internet access may be limited in developing countries, internet-based training offers many possibilities and benefits, especially if that internet-based training can be acquired offline using mobile technologies.

Setting aside the obvious challenges of infrastructure, there are many reasons for the development of internet-based education in global health:

1. Facilitates easy access to updated information and training materials as new research and new case studies are made available;
2. Is low cost for the education provider, and also for the user who already has access to a smartphone or laptop;
3. Provides distance learning opportunities for those who cannot travel easily;
4. Reduces the cost of training workshops that traditionally involve per diem, hotel, and travel expenses;
5. Provides additional opportunities for collaboration among similar professionals to learn and problem-solve among peers;
6. Allows greater opportunity for the user to work through a challenge at work in real time;
7. Provides more flexibility for the user in the time in which to learn what they want or need to learn.

During the past 15 years, there has been a rapid development of virtual training resources in all sectors around the world. These resources include virtual meeting and presentation software such as Webex; cloud-based learning management systems such as Adobe Captivate Prime, Docebo, Matrix, Kajabi, and Moodle that turn your materials into online classrooms; content creation software such as Articulate Storyline to dynamically and interactively present your content; and countless other services and applications to host, sell, and promote your online classroom. Other developments have provided fuel to the proliferation of online training – namely, WYSIWYG (what you see is what you get) editors that allow users with minimal knowledge of computer coding to create professional-looking products. And of course, we cannot forget to mention the use of YouTube in providing easy-to-access and free-to-host video instruction.

All these resources allow virtually any organization, government, or individual with a modest budget to create web-based training on any topic. However, some hidden costs may prevent some from becoming a global health training provider: "Cost of software, facilitator-training requirements, costs of the instructors' time for developing new programs, and maintenance of the software, updates, and cost of providing learner support within the training platform. Therefore, unless an organization already has eLearning programs, it may not be possible for some organizations." [2]. Yet, the main point to take away here is that with cloud-based technologies, there is a greater opportunity to provide up-to-date information through internet-based training programs so that healthcare workers in developing countries can access the latest information to do their work effectively and efficiently.

Use of Internet-Based Education to Provide Training to Health Workers in Developing Countries

Traditional direct classroom-type training methods have been the standard and continue to prevail because of poor infrastructure, particularly in rural areas in developing countries, to support widespread internet-based learning. However, that limitation is changing as more and more developing country populations have access to mobile phones and are increasingly exposed to wi-fi and internet connections in areas serviced by electricity.

With the development of technological solutions that provide inexpensive learning platforms, some great resources that have been developed are available free for those healthcare providers with an internet connection. Many of these free internet-based resources are for global health professionals, most notably the Global Health E-Learning Center created by the United States Agency for International Development (USAID) flagship knowledge management project, K4Health. Others include courses from WHO, Fogarty Center at NIH, Johns Hopkins University, RGH, and Coursera. These sources offer free or low-cost training that is available to more and more healthcare providers. Since 2005, the Global Health eLearning center alone registered more than 97,000 learners from 246 countries who took the 50+ available courses. "Approximately 19% of learners are USAID staff (the original primary audience), while the remaining 81% represent developing world public health professionals" [3].

Where Are the Challenges in Internet-Based Learning?

Some of the training materials and courses in global health available via the internet are essentially means of sharing massive amounts of information and often lack the teacher-to-student interaction, or peer-to-peer interaction, that would ensure learning and application, not just knowledge transfer. More and more universities are offering blended courses (a mix of internet-based and person-to-person classes); however, cost and the need for physical presence for some learning activities create barriers for the healthcare providers and other health professionals in developing countries. As mentioned earlier, more opportunities are available now to access online training, and with the rise in mobile technology and access to the internet, there are more options to develop low-cost, interactive learning solutions.

In Table 1 we list questions that internet-based course developers and instructors should ask themselves to assess the usefulness and applicability of a course[1] (Wong 2010). These questions help to highlight the challenges of creating internet-based

---

[1] Text.

Table 1 Questions for internet-based course developers and instructors [4]

1. How useful will the prospective learners perceive the internet technology to be? For example, in any particular context and compared to what is currently available to them, to what extent will this technology:
(a) Increase their access to learning?
(b) Provide consistent, high-quality content?
(c) Be a convenient format in which to receive their education?
(d) Save them money?
(e) Save them time?
(f) Link to course assessment?
2. How easy will the prospective learners find this technology to use?
3. How well does this format fit in with what learners are used to and expect? Achieving interactive dialogue:
4. How will high-quality human–human (learner–tutor and learner–learner) interaction and feedback be achieved? For example, what use will be made of
a. Structured virtual seminars?
b. email, bulletin boards?
c. Real-time chat?
d. Supplementary media (e.g., video, audio, phone calls, videoconferencing)?
e. Course assessment and feedback on performance?
5. How will high-quality human–technical interaction and feedback be achieved? For example, what use will be made of
(a) Questions with automated feedback?
(b) Simulations?

Source: Reprinted from Wong, G., Greenhalgh, T., Pawson, R. (2010). Internet-based medical education: a realist review of what works, for whom and in what circumstances. BMC Med Educ 10:12. https://doi.org/10.1186/1472-6920-10-12, licensed under the terms of the Creative Commons Attribution License (http://creativecommons.org/licenses/by/2.0)

courses and explain how the cost of developing an internet-based course can be quite high. More importantly, these questions also help to explain some of the challenges to develop online training programs and why there are so few data, if any, about learning outcomes at this time, despite the numerous calls for more information. There are simply too many variables in a field that is constantly changing and developing. What is clear from current existing data, however, is that as in any classroom training, internet-based training courses must factor in the needs and priorities of the learner. When we envision healthcare professionals as the target learning group, we must therefore consider the following specific challenges.

What Are the Challenges/Barriers Faced by the Global Healthcare Workforce When Using Technology to Improve Their Knowledge and Skills?

The greatest challenge for any healthcare professional may be the lack of time to complete any training. "The introduction of e-learning can represent an intrusion into the personal time and resources of a trainee" [5]. According to one study of eLearning, the "most common disadvantages reported by learners were: more time-consuming; lack of student-teacher interaction and tutor support, feelings of isolation, being unable to clarify doubts with a tutor, and lack of in-depth group discussion" [6]. Internet-based training materials, especially those that were simply transferred from traditional university course content, focus on knowledge transfer and not on improving student performance. The main barrier to success is that the courses do not always focus on application of knowledge. Unfortunately, the most difficult step in learning is to apply the knowledge to your own specific situation, which is unique to you. It is necessary to include experiential components to access the learner's own experience, while also asking them to perform tasks and then report on what they learned. Experiential learning provides healthcare providers with tools and strategies that pertain to their specific situation while learning how to adapt to future challenges of a similar nature.

Personalization of learning rather than the "one size fits all" approach is becoming a significant aspect of formal learning that provides students with a learning path based on their interaction with learning components. Content curating for learning, for instance, is the process of sorting data on the internet and presenting it in a way that is meaningful and easy to process. Such content can be used to support formal (traditional) training or as part of formal learning. Although the provider can establish learning paths, the learners control customizing and reconfiguring the way they want to learn. Therefore, content curating provides ready-to-use, real-life materials so the learner has a larger role in contributing to their own learning [7]. A source for many curated programs is YouTube, with endless presentations, videos, and speeches that provide endless resources for curated content.

Case Study

How to overcome these challenges? The experience of Realizing Global Health (RGH) with online training and coaching as a response to the need for personalized global health standardized training for healthcare providers in developing countries.

In 2005, Dr. Beracochea started a new consulting company to accelerate achieving the Millennium Development Goals (MDGs). She focused on developing ways to improve health systems so developing countries could implement better health promotion and disease prevention and treatment programs. Having healthcare professionals who are confident and capable of doing this type of work was a priority.

She realized that the usual training approach of healthcare providers leaving their place of work for a hotel for one or two weeks to acquire new knowledge was not practicable at a global scale.

The world needed better health teams to deliver quality healthcare consistently, and consistently to every patient every day everywhere, and to achieve the health MDGs. The main strategy to achieving MDGs was to ensure that services are available where most needed, and that quality of care is maintained consistently wherever care was delivered or whoever was the provider. She researched an effective approach regarding online education, but most information represented developed countries and not developing countries. Therefore, the RGH team created its own approach. Here we explain how we did it and the lessons learned so far.

First, we defined a number of principles the training had to meet, as summarized in Table 2.

- The approach had to be simple so it could be replicable and scalable at the global scale. Each online program was designed to help participants, mostly healthcare providers, to take action, starting with simple tasks, or "baby steps" such as writing a career mission and then building towards more complex actions and behaviors, such as using a checklist to meet daily performance targets. Simple training is not easy to do but makes programs clear and easily replicable with sustained quality.
- The approach had to help close the "Know–Do Gap." Based on Dr. Beracochea's study of primary healthcare providers in Papua New Guinea [8] and our own observations, we had realized that people do not always do what they know; that is, knowledge is always better than practice. For instance, healthcare providers reported that they know they should wash their hands before examining a patient or weighing a baby, but when the same provider was observed, they did not do it consistently.

Table 2 Design checklist of principles of online training in Global Health

Simple: starting with "baby steps" to make change of work routines easy and build self-confidence
Know–Do gap: training must reduce the gap between what people know and what they do
Motivation and inspiration to do well are pillars for improved performance
Professional ethics are part of the learning experience
The health system is addressed as a whole and introduces implementing standard operating procedures that improve the whole system
All sectors and every location within a country differ and therefore health professionals should adapt procedures to local circumstances without compromising quality of care
Each location in the country also differs in ability to provide electricity or internet access, which affects the use of technology in training, so low-tech options must be available
Two-way online training creates continuity in the learning process to build new work habits, and changes mindset and attitudes to ensure continuous and measurable change and improved performance results (see scorecard in the Appendix)
Be affordable at global scale

- The foundation of the RGH approach is on motivation and inspiration to change so the training participants can be motivated to do well and be inspired to meet standards consistently. For that reason, the RGH online programs are based on a story that inspires participants to change and motivates them to take risks and aim for more ambitious performance targets. The story sets the context for what the participant is to do and models leadership behavior and innovation. The RGH programs also model being a "professional" and professional ethics as well as sound medical performance. These training programs also build inspiration and motivation skills by having coaches actually personally encourage the participants to do what the characters in the story do to overcome challenges, including promoting self-motivation, motivating others, and finding inspiration in one's own work every day.
- The RGH internet-based training is "systemic," that is, the goal is for the whole health system to work better, achieve bigger coverage targets, improve quality, and protect and support healthcare providers every day. For that reason, participants understand the impact they make on the health system and how to help make it work better. They learn that every sector of the health system needs to implement standard operating procedures (SOPs), and healthcare providers are those who put the SOPs in place and make the system work for all involved. In addition to clinical skills, information systems, monitoring, and evaluation skills are part of the curriculum of every program as part of the systemic approach and also integrate accountability and self-monitoring habits. Scorecards and other tools are used to make informed decisions and take action as well as report progress and challenges using the new SOPs regularly.
- The learning approach also had to be flexible so every healthcare providers could apply the learning of the SOPs to his or her unique circumstances. For example, the degree of development and gaps of the participant's health system, resources he or she can access, and availability of transportation and electricity, water, and sanitation vary from place to place. So, the training had to be flexible to work in different situations. However, in global health, one size does not fit all, so we made the online programs simple, not easy but simple, so that the participant could fit their own situation into the context of the program. Every provider, health system level, sector, and every location within a country differs, and therefore the participant needs to learn how to address these differences across and within their country's health system. Participants are thus helped to interpret and to adapt SOPs to produce the desired improved results to achieve global health goals and local targets of their own facility or program.
- Each location in each developing country also differs in the ability to provide continuous electricity supply or internet access, thus affecting the use of technology for staff training. So, the approach had to be offered through a range of low-tech tools, starting with just sending lessons by email. Lessons and assignments are downloadable and available offline.
- The RGH approach was to build a long-term relationship too, turning trainer and participant into distance collaborating colleagues. This two-way online training approach was designed to create continuity in the learning process to build new

work habits as well as lifelong collaboration. We had seen the limited impact provided by other forms of in-person and online training. Therefore, we realized that professional development is not an unpredictable number of intermittent events, but a well-planned and executed continuous professional development process that should accompany the healthcare provider throughout their career. In this way, training can also create lifelong friendships that support each other, help us change both our own mindsets and attitudes and those of our students to ensure continuous and measurable change, so that improved performance results are sustained and individual expectations are exceeded. (See Sample Scorecard in the Appendix.)

• Finally, the training approach needed to be affordable at the global scale so that every year the critical number of leaders and healthcare providers, and better performing facilities and health teams, would increase and achieve measurable results. Global impact could then be measured in terms of the country's health indicators and global MDG targets then and now, the targets of the SDG agenda, and particularly with SDG3, which called for universal health coverage.

In short, all these traits of our online programs combined with high motivation have created what we called our low-tech/high-touch RGH approach.

Why We Started RGH Programs

We wanted something simple, not easy or simplistic, but simple, that could be rapidly scaled up. We started by defining the characteristics of our training in opposition to what was considered the usual training in global health:

1. The training was to be low cost to facilitate access at a large scale.
2. Training was also to be delivered by email daily to build professional relationships with participants as colleagues. Many of the relationships persist to this day.
3. The programs were not to take time from work and from valuable patient care.
4. We designed them so they could be undertaken while still working full time. Therefore, there was no need for per diem. The main incentive is job satisfaction and the desire to demonstrate improved results and, consequently, possible opportunities for career advancement.
5. The lessons were short and focused on helping the participant take one immediate action. We called them "knowledge bites" to ensure each lesson included one bite as opposed to training that has too much information that cannot be retained or used.
6. The programs were needed for healthcare professionals and community leaders with various backgrounds in public health. So, we emphasized the value of personal experience and their strength of character as the point of departure; we used personalized coaching through individual emails to each participant to

help them see the relevance of what they were learning in the context of their own unique circumstances and situation.

7. The content was focused on principles that participants would adapt to their unique situation with the help of a coach and not rely so much on technical information.

8. Understanding the context, gaining support from local authorities, and not giving up in the face of challenges along the way was more important than demonstrating having acquired technical knowledge. Resourcefulness was the most important resource, and the coaches' job was to be encouraging in helping participants figure out alternative courses of action and options to overcome the inevitable challenges.

9. Role models of professional behavior were presented in story format to demonstrate professionalism, integrity, honesty, and accountability; that is, complex ethical and moral principles not usually taught in global health training.

10. The relationship between coach and program participant was always focused on what was working as opposed to what was not working, or what was wrong. In this way, participants learn to value what they do as a stepping stone towards a larger goal.

11. The coach was to help the participant build on what existed and make the best of any, and whatever, resources were available. No additional resources were envisioned at the start. It was the participant's responsibility to demonstrate results first and then look for additional resources.

12. Finally, we wanted participants to be immersed in a new healthcare delivery setting with written operational procedures and set quality standards, and to see themselves as beacons of change to make accepting the status quo unacceptable. That is why they had to take daily lessons and also be in touch with their coach daily. In short, we wanted them to demonstrate leadership and desire to be better leaders, and that does not happen by attending a 3- or 5-day workshop. Change happens when we decide to change. Getting participants to commit to change and act was the ultimate success for us.

There was a technical content, too, but it was part of the SOPs that simplified the complex process of delivering quality healthcare consistently and efficiently. The programs were designed to encourage people to take action, starting with basic hygiene such as consistent handwashing, and then moving on to more complex actions such as new SOPs for maternal and child healthcare, family planning, and medicine dispensing. Coaches would ensure that participants' answers would be relevant. In many cases, there was not a right or wrong answer to the activities, but we focused on helping participants realize their desired result should be, or what the situation was that needed to change. We encourage the participants to use their own experience to figure out how to initiate the smallest change, starting with one person, one patient. In this way, we were able to value subjective views and experience, and not just objective right or wrong answers. The training was to help participants have confidence in themselves and realize that people often have the knowledge they need to take action and improve their own situation and performance. They just needed "a bit" of help to assist them with applying what they know. Consequently, coaches were trained to encourage, motivate, and inspire their "coaches" to apply their knowledge to act differently and get different results.

To this day, RGH still focuses on the same principles. We have not had to question these or change them. The challenge has been to ensure consistency across different donors and funding sources, which have varied agendas and principles. The technology and the tools for reaching more healthcare professionals through our programs have improved, but the principles for designing our online training have not altered. Today RGH continues to evolve and take advantage of the changing technology. We provide courses that take advantage of two-way communication systems so that coaches can advise the learner on how to apply what they learn in real time; courses are available on all mobile devices to provide more flexibility and reduce the need for expensive computer hardware, and we use multimedia presentations, but we can still offer programs via email only, for those in low-bandwidth areas.

The popularity of social media and mobile technology allow for more teacher-to-student and peer-to-peer interaction, which is essential for the development of teamwork needed to communicate and develop strong health systems. Better forms of communication, real-life problem solving, and real-time data acquisitions are all technological advances that are rapidly improving the quality of education and the opportunity for health professionals to learn and practice new tools and strategies.

How Did the First Distance email-Based Training Work?

Following are some examples of various programs and how we applied the principles and our results.

Case Studies

- **7-day MPH (Master Public Health).** This program was designed to master basic public health skills and awaken and develop leadership skills while giving practical basic public health skills for participants to implement short public health improvement projects. For 7 days, participants would receive an email with a chapter of a story that followed the career of a district health officer as he made changes to improve the health status of the people in his district. Along with the story chapter for that day, they received a "Learning Lesson" that included a number of "knowledge bites," that is, short content on important and essential public health concepts, as well as tools, links to additional information, and resources on the topic of the day. They received a "work guide" that included some questions for them to reflect and decide what actions they would take to elaborate their improvement project. They would email their completed work guide to their coach who would then reply within 24 h with encouraging feedback and practical advice. A coach's training manual was created that included common scenarios and how to reply to students' questions and challenges. Coaches-in-training were monitored until they demonstrated having mastered the desired degree of competence. From 2007 to 2010 more than 800 participants from more than 40 different countries took this program. Their success stories are too numerous to describe here. What is important and empowering is that the success was theirs, not that of a donor. They had ownership of the results because they had taken the leadership to change how they worked and improve their performance. For example, a client had all their field staff take the training and each of them designed new projects and were able to demonstrate results. Their satisfaction with their jobs increased as a result of having a coach who helped them make decisions, someone who was not their boss and who did not take any credit for their progress. A new version of this program is now being developed because many of our participants have encouraged us to do so, and although the program has not been offered in more than 5 years, we still get requests for this program from health providers who want to improve how they work and to move ahead in their careers. Our goal is to empower our previous participants to continue teaching this program in schools of medicine, nursing, and other settings.

- **The HFAN Program.** The Health for All NOW program was the next generation of programs. Building on the success of the 7-Day MPH, a more clinical program was developed based on the same setting: a clinic or health center in some developing nation. This time we focused on healthcare management aspects of what it takes to manage a clinic or health center and put standard operating procedures in place. Measuring indicators and accountability using a Health Facility Scorecard were crucial. Participants were asked to implement a new standard operating procedure using a process checklist and monitor its performance using one or two indicators. More than 200 participants have taken this program by email. An online version using a cloud-based technology has been developed, and donors have sponsored a number of healthcare providers.

- **The HOSW Program.** How to Organize a Successful Workshop was a newer iteration of the coaching-supported blended form of instruction offered at RGH. This course, developed at the request of a client, took advantage of a cloud-based learning management system (LMS) to provide the written content and instructional videos to participants from various organizations in Lebanon. We also provided participants with a digital textbook through Amazon, and used Skype and email to provide direct interaction with the coach. Using these tools, we provided an array of resources to the participants while working with them closely to develop individual workshops that met their own personal and professional goals. The course proved that we could teach others how to develop training online, as well how to plan and conduct a workshop that helps improve the performance of the participants' organizations.

- **Improving Healthcare in Developing Countries.** Throughout the years, we have realized that our approach to training is not for everyone. Some people just want information, although they do not use it; some want ready-made solutions and look for excuses for why it would not work in their country; and some just want the opportunity to get a few days off and some per diem money. For that reason, we have created a free introductory program that helps prospective training participants to try our experiential training and find out if it is right for them. This program applies all the principles we have described here and is focused on what the participants need to know about global health to decide what actions to take, what strategies they can use, and how to use them to make an impact in their jobs or communities. This program was launched in September 2017 and is being evaluated. We encourage you to try it and let us know what you think.

- **Global Health Career Coaching.** Another by-product of the original 7-Day MPH program was the need to streamline coaching to improve the career of healthcare providers and global health professionals in general. Our experience coaching global health professionals at various stages in their careers to achieve their career goals through our online programs helped us develop three career coaching programs to help global health professionals with their career decisions. The **Career Moves Program** helps participants decide their next career moves. It helps with defining career goals, editing the CV accordingly, and getting the help needed to get ready or actually make their next move. The **Career Success Program** helps participants to utilize their strengths to succeed in their career. They take stock of their experience and how to best demonstrate real success on their terms, and to reach more of their audience in developing countries. The **Career Transitions Program** assists participants make bold career moves to reach the next stage in a successful global health career.

All these programs are personalized and tailored to specific career needs, but they all use the same coaching principles we learned when coaching the participants of the first 7-Day MPH program: encouragement, emphasis on small incremental progress, not perfection, and problem-solving assistance are the main tools a coach needs to help another colleague to apply increased leadership skills and succeed.

Conclusion: What Does All This Mean for Internet-Based Learning in Global Health?

What is the future? Training is an effective way to transfer the expertise of one professional to another to improve global health. However, training is not effective if it does not reach all the healthcare providers who need to improve and save more lives. Also, technical knowledge is not the only thing we need to transfer to improve global health. We need to transfer attitudes and skills and practice principles that really empower health professionals in developing countries to implement the changes and improvements their health systems require; eventually, this needs to happen independently from donor support. Training, if successful, needs to demonstrate that such support will not be necessary in the future. All training funded by donors need to be sustained by local institutions, such as nursing and medical schools, to be part of the country's continuous education program. We believe that future training will meet this requirement and follow the principles listed in Table 16.2. Any training not sustained by local institutions may be well intentioned and help a few people, but it will not be replicable and will not be sustainable.

In our experience, we have observed that health professionals in developing countries are just as capable as, and usually more resourceful than, their counterparts in developed nations. They have to be more resourceful because they face more challenges and limitations. On the other hand, health professionals from developed nations have access to more and up-to-date information and seem to be more determined to never give up and to figure out a way to solve problems. Training needs to build on these strengths so that health professionals from both developed and developing nations can work together to save more lives and achieve universal health coverage. We envision creating a group of coaches who will never give up until they figure out a way to help their students succeed to make great leaders. Most of our graduates have grown professionally to become health professionals who listen and adapt their coach's advice to their own situation and then take action to change how they work. They have become great leaders and agents of change.

Our experience has shown us that it is the in-service training that must change to achieve not only better results, but also sustainable results, and to never undermine the country's ownership of any results or improvements achieved. Donors should not focus on attribution and taking credit for what they do. Instead, they need to account for their contribution, and sponsor larger numbers of health professionals to implement change in their country, supported by coaches who do not take the credit for their students.

We look forward to a future where donors fund and track the results of a large-scale, in-service training program of health professionals. This program will lead to an increasing number of clinics, health centers, and hospitals where these health professionals are using standard operating procedures to meet quality standards of care consistently. In this way, donors will support country leaders to improve how they manage their own programs, deliver services, and measure and account for their performance indicators. Fortunately, the tools and the technology are available to accomplish this goal. We plan to continue the evolution of internet-based training pedagogy to ensure that we reach the largest number of health professionals and provide customizable courses that meet the needs of the entire health system, and not the success of only an individual project or donor. We hope that some of those reading this chapter will become coaches and go on to create new and innovative programs. Why not you?

Appendix. Sample Health Scorecard

Month: _____ Year:____ Facility:_____.

Clinic No. 1: Annual target/objective indicator	Monthly average score or result	Score/ result this month	Progress to date	Action
1. Newborns delivered and visited in the first week	98/75	91/90	99% coverage	Improved schedule of home visits to ensure newborns are priority #1.
2. Immunize 900 infants and children	75	85	785	No action required
3. Provide antenatal care to 300 mothers	25	32	216	No action required
4. Monitor and investigate every maternal death	0	0	0	No action required
5. Monitor and investigate infant deaths	0	1	1	Traffic accident. Completed home visit and audit report.
6. Treat all new malaria cases	12	34	137	Planning for bed net re-impregnation month.
7. Treat and follow up all new and existing tuberculosis cases	2	3	27	All patients are on treatment.
8. Treat and follow up all new and existing HIV infections	3	2	23	All patients are in support program and referred to the PLWHA association
9. Supervise all deliveries (percentage of supervised deliveries)	80%	82%	81%	201 births in the district this month
10. Monitor and follow up low birth weight babies	0	3	19	All cases come from rural areas; team is working to improve referrals and antenatal care service at Aid Posts.
11. Report all adult deaths	3	1	17	One AIDS death; orphans are HIV− and in family custody and are visited every week to help overcome grief.
12. Number of home visits to follow up	80	78	632	All patients who defaulted treatment or missed antenatal visit were visited this month
Total indicators:	Coverage area:	Indicators on target:	Progress:	Number of emergency actions to be taken:
12	All 14 villages in coverage area have met their monthly targets	11	On track to meet annual objectives	None. All issues resolved

References

1. Otto K, et al. Information and communication technologies for health systems strengthening: opportunities, criteria for success, and innovation for Africa and beyond. In: Lutalo M, editor. Health, nutrition and population (HNP) discussion paper. Washington, DC: World Bank; 2015.
2. Piskurich GM. Online learning: e-learning. Fast, cheap, and good. In: Performance improvement. Medford: Wiley; 2006.
3. Knowledge for Health (K4H) Project. Building M&E capacity through eLearning collaboration. Washington, DC: USAID; 2013. https://www.globalhealthlearning.org/sites/default/files/page/CollaborationSpotlight_FINAL_v3_July2013.pdf
4. Wong G, et al. Internet-based medical education: a realist review of what works, for whom and in what circumstances. BMC Med Educ. 2010;10:12.
5. Ruggeri K, et al. A global model for effective use and evaluation of e-learning in health. Telemed J E Health. 2013;19(4):312–21.
6. World Health Organization. In: Najeeb Al-Shorbaji, et al editors. eLearning for undergraduate health professional education: a systematic review informing a radical transformation of health workforce development. Geneva, Switzerland; 2015.
7. Pandey, A. eLearning trends and predictions for 2017. Retrieved July 09, 2017, from eLearning Industry.2017,January10.https://elearningindustry.com/elearning-trends-and-predictions-2017
8. Beracochea E, Dickson R, Freeman P, Thomason J. Case management quality assessment in rural areas of Papua New Guinea. Trop Doct. 1995;25(2):69–74.. Retrieved July 09, 2017 from https://www.ncbi.nlm.nih.gov/pubmed/7778198

Chapter 17: Global Public Health Disaster Management and Technology

Erica L. Nelson, Nirma D. Bustamante, and Sean M. Kivlehan

Introduction

Disasters are sudden, tumultuous events that disrupt communities and cause human, material, economic, and ecological losses, as well as exacerbating preexisting sociopolitical circumstances. When invoked, the word "disaster" conjures up images of the 2010 Haitian earthquake, or the 2004 Indian Ocean tsunami, with more than 250,000 casualties each and bleak landscapes of devastated communities, infrastructure, and ecology. Disasters are varied, caused by natural or manmade hazards, diverse in degree and type of impact, yet they are all united by the overwhelming destruction that the United Nations International Strategy for Disaster Reduction (UNISDR) defines as "exceeding the ability of the affected community or society to cope using its own resources." [1]. Integral to the practice of global public health is an acknowledgement of the inevitability of such events, the potential impact on community and infrastructure, and the means by which to mitigate, prepare for, respond to, and recover from them.

E. L. Nelson
Department of Emergency Medicine, South Shore Hospital, South Weymouth, MA, USA

Harvard Medical School, Boston, MA, USA

Harvard Humanitarian Initiative, Cambridge, MA, USA

N. D. Bustamante
Department of Emergency Medicine, Brigham and Women's Hospital, Boston, MA, USA

Harvard Medical School, Boston, MA, USA

S. M. Kivlehan (✉)
Harvard Humanitarian Initiative, Cambridge, MA, USA

Department of Emergency Medicine, Brigham and Women's Hospital, Boston, MA, USA

Harvard Medical School, Boston, MA, USA
e-mail: sean.kivlehan@gmail.com

© Springer Nature Switzerland AG 2020
P. Murthy, A. Ansehl (eds.), *Technology and Global Public Health*,
https://doi.org/10.1007/978-3-030-46355-7_22

Disaster management, disaster medicine, and the multiple technologies that have evolved to contribute to these efforts constitute a vast body of knowledge that cannot be thoroughly discussed within this chapter. However, beginning to gain an understanding of disaster management and the technologies that are being employed throughout its cycle is integral to the discussion of technology within global health.

During the past two decades, disaster response has grown from isolated post hoc reactions to hazards to a tremendous field that acknowledges a common cyclical pattern surrounding disaster timelines. This cycle is disaggregated into four reactionary stages: preparedness, response, recovery, and mitigation. Although awareness of all phases is necessary during programmatic design and impact evaluation, each phase requires unique perspectives, data, initiatives, and, therefore, technology.

In its nascence, the field of disaster response technologies focused on tactical and medical objects, such as tourniquets, radio equipment, and extrication devices. With a broader scope, a more sophisticated understanding of disasters and the emergence of powerful yet readily available technology, disaster management science can leverage computational sciences, mobile communication devices, and the internet for a more holistic, coordinated, and useful response. At the leading edge of disaster management technology is an emphasis on data collection, analysis, and dissemination. Tools such as geoanalytics, modeling and optimization, simulation, information and communication technology (ICT), and crowdsourcing have been developed to create faster real-time information streams, bolster the agencies of affected communities, produce more sophisticated and useful initiatives, and improve disaster management coordination.

Disaster Preparedness

Early integration of geospatial information into disaster preparedness came in the form of creating simple maps that depicted background reference information including landforms, political boundaries, and roads. These "basemaps" were later superimposed with post-event hazard data to understand the degree of impact, as exampled by the 1906 San Francisco Fire Map Basemaps, which continue to be invaluable in disaster management, and explicitly disaster preparedness and mitigation, as they are canvases for the assessment of vulnerabilities and response planning.

Mapping "vulnerability" – those complex sociopolitical, human–environment interactions that render communities at risk to a hazard – confers true insight into potential impact and anticipated needs post disaster [2]. Generally, vulnerability mapping included basic demographic (i.e., percentage of under-five population, gender, etc.), economic, and structural considerations. However, the conversation of vulnerability is evolving. Since Hurricane Katrina, for example, American public health experts have acknowledged the impact of chronic health conditions, such as diabetes, asthma, and physical disability, on post-disaster needs and morbidity and mortality. Recommendations now suggest that disaster preparedness organizations inventory population basemaps that include chronic health and disability data [3].

However, in many developing countries, there is a scarcity of accurate, up-to-the-minute spatial data regarding the population, let alone critical facilities, healthcare infrastructure, or population vulnerabilities. Remote sensing, utilizing satellite or other aerial imagery platforms, is now crucial in creating and augmenting basemaps by combining layers of infrastructure, hydrography, elevations, and forest cover into an orthoimage file These high-resolution aerial images combine the visual attributes of photographs with the spatial accuracy of maps, such that feature displacement and scale variations caused by terrain and technology are rectified to create accurate disaster planning basemaps.

Along with hazard and response modeling, as is discussed in the next section, geoanalytics allows a more sophisticated understanding of geographic susceptibility, and community and infrastructural vulnerability, that is critical to developing safe access routes, adequate resource inventories, and other disaster response algorithms.

Modeling and Simulation in Disaster Preparedness

Disasters originate from diverse geophysical, climatological, technological, biological, and sociopolitical variables that impact populations not only by the magnitude of the disaster itself, but also secondarily to the infrastructural foundation and inherent vulnerabilities of the affected population. Effective preparedness requires accurate understanding of both the potential hazard and the preexistent demographic, infrastructural, sociopolitical, economic, and medical characteristics of the communities they affect to (1) amass appropriate food and water resources, medical inventories, volunteer and non-volunteer response personnel, and equipment, and (2) create warning, evacuation, search and rescue, and other response and recovery plans.

Geographic Information System (GIS) modeling and simulation is a valuable tool for emergency preparedness and management. Such modeling has the capability of simulating emergency scenarios in various situations with temporal attributes. Also, it can aid emergency managers in making critical decisions by using spatial analysis for (1) risk and threat assessment, (2) scenario modeling, (3) situational awareness, and (4) resource allocation.

Hazard modeling imports multivariate geospatial, climatological, meteorological, temporal, and infrastructural data into a computational model or simulation, superimposed upon a GIS platform, to determine the likelihood of disaster impact. Explicitly, modeling can be utilized to predict flood inundation, coastal surge heights, seismic vulnerability, landslide susceptibility, smoke plume distribution, and infectious disease transmission. Vulnerability, that is, the capacity to anticipate, cope with, resist, and recover from a hazard, can also be mapped [4]. When hazard predictions and vulnerability demographics are simulated, risk can be estimated. Quantitative methods, including complex analytical and measurement methods, causal inference, structural equation modeling, and decision theory, are commonly used in public health research to create these predictions [2].

One such example of hazard modeling is that of the U.S. SLOSH Program, or the Sea, Lake and Overland Surges from Hurricanes Program, which is utilized not only to forecast weather but also to determine which communities are susceptible to surge flooding and inform disaster preparedness programs. Systems such as Sahana Asia have been developed to simulate disaster mitigation and preparedness activities to manage disaster data that support early disaster warning and mitigation in advance [5]. Interdisciplinary efforts, as evidenced by the U.N. Development Program's Disaster Hotspots project, are now conjoining hazard modeling and operational research to provide decision support for evacuation routing, resource allocation, medical response infrastructure, and supply chain schema in response to earthquakes, flood, wildfires, and landslides.

Virtual Reality Simulation

The chaotic nature of disaster response requires sufficient preparation and familiarity with the sequence of events, communication, and skills to respond effectively and efficiently. New technologies, programs, and applications are making high-fidelity simulation within disaster preparedness more accurate, and hence more reliable for training.

Virtual reality (VR) simulation incorporates real event elements (large crowds, infrastructure, visual/auditory cues) into training scenarios to prepare personnel to respond within the high acuity, chaotic, and stressful environment of a disaster or public health emergency. Mass casualty triage training can incorporate VR-based scenarios that respond to user inputs and provide instant feedback through the use of avatars. A recent study comparing triage performances during disaster simulation exercises using VR and standardized patient drills evidenced the efficacy and feasibility of VR as an alternative for training in disaster triage [6]. Furthermore, VR-based training can be cost-effective when compared to more traditional training models if one considers the number of learners that it can potentially reach, the range of applications, and the ease of repeated use [7].

Programs such as SimulationDeck, a secure web portal that replicates online communication tools used during an acute disaster, allow professionals to simulate mass information campaigns as they would after a disaster, to evaluate their efficacy, and to address challenges before the true event. Because of the extensive use of social media for communication and emergency management, SimulationDeck is becoming more important for organizations to emulate the use of the medium for responder training. Social networks such as Facebook and Twitter, as well as agency websites and blogs, are simulated to train responders in disseminating accurate and coordinated public information during an emergency [8].

Disaster Response and Recovery

During the response phase of a disaster, geoanalytics and remote sensing are increasingly critical in impact assessment and response support. It is not just formal or planned systems that provide this information: the rapidly increasing penetrance of mobile technology and internet access puts social media such as Twitter and Facebook among the earliest primary sources of information following a disaster. Capitalizing on this flood of information arriving directly from the ground and quickly curating it into actionable and reliable information is a key function in disaster response. Crowdsourcing has emerged as one mechanism to perform this and can be defined as an online-distributed, problem-solving production model that leverages the collective intelligence of online communities for specific purposes [9].

Understanding spatial relationships through geoanalytics enables public health and disaster management personnel to assess risk as a factor of distance, create flow-through networks for response programs, better disseminate needs assessment data, coordinate multi-team, cross-departmental response initiatives, and perform impact analysis. Geoanalytics contributes significantly to each of the phases of disaster management.

GIS are composed of the hardware, software, and management systems that gather, store, manipulate, and display geographically referenced data to create an accessible visual database. "Geoanalytics," or "geospatial analysis," is a computational science that applies inferential statistics to geospatially tagged data to evaluate patterns and relationships that might not have been otherwise observed had spatial characteristics not been appreciated. Both tools emphasize the "where" variable of any question, but geospatial analytics goes beyond simple mapping and generates spatial hypotheses to make valid scientific inferences. In the context of disaster management, geospatial methodologies transcend disaster management phases to both understand the pre-disaster state of a community and assess the evolving impact of the hazard.

One of the first major events in which remote sensing imagery was utilized for day-of-response efforts occurred on September 11, 2001, after the attacks on the World Trade Center in New York City. Satellite and aerial imagery, LIDAR (light detection and ranging) imagery, and data from handheld electronic devices that combined Global Positioning System (GPS), internet, and GIS databases were combined to support search-and-rescue efforts, response planning, and information dissemination [10]. After the 2004 Indian Ocean Tsunami, the U.N. Humanitarian Information Center utilized ArcGIS to augment incomplete basemaps with thematic layers characterizing infrastructural damage, displaced populations, and response organization distribution in an effort to improve supply chains, monitor for communicable diseases, determine field hospital and mobile resource locales, and inform disaster recovery planning [11]. Within 5 days of the 2010 Haiti Earthquake, more than 15 organizations from eight countries uploaded satellite data to the freely accessible United Nations Platform for Space-based Information for Disaster Management and Emergency Response (UN-SPIDER). The Haitian Earthquake

Data Portal was launched and publishing GIS data within 48 h, and more than 3 million Haitian cell phone users were rebuilding maps and contributing to needs assessment efforts.

Mobile Technology and Phones

Information and communications technology (ICT) has been identified by the United Nations as useful in every phase of disaster preparedness. ICT includes traditional media, such as radio and television, and new media such as cellular, internet, and satellite [12]. Traditional media represented a significant improvement in the speed of information dissemination when compared to its print predecessor, but new media are rapidly displacing all prior forms of mass media as the preferred source of current news. Mobile technology, internet access, and the rise of social media allow for growth that is changing the way information in disasters is gathered, analyzed, and disseminated [13].

Global mobile phone penetration was 67% in 2019 with 5.2 billion subscribers, and this is expected to rise to 70% with 5.8 billion subscribers in 2025 [14]. The gap in internet access between developing and advanced countries has been closing rapidly over the past decade. In 2015, the global median of internet access was 67%, but this is composed of medians of 54% in developing countries and 87% in advanced countries. Smartphone ownership in developing countries is rising extremely rapidly, nearly doubling from 2013 to 2015 to 37%. This growth is fueling the increased use of social media in these regions [15].

However, mobile devices are no longer only used for communication. Given their growing affordability and accessibility, cell phones, tablets, and laptops are being used across the world to (1) collect and share data, (2) implement programs, (3) aid in the provision of medications and healthcare, and (4) assist in acute disaster settings. Applications such as stock management, disease surveillance, identification and tracking of patients, awareness campaigns, and their use as medical devices have transformed health delivery and evaluation [16].

Mobile data collection systems allow for the customization of surveys to collect specific data with photographs, information from a list selection, voice recordings, and GPS coordinates. Free and open tools such as Kobo Toolbox allow the user to build forms and collect, analyze, and manage data. Because of its offline capabilities, Kobo Toolbox has been adopted as the preferred electronic data collection tool by the United Nations Office for the Coordination of Humanitarian Affairs (OCHA) to improve standardization, reliability, and ease of access during humanitarian crises [17].

Social Media

Persons affected by a disaster now have increased access to social media, and it is becoming a tool for early information gathering and dissemination. Typically, the first reports from an area affected by a disaster come from posts to Twitter or Facebook by the affected population. Sometimes this information can be overwhelming and conflicting, and verification may be difficult or impossible. Best practices have developed to guide response planning by mapping social media posts on Twitter, Facebook, and other media onto heat maps and interconnected diagrams. Facebook rolled out its "marked safe" feature in 2014 to allow individuals to communicate their status after a disaster, thereby easing some of the pressure on cellular networks during the acute phase.

Realizing the key role of social media in disasters, some public health agencies have integrated a formal Social Media Monitoring Team into their Incident Command System with some success [18]. Larger organizations have begun building out operations in this sector as well, with examples including the American Red Cross's Digital Operations Center (DigiDOC) and the Federal Emergency Management Agency (FEMA) "Watch Centers." [19, 20].

Early Warning Systems

The broad penetration of mobile technology paired with GIS technology included in smartphones has revealed new avenues into building early warning systems. Systems relying on minimal user input and passive analysis of existing data can be analyzed and applied to disaster-related functions, such as natural disasters and infectious disease outbreaks.

An example of a minimal user input system is the U.S. Geological Survey (USGS) "Did You Feel It?" earthquake mapping application. This application combines user responses and their location with actual seismic data to provide more detailed earthquake impact maps than were previously available. MyShake is a crowdsourced early earthquake warning program that detects shaking on a user's smartphone, sends this information to a processing center, and uses algorithms to determine whether an earthquake is under way. Using the GPS information from the phones and the intensity of shaking, the app can then send early warning alerts to an area's users that provide the precious seconds to minutes needed to reach safety. Furthermore, these data can be routed to public transportation systems and utilities to active emergency shutdowns before the seismic waves arrive [21].

Google Flu Trends analyzed usage of search terms from users that may be flu related and mapped this geographically and temporally to track flu outbreaks. Comparisons of this with actual Centers for Disease Control (CDC) data initially correlated well for influenza-like illness, but later estimates showed the algorithm to be overestimating laboratory-confirmed influenza rates by 50% and missing smaller outbreak peaks [22, 23]. Despite this failure, surveillance systems that use large data for historical mapping or prediction hold substantial promise for developing the early warning systems of the future. One successful example is the Short-term Inundation Forecasting for Tsunamis (SIFT) developed by the National Oceanic and Atmospheric Administration (NOAA) Center for Tsunami Research, which predicts the amplitude and travel time of a tsunami following an earthquake based on combined historical and real-time numerical models [24].

Flood, fire, and volcano early warning systems are also burgeoning, as evidenced by the Dartmouth Flood Observatory (DFO) River Watch flood detection and measurement system, Sentinel Asia early flood warning, and the Moderate Resolution Imaging Spectroradiometer (MODIS) data used for many international fire SensorWeb early warning systems. South Africa's Advanced Fire Information System (AFIS) integrates these data with vector information to calculate the fire trajectory and automatically warn the population of fire migration via mobile phone messaging.

Mapping

GIS developed through crowdsourcing is useful in a non-disaster setting with programs such as the navigation application Waze, but in disaster settings it can be a real-time, dynamic source of information on the ground, made possible by the GPS functionality built into modern mobile technology. Ushahidi, an open source mapping platform, was used to create crowdsourced maps of the 2010 Haitian earthquake and the Thailand floods. Another open source platform, GeoChat, has been used to track influenza outbreaks and alert exposed populations in Cambodia [25]. These applications and others utilize human input and can also harvest information from social networks and other sources of information, such as city infrastructure and utility maps.

During the 2013 Typhoon Haiyan in the Philippines, the online open source map program OpenStreetMap was used to rapidly develop street maps of affected regions. This source provided maps of previously unmapped regions for humanitarian workers and also classified structural damage to buildings through a tagging system. However, later ground surveys showed this approach of using satellite data to determine structural damage is less reliable than traditional methods. Ongoing work in this area is focusing on training volunteers to better recognize damage and providing access to pre-disaster images for comparisons [26].

Geoanalytical integration into disaster management can be even more tangible than assessment needs and humanitarian coordination. GIS-linked data are now informing computer-aided dispatch (CAD), a system that utilizes geospatially tagged data regarding infrastructure, incident distribution, mobile and immobile resources, and real-time response unit information to improve disaster response logistics [27]. Through advanced vehicle locating, responder interface, and real-time tracking of the event, CAD identifies the most appropriate and available resources required to reduce response times, increase responder safety, and enhance situational awareness. These systems have been utilized in coordinating fire-fighting efforts, hazardous spill response, and emergency medical service dispatch [28].

Disaster Recovery and Information Dissemination

Disaster recovery constitutes the actions required for a community to resume critical functions following a disaster. Disaster recovery is as complicated a task as disaster preparedness and requires a sophisticated understanding of infrastructure, resources, and population casualties combined with community priorities, vulnerability, and future risk. Key facilities and societal functions must be given priority for reconstruction. Pathways between the damage perimeter and those facilities must be identified, and hazard modeling must be employed to mitigate future destruction. Geoanalytical databases are ideally suited for the amount of data and the data manipulation needed for these efforts. Aerial imaging by unmanned aerial vehicles (UAVs) can also be valuable in recovery programs. In the Philippines, Medair utilized two-dimensional (2D) and three-dimensional (3D) terrain models produced from high-resolution aerial images collected by UAVs to inform post-Typhoon Yolanda recovery efforts. In consultation with the local government, low-cost drones were flown over Tacloban and Leyte to provide information to first responders and community leaders regarding areas of greatest need [29, 30].

Notwithstanding the tremendous potential, geoanalytics and remote sensing, be it by drones or satellites, have their undeniable pitfalls. Critical to the adoption and optimization of these geospatial technologies is an international consensus regarding international law, shared data dictionaries, functional collaboration, and open but safe information sharing. The overwhelming tonnage of data combined with incompatible technological lexicons and a lack of universality surrounding operational datasets have left the geoanalytical community fractionated. Arguments pertaining to accessibility and affordability of GIS technologies in austere environments are valid. Also, the lack of infrastructure in disaster response mechanisms to validate and analyze the volume and velocity of such innumerable sources is quite a legitimate obstacle.

In the past decade, however, geoanalytics, remote sensing, and the utilization of these data have continued to evolve. The resolution of satellite images and aerial photographs has improved drastically, thus expediting routing of escape, rescue, or relief distribution. Public domains such as Google Maps and numerous geoanalytical volunteers, facilitated by mobile applications and open source platforms such as Ushahidi and OpenStreetMaps, have moved disaster response from the domain of select professional groups to communities, both local and international. International organizations and nongovernmental organizations have launched online dissemination mechanisms for better response coordination, such as HumanitarianResponse. info, the Center for Research on the Epidemiology of Disasters Emergency Events Database (EM-DAT), the Global Disaster Alert and Coordination System (GDAC)

Virtual Onsite Operations Coordination Centre (OSOCC), the MIT/Harvard Data Portal, and the Sahana Free and Open Sources Disaster Management System. The disaster response community is beginning to address the complexities and pitfalls of such large amounts of data by forming working groups, such as that on Applied Technologies which operates under the auspices of the Humanitarian Action Summit.

Cloud Repository Services

For information systems to be of use, it is necessary to integrate large amounts of data from different sources. Cloud-based services have emerged as a potential platform for disaster settings. This model allows for on-demand, internet-based access to a shared pool of computing resources, including networks, storage, and applications. Resource virtualization, large-scale pattern recognition, high reliability, generality, and scalability, as well as low-cost and on-demand services, allow cloud-based services to link numerous computers and services during a crisis.

Governmental and nongovernmental organizations can now store their information and data across different servers around the world. By its ability for continuous syncing capabilities as well as creating multiple copies of a data set, cloud computing provides the ease of tracking down important information quickly as well as swift recovery of critical information. Even when disasters interrupt internet access, which is not infrequent, lack of connectivity is somewhat temporary in comparison to when disasters destroy local computing infrastructure completely. As soon as internet access is regained, data sets can be retrieved through cloud-based services. Furthermore, cloud computing information is usually hosted in well-protected data centers, away from the conflict or disaster setting [31]. Within the field of geospatial data, it provides a potential solution to its complex structure, the massive amounts of data, and high levels of computing requirements during an acute crisis [32].

Information Dissemination

The compilation and analysis of crowdsourced information is only as effective as its reliability and dissemination. The Sahana Foundation developed an avenue to publish different sets of data sources by means of Linked Open Data (LOD) technology and to interconnect them with other sources on the LOD cloud. Data verification remains a challenge, particularly in the most acute phases of a disaster, but efforts have been made to improve this aspect. There are various approaches to the compromise of these competing goals: aggregating information and only considering clear patterns, small-scale manual verification of key reports, or crowdsourced fact checking [33]. However, there is an inverse relationship between verification and timeliness. For example, social media reports relevant to a disaster are frequently the most rapid form of reporting, but can be incorrect, self-serving, or even malicious.

Independent verification is time- and resource consuming, both of which are precious commodities in an evolving disaster.

Compiled information should be quickly and openly accessible to all who may need it. The humanitarian information portal ReliefWeb is one example of a disaster-oriented aggregator and disseminator of information from and to responders, planning agencies, funders, and the affected population. It is operated by the United Nations Office for the Coordination of Humanitarian Affairs (OCHA) and updated continuously with situation reports, maps, and even humanitarian-related job postings. Virtual organizations, such as Humanitarian Road, are also transforming this platform. Virtual organizations are geographically distributed organizations with members bound by a common interest who communicate and coordinate their work through information technology [34]. Created in 2010, Humanitarian Road and its volunteers use internet and mobile communications to collect, verify, and route information online during sudden-onset disasters. They have responded to crises all over the world to collect public safety information and to direct the public to government and international aid agencies that can provide assistance during a disaster [35].

The collection and organization of data is important; yet, during a disaster, it is the dispersal of data to those on the ground that becomes crucial. Two such technologies are making communication during disasters more reliable and direct. Intellistreets, for example, is an emerging technology that uses streetlight poles with wireless technology to provide emergency alerts and information during a disaster to the public. Another example is iDAWG, a device being developed with the objective of maintaining communication between different relief services without relying on cell towers or internet networks [8].

The remote sharing of information among providers is also becoming more accessible. There are several reliable open online data sources (Table 1) that provide a strong foundation for data collection and dispersal during an acute crisis, providing an invaluable resource to responders and researchers alike.

Next Steps

The evolution of technology within the field of disaster management has accelerated tremendously in the past decade, with geoanalytics, modeling and optimization, simulation, ICT, crowdsourcing, and social media completely changing the way data are collected, analyzed, and disseminated. Inevitably, there is much to be done to standardize, integrate, and optimize the utilization of these tools. Geospatial databases must be able to interact with each other, requiring common dictionaries and open application program interfaces (APIs). Operational algorithms for data collection and analysis should be studied, creating empirically validated best practices and standard operating procedures. Conversations about data ethics in post-disaster environments should take place during all levels of policy and programmatic discussion. Infrastructure needed to ensure reliable and equitable access to technologies

Table 1 Open online data sources

Relief Web	http://reliefweb.int/	The leading humanitarian information source on global crises and disasters. It is the specialized digital service of the U.N. Office for the Coordination of Humanitarian Affairs (OCHA).
The Humanitarian Data Exchange (HDX)	https://data.humdata.org/	An open platform for sharing data with the goal of making humanitarian data easy to find and use for analysis.
UNOSAT	http://www.unitar.org/unosat/	The United Nations Institute for Training and Research (UNITAR) Operational Satellite Applications Programme (UNOSAT) is a technology-intensive program that delivers imagery analysis and satellite solutions to international organizations within and outside the UN system for humanitarian relief, human security, and strategic territorial and development planning.
MapAction	https://mapaction.org	Provides crucial data from the scene of the disaster quickly in the form of maps, which aid agencies in making informed decisions and delivering aid to the areas of highest need.
Open Street Map	https://www.openstreetmap.org	Continuously being built by a community of mappers, it provides mapping data about roads, trails, cafés, and railway stations all over the world.
Healthsites	https://healthsites.io	Database created with the goal of making the location of every health facility in the world available in addition to their respective associated services and resources. Using these accessible baseline data, additional data can be uploaded, managed, and made easily available during a disaster.

and data should be maintained. Data dissemination mechanisms should harness the fast uptake of smartphones, social media, and the development of organizational dashboards to improve disaster management coordination. From the engineering logistics of electricity and WiFi availability to the theory behind data ethics, to the academic evaluation of geoanalytical and remote sensing techniques, there is much to be done within disaster management technologies.

Case Study

You work for Disastech International, an NGO that focuses on using technology in disaster preparedness and response. A 7.9 magnitude earthquake has just hit off the coast of Chile, near Santiago. Fortunately, your NGO specializes in these types of natural disasters and is able to use its experience and technology to respond. Because Chile sits on the arc of volcanos and fault lines circling the Pacific Ocean, there was immense damage to the population of more than 6 million. Yet, Disastech has been using GIS to create basemaps of the city, including the vulnerable areas that are the hardest hit. Your basemaps include basic demographic, economic, and geospatial information that provided the foundation for a hazard modeling map of the city. Furthermore, because of the extensive expertise of your NGO, you have detailed topographic, 3D models of the region using UAV imagery. Using these maps, you can provide the international community with information about high-risk areas where there are likely to be the greatest numbers of victims and survivors. Your previously prepared maps can be used to evaluate the most probable routes to deliver aid and logistical supply chains. You are also able to provide the locations of the previously established health facilities for injury referral.

Because of the scale of the earthquake and the population density that was affected by it, social media and mobile technology become the first line of information output after the disaster. Capitalizing on the flood of information from posts through Facebook and Twitter, Disastech is able to identify the hotspots where the highest impact occurred. You forward the information you collected to UN-SPIDER. Additionally, hours after the earthquake hit, Disastech deployed a team to complete a rapid assessment using Kobo Toolbox, information that will be forwarded to UN-OCHA, which is coordinating the international response. In addition to the local response, Disastech has been in constant communication with SIFT to help alert neighboring countries in the Pacific. In the next 24 h, you update your previously prepared basemaps with up-to-date information on the neighborhoods most affected, hotpots of victims, best routes for health referrals, and the regions needing the most aid. You update this information every 24 h. To begin reconstruction planning, 1 week after the earthquake hits, you use satellite imagery, social media, and UAVs to deliver detailed city maps to the Mayor of Santiago that include the hardest hit infrastructure and safest pathways around the city.

References

1. United Nations Office for Disaster Risk Reduction (UNDRR). https://www.unisdr.org/we/inform/terminology. Accessed 10 Jan 2017.
2. Testa MA, Pettigrew ML, Savoia E. Measurement, geospatial, and mechanistic models of public health hazard vulnerability and jurisdictional risk. J Public Health Manag Pract. 2014;20(Suppl 5):S61–8.
3. Aldrich N, Benson WF. Disaster preparedness and the chronic disease needs of vulnerable older adults. Prev Chronic Dis. 2008;5(1):A27.
4. Jha MK. Natural and anthropogenic disasters: vulnerability, preparedness and mitigation. 1st ed. Dordrecht: Springer; 2010. https://doi.org/10.1007/978-90-481-2498-5.
5. Sahana Foundation. Software features. https://sahanafoundation.org/eden/features/. Accessed 10 Jan 2017.
6. Andreatta PB, Maslowski E, Petty S, Shim W, Marsh M, Hall T, Stern S, Frankel J. Virtual reality triage training provides a viable solution for disaster-preparedness. Acad Emerg Med. 2010;17(8):870.
7. Hsu E, Li Y, Bayram J, Levinson D, Yang S, Monhan C. State of virtual reality based disaster preparedness and response training. PLoS Curr. 2013 April 24; 5: https://doi.org/10.1371/currents.dis.1ea2b2e71237d5337fa53982a38b2aff.

8. Pittman E. 3 emerging technologies that will impact emergency management. In: Emergency management: preparedness and recovery. 2012. Available from: http://www.govtech.com/em/disaster/3-Emerging-Technologies-Emergency-Management.html. Accessed 08 July 2017.
9. Brabham DC, Ribisl KM, Kirchner TR, Bernhardt JM. Crowdsourcing applications for public health. Am J Prev Med. 2014;46(2):179–87.
10. Kawasaki A, Berman ML, Guan W. The growing role of web-based geospatial technology in disaster response and support. Disasters. 2012;37(2):201.
11. Ciottone GR, Biddinger PD, Darling RG, Fares S, Keim ME, Molloy MS, Suner S. Ciottone's disaster medicine. Philadelphia: Elsevier; 2016.
12. Wattegama C. ICT for disaster management. United Nations Development Program – Asia-Pacific Development Information Programme. 2007.
13. Barthel M, Shearer E, Gottfried J, Mitchell A. The evolving role of news of Twitter and Facebook. Pew Journalism and Media Web site. http://www.journalism.org/2015/07/14/the-evolving-role-of-news-on-twitter-and-facebook/. Updated 2015. Accessed 10 Jan 2017.
14. Groupe Speciale Mobile Association (GSMA). The mobile economy 2020. GSMA Mobile Economy Web site. https://www.gsma.com/mobileeconomy/wp-content/uploads/2020/03/GSMA_MobileEconomy2020_Global.pdf. Published 2020. Accessed 05/21, 2020
15. Poushter J. Smartphone ownership and internet usage continues to climb in emerging economies. Pew Global Attitudes & Trends Web site. http://www.pewglobal.org/2016/02/22/smart-phone-ownership-and-internet-usage-continues-to-climb-in-emerging-economies/. Updated 2016. Accessed 01/10, 2017.
16. Fava P. Mobile health technology: key practices for DRR implementers. Cooperazione Internazionale Report. 2014.
17. Vinck P. Kobo toolbox. http://www.kobotoolbox.org/#block-views-skills-and-services-block. Updated 2017. Accessed 01/10, 2017.
18. Hadi T, Fleshler K. Integrating social media monitoring into public health emergency response operations. Disaster Med Public Health Prep. 2016;10:775.
19. Markenson DHL. American Red Cross Digital Operations Center (DigiDOC): an essential emergency management tool for the digital age. Disaster Med Public Health Prep. 2014;8(5):445–51.
20. Thomas C. FEMA to monitor social media during disasters. operation dragon fire. National Voluntary Organizations Active in Disaster Web site. http://odf.nvoad.org/fema-to-monitor-social-media-during-disasters/. Updated 2016. Accessed 01/10, 2017.
21. Kong Q, Allen RM, Schreier L, et al. MyShake: a smartphone seismic network for earthquake early warning and beyond. Sci Adv. 2016;2:e1501055.
22. Ortiz JR, Zhou H, Shay DK, et al. Monitoring influenza activity in the United States: a comparison of traditional surveillance systems with Google flu trends. PLoS One. 2011;6(4):e18687.
23. Lazer D, Kennedy R, King G, et al. The parable of google flu: traps in big data analysis. Science. 2014;343(6167):1203.
24. National Oceanic and Atmospheric Administration (NOAA) Center for Tsunami Research. Tsunami forecasting. http://nctr.pmel.noaa.gov/tsunami-forecast.html. Updated 2017. Accessed 01/10, 2017.
25. Kamel Boulos MN, Resch B, Crowley DN, et al. Crowdsourcing, citizen sensing and sensor web technologies for public and environmental health surveillance and crisis management: trends, OGC standards and application examples. Int J Health Geogr 2011;10:67-072x-10-67.
26. Zastrow M. Crisis mappers find an ally. Nature. 2014;515:321.
27. Caunhye AM, Nie X, Pokharel S. Optimization models in emergency logistics: a literature review. Socio-Econ Plan Sci. 2012;46(1):4.
28. ESRI. Geospatial computer-aided dispatch. White paper. ESRI, Redlands, CA. 2007.
29. Gilman D. Unmanned aerial vehicles in humanitarian response. OCHA Policy Development and Studies Branch Occasional Policy Paper. June 2014;10.
30. Smith N. Post-disaster mapping with aerial imagery. Development Seed Web site. https://developmentseed.org/blog/2015/08/12/post-disaster-imagery/. Published August 12, 2015. Updated 2015. Accessed 01/08, 2017.

31. Velev DZD. Principles of cloud computing application in emergency management. In: International Conference on E-business, Management and Economics, 2011.
32. Ge X, Wang H. Cloud-based service for big spatial data technology in emergency management. In: International Conference on Geo-spatial Solutions for Emergency Management and the 50th Anniversary of the Chinese Academy of Surveying and Mapping, 2009.
33. Mehta AM, Bruns A, Newton J. Trust, but verify: social media models for disaster management. Disasters. 2017;41(3):549–65.
34. Anuju M, Carley K. Network structure in virtual organizations. J Comput-Mediat Commun. 1998;3(4). https://onlinelibrary.wiley.com/doi/10.1111/j.1083-6101.1998.tb00079.x
35. Starbird KPL. Working and sustaining the virtual "Disaster desk." Proceedings of the 2013 conference on the computer supported cooperative work, 2013:491.

Chapter 18: Employing Data Science Technologies Towards Shaping a Sustainably Healthy Future: The Efforts in Contemporary Taiwan

Chih-Wei Chen

Introduction

In the past decades, humans have conquered a series of fatal diseases and significantly improved health levels and hygiene conditions for human society. However, with rapid urbanisation and development, human society is facing new challenges such as the aging society, reduced birth rate, and chronic diseases, which further result in urban decay and reduced numbers of labourers in rural areas. Globalisation also increases the risks of epidemics spreading around the world. Facing these increasingly severe threats, humans are continuously endeavouring to improve public health conditions and control diseases in human society.

In the contemporary digital era, data science technologies have been developed at an unprecedented speed as well as spread to every domain of human life. Hence, public health conditions could be upgraded by applying the smart tools of data science technologies, such as spatial information, large data, data visualisation, and so on, on the basis of the Geographic Information System (GIS). Thus, technology can provide dynamic and interactive exchanges on data and information amongst industries, government, and academia for cooperation and collaboration in a more efficient approach towards shaping a sustainably healthy future.

The employment of smart tools could significantly improve communication efforts amongst cross-domain and multi-level stakeholders to understand the current situation, identify the problem, and further make action plans to promote the public health conditions comprehensively and systematically. Smart tools provide technical support for a decision support system (DSS) to make fact-based decisions.

C.-W. Chen (✉)
Royal Geographical Society (with IBG), London, UK

University College London (UCL), London, UK
e-mail: chihwei.chen@udm.global

© Springer Nature Switzerland AG 2020
P. Murthy, A. Ansehl (eds.), *Technology and Global Public Health*,
https://doi.org/10.1007/978-3-030-46355-7_23

Consequently, on the basis of data science technologies, a brand-new concept, the "Smart Health Network System," could be proposed for the public health system, possessing great potential to improve health conditions for all people at all ages. More efforts to provide open data, upgrade digital infrastructure, and ensure cybersecurity, however, are still necessary to support the establishment of the Smart Health Network System (SHNS) towards shaping a sustainably healthy future.

Global Trend Towards Healthy Lives and Well-being

In 2015, the United Nations officially launched the 17 Sustainable Development Goals (SDGs) to address the issues and challenges that humans are facing in today's world, especially SDG3, which emphasises the importance of ensuring healthy lives and promoting well-being for all at all ages, as well as detailing nine targets towards the achievement of that vision [1].

To measure the progress of SDGs in detail and make accurate comparisons in support of future policies and action plans, the Inter-Agency and Expert Group on SDG Indicators (IAEG-SDGs) developed a global indicator framework, which was adopted by the General Assembly of the United Nations. This framework was contained in the Resolution adopted by the General Assembly on Work of the Statistical Commission pertaining to the 2030 Agenda for Sustainable Development to ensure the accountability of statistical data, monitor the progress of sustainable development, and feedback to policymakers [2]. Moreover, the global indicator framework is implemented by using data science technologies to develop tools, such as the SDG dashboard, Urban Data Platform, CitySDK, and so on, which could obtain, store, process, and analyse data to visualise the SDGs progress from both time and spatial perspectives as well as assist in making further concrete and effective action plans.

The SDG dashboard relies on the unified data platform to visualise the analysis and monitor future environmental demands and economic potentials, as well as feedback on the progress of data collection and collation [3], which has been utilised by the United Nations, the USA, the UK, and other countries [3–5].

The Urban Data Platform, which provides a platform to visualise data and information for European cities and surrounding regions, was jointly launched by the Joint Research Centre (JRC) and the Directorate General for Regional and Urban Policy (DG REGIO) of the European Commission [6]. In particular, the indicator for SDGs could be intuitively observed in different European Union (EU) countries (from the spatial perspective) along with the changing decades (from the time perspective) simultaneously.

CitySDK, first established by the EU, is a software development kit and an applicable cross-domain smart city development program that was issued by the Seventh Framework Programme [7]. Then, the U.S. Census Bureau drew on the experiences of EU CitySDK to establish the US CitySDK jointly with other agencies in the US federal government to make its authoritative data as open data in terms of the nation's people and economy. Their intent was to make the Census data more accessible, and to assist policymakers and officers in allocating resources and investments more reasonably, as well as to help business leaders optimise their operations [8].

Taiwan's Efforts for the Improvement of Public Health

Coming back to Asia, drawing on the experience of UN SDGs and combining with local conditions, Taiwan's government has developed localised SDGs (18 goals, 143 targets, and 342 indicators) to promote sustainable development in Taiwan and communicate with the world through this shared language, wherein SDG3 highlights the goal to ensure and promote healthy lives and well-being for all persons at all ages [9].

Therefore, according to the US and the UK, the open data program of National Reporting Platform (NPR) is applied and features the functions of data visualisation, reliability index, data interpretation, and data link. Moreover, the functions of the SDG data management and application platform include data search in a logical form, data establishment, data return with visualisation management, data analysis, and application from the spatial perspective.

During the process of SDGs analysis and implementation, the data used should be assessed in terms of the necessity, reliability, compatibility, accuracy, applicability, time efficiency, and other indices. The data science technologies that are used include spatial data to facilitate the vitalisation and application of national sustainability-related data, which are then effectively linked to the United Nations to enhance global connection.

Hence, the GIS as an essential smart tool has been widely applied, incorporating data science technologies such as data process and analysis, data visualisation, application of large data, and spatial and information platforms, to dynamically present the changes and differences of data and information from both time and spatial perspectives. Meanwhile, such tools provide a platform for the government and civil society to interact and use the system efficiently.

To support promotion and implementation of the policies as well as achieve the vision towards healthier life for all, Taiwan has also been actively exploring and harnessing data science technologies to develop smart tools via research and design (R&D) to facilitate communications and interactions amongst industries, government, and academia, as well as individuals.

Today, Taiwan expects to combine digital technology, such as the GIS, with a series of data science technologies (e.g., data analysis, data visualisation, large data, spatial information platform) that allow the best use of geospatial information to develop a decision support system (DSS). This system will assist the central government in implementing and monitoring the SDGs, with feedback for further policy making, as well as promote and implement public health-related policies and action plans to strive for the goal of "leave no one behind."

Taiwan Practice Experience: Data Science Technologies in Contemporary Health Policy

Since 2005, the National Geographic Information System (NGIS) has had a key role.

To accurately assess the resource allocation ratio for different regions or programs at the beginning of planning for various sustainable policies, the United Nations Global Geospatial Information Management (UN-GGIM) has strived to promote the geospatial information to be listed as the vital tool while measuring the SDGs indicators, meanwhile believing that the chairperson of each country must understand every indicator-related activity in terms of where it happens to allow the SDGs to have practical meaning [10].

Taiwan has been developing the NGIS for more than 20 years, and today it is essential as the shared geospatial information platform, which takes the UN SDGs as the foundation for data collection and collation with the assistance of data visualisation, to produce related data and information through data processing and information exchange to further facilitate the interactions amongst industries, government, and academia, as well as communicating with the world to shape a smart and sustainable future together [11].

The NGIS has been developed to provide information regarding 12 themes, including natural environment, transportation network, and socioeconomic, by incorporating geographic information both overground and underground (topography, geology, hydrology, land ownership) as well as the attributes (text and symbolic) into the database, allowing users to overlap the theme maps on the basis of their demand, which could facilitate government management, planning, and policy making [11].

To lay a solid foundation for using the NGIS to assist the promotion and implementation of SDGs, the data inventory is further processed, the reliability of the collected data is assessed, and then an analysis platform is built for SDG data management and dashboard. The development and application of related SDGs data are further promoted to the organisations that are responsible for data via the education and training approach.

The promotion policy for the entire NGIS is made through cooperation between departments and councils to enhance the content and quality of geospatial data, draw geographic data relating to national development, and improve the smart ability of the NGIS to analyse and respond to problems towards shaping a smart and sustainable nation.

Regarding SDG3, 'health for all,' Taiwan has investigated the locations and functions of medical and healthcare centres and related organisations that provide medical treatment in terms of epidemic disease, chronic disease, and long-term care. All levels of medical organisations and most of the diseases in local areas are covered. Such information is then visualised through the GIS to assist the citizens in choosing the most appropriate medical organisation for treatment, while assisting local government in making systematic plans to allocate resources for medical organisations so as to meet the demands of citizens.

In detail, the GIS is an important tool for stakeholders and individuals to interactively and intuitively visualise useful information (e.g., location, scale, and principal functions of hospitals or healthcare centres), especially to direct patients to find the right place with the best approach (e.g., choose appropriate medical and healthcare centres based on personal health situations and demands, as well as choosing the most convenient transportation route).

In 2015: Epidemic Prevention of South Taiwan, Tainan City

According to the World Health Organisation, dengue is a viral disease transmitted by mosquitoes that is widespread throughout the tropics. Today, severe dengue has become a major cause of serious illness and death in adults and children, especially in the Americas, Southeast Asia, and the Western Pacific regions. No effective and specific treatment for dengue is available; therefore, prevention and control of dengue is essential through early detection and access to proper medical care [12].

Threatened by the fatal dengue fever, Taiwan has made every effort to prevent and control the spread of this disease, especially in Tainan City, which devised the strategy to employ "Geographic Information System for Dengue Prevention and Control," [13] which requires practical experience, such as swiftly and accurately analysing the data and providing sufficient support for policy making through prompt recording of prevention and control actions. Moreover, the system provides possibilities to search, track, monitor, and store documents from the geospatial perspective, allowing the Centres for Disease Control to understand the current situation, predict the possible future trend, and make efficient prevention action plans. The operation of the system has significantly reduced the manual administrative work procedures of the past, but made swift statistical analysis and improved the timeliness and accuracy of the information for an epidemic. System operation is then be assisted by the analysis of each major element of the epidemic through large data technology, including weather conditions, community conditions, activity areas for the confirmed case, hidden disease sources, egg trap monitoring, and so on, to provide the epidemic prevention staff with more accurate and effective prevention and control.

Beyond the successful application of GIS in dengue prevention and control, to address the increasingly severe issue of the dengue epidemic around the world and strengthen the regional epidemic prevention network, Tainan City shared their experience with neighbour countries who are also facing serious threats from dengue, such as Indonesia, which is an infected area that has brought approximately 8% to 31% of dengue fever to Taiwan in the past 4 years, according to the data from the Centres for Disease Control at the Ministry of Health and Welfare [14, 15].

Today (2019): Cross-Domain Applications: the Taiwan Economic Society Analysis System (TESAS)

Beyond the public health domain itself, efforts to facilitate overall improvement are also made through cross-domain collaborations, wherein data science technologies could bridge the gaps amongst domains through data process and analysis, information integration, data visualisation, etc. to address the issues arising from the ageing society, urban decay, and other concerns. Hence, the successful promotion and implementation of smart and sustainable health lie in the foundation of up-to-date and reliable data.

For example, the Taiwanese government uses GIS to map and compare the location of healthcare centres and transportation routes to discuss improving the structure of medical and healthcare centres as well as the transport system in the city to provide a better experience for people to be treated comfortably and in a timely manner. In detail, the structure of medical and healthcare centres is not comprehensive (e.g., insufficient hospitals but too many patients, fewer clinics to fulfil the demands from patients with prevalent disease and chronic disease); also, the transport system is limited by the coverage and could not ensure all the patients can access the proper healthcare centre, as well as not being sufficently convenient for aged people. However, the combination of different datasets in terms of medical and healthcare centres as well as the transport system could assist the researchers and policymakers to determine whether the medical and welfare centres in the city can support all the ageing people, and whether the transport system is convenient enough for ageing populations to access the needed centres. After investigation and analysis, government agencies could make further appropriate decisions to improve public health conditions.

In turn, facing such issues as ageing society, low birth rate, and urban decay, the Taiwanese government has been actively promoting the Regional Revitalisation Policy and developing the Taiwan Economic Society Analysis System to provide the required technical resources and digital environment [16]. Moreover, the model of the Taiwan Economic Society Analysis System (TESAS) gathers the forces and consensus of local citizens, reproduces public memory, and provides a channel for professionals and web users to understand local areas in promoting public health from the national level to township level.

Bearing all the efforts of using data science technologies to improve medical and health conditions, the brand-new concept "Smart Health Network System" could be proposed to shape the new vision of public health, as well as make comprehensive and revolutionary progress in public health in Taiwan towards the aim of health for all at all ages (Fig. 1).

Beyond the efforts within the nation, Taiwan also actively takes global responsibility to share its successful experiences with neighbouring countries through the National Policy: New Southbound Policy [17], and further to turn to a new dialogue with the world to improve public health conditions and achieve universal health coverage [18], as an echo of the UN SDG 17 global partnership.

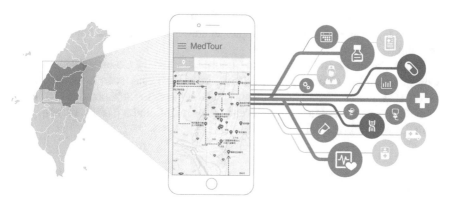

Fig. 1 Concept of the Smart Health Network System (SHNS) in Central Taiwan

Contemporary Challenges and Solutions for the Smart Health Network System

However, in the progress towards the development of the Smart Health Network System (SHNS), data science technologies as the primary tools not only create great potential and opportunities but also bring huge challenges, such as the demands of open data, upgrading infrastructure for digital tools, and ensuring cybersecurity. Hence, further efforts are still indispensable to build an active and safe environment for the SHNS in the contemporary digital era.

Open Data

Living in the contemporary digital world, people are increasingly aware of the importance of data, because data are the basic unit and fundamental core for digital technologies in building a smart and sustainable city. Moreover, the demand for open data is increasingly apparent to facilitate information exchange amongst departments and stakeholders, allowing further collaborations for innovation and improvements. Furthermore, open data contribute greatly to using data science technologies by providing broadened accessibilities for people and increased possibilities for innovation and stimulation of the economy.

Hence, the United Nations launched the Open SDG Data Hub to facilitate fact-based decision making by promoting the explorations, analysis, and application of data [19]; meanwhile, the UK developed the Find Open Data to assist stakeholders in building products and services by allowing citizens to find data published by multiple stakeholders including central government, local authorities, and public bodies [20].

The Taiwanese government also launched the Government Open Data Portal [21], which includes 18 major categories such as Living Safety and Quality, Elderly

Care, Birth and Adoption, and so on, to promote cross-department data exchange, improve the efficiency of policy implementation, and meet the requirements of the public.

Moreover, the Centres for Disease Control launched the Communicable Disease Control Open Data Portal [22], which includes such categories as dengue fever, HIV/AIDS, biosafety, and tuberculosis, allowing users to understand the values of open data through interactive graphs and tables, maps, and a dashboard, as well as to find useful information.

Infrastructure

If data are regarded as the basic unit and fundamental core of data science technologies today, the digital infrastructure should be the carrier for data and information to be stored, transferred, processed, analysed, and managed. Continuous access to the internet for data and information, especially in high-impact areas such as public health, as well as government services, makes the digital infrastructure increasingly essential. Thus, failure to build a robust digital infrastructure could have disastrous consequences.

According to the World Economic Forum, the digital infrastructure consists of networks, data/protocol, devices, and services/storage and acts as communication service providers, digital service and product providers, as well as hardware manufacturers to facilitate the work for policy makers/regulators, industry participants, and other end users [23].

According to US experts, "any new project in the US should be equipped with digital infrastructure." [24] Meanwhile, the UK launched the Digital Infrastructure Investment Fund (DIIF) in 2017 to invest £400 million with the expectation to revolutionise Britain's digital infrastructure and unlock £1 billion for full fibre broadband [25].

In the development of digital infrastructure for a smart city, Taiwan aims to build a data hub that includes functions of electronic content, to obtain, process, transfer, provide services of data searching (allow effective data exchange in a more open framework), service development (allow local government and stakeholders to develop local services on the basis of local conditions), experience sharing (allow smooth operation of the city through systematic thinking and sharing with local citizens to interpret data), and data creation (allow further creation of data from daily life and government services).

In this aspect, the Taiwanese government also unveiled a plan to invest NT $46 billion over 8 years, starting in 2017, to improve digital infrastructure and bridge the gap between urban and rural areas [26].

Cybersecurity

As data information is being increasingly used in official matters such as government, healthcare, and education, cybersecurity becomes essential for a consistently healthy environment for the employment of data science technologies. In recent years, data applications throughout the world were threatened by cybersecurity issues, especially the massive cyberattack that swept across the world in 2017, in which the National Health Service (NHS) in the UK was one of the public health organisations affected, [27] reawakening people's awareness of the need for data security. In response, in 2018 the European Commission launched the General Data Protection Rule (GDPR) to build stronger protection for personal and business data to ensure a secure environment for data users [28].

The Taiwanese government launched the National Centre for Cyber Security Technology to establish a secure environment for data and information, improve the protection and management of data and information security, share diverse information, and strengthen international communication on cybersecurity [29].

Conclusion

In conclusion, with data as the fundamental core, data science technologies have become the essential pillar of today's development, especially in the public health domain. On one hand, data science technologies are being used to evaluate the current situation and progress towards the achievement of SDGs through indicators, as well as to develop a decision support system (DSS) to facilitate the development of public health systems and improve health conditions. Moreover, data science technologies are also used to perform cross-domain investigations and integrate information to comprehensively upgrade the public health system to address social issues, such as the ageing of society, to achieve the vision of health for all. However, the use of data science technologies could not persist without the strong support of open data, digital infrastructure, and cybersecurity.

On this basis, Taiwanese experiences in developing the Smart Health Network System to promote public health conditions towards shaping a smart and sustainable future for all at all ages are valuable and worth referencing. More importantly, let us go back to the UN SDGs and focus on the most essential goal, number 17, whose fundamental concept is global partnership. Indeed, shaping a sustainably healthy future is like the slogan "Leave No One Behind," which is widespread amongst people around the world, and requires everyone's efforts irrespective of the hindrances of national borders and races, while endeavouring for a more sustainable future together.

References

1. United Nations. Sustainable Development Goal 3: Ensure healthy lives and promote well-being for all at all ages. 2015. https://www.un.org/sustainabledevelopment/health/.
2. United Nations. Global indicator framework for the Sustainable Development Goals and targets of the 2030 Agenda for Sustainable Development. https://unstats.un.org/sdgs/indicators/indicators-list/
3. Sustainable Development Solutions Network. SDG Index and Dashboards Report 2018. Global Responsibilities: Implementing the goals. 2018. https://dashboards.sdgindex.org/#/
4. United States Government. U.S. National Statistics for the U.N. Sustainable Development Goals. https://sdg.data.gov/
5. Office for National Statistics. Office for National Statistics. https://www.ons.gov.uk/
6. JRC, DG REGIO. Urban Data Platform. https://urban.jrc.ec.europa.eu/#/about
7. European Commission. CitySDK. https://www.citysdk.eu/
8. US Census Bureau. CitySDK. https://uscensusbureau.github.io/citysdk/
9. Executive Yuan. Taiwan's Voluntary National Review–Implementation of the UN Sustainable Development Goals. https://www.roc-taiwan.org/uploads/sites/104/2017/09/Taiwan-VNR.pdf
10. UN-GGIM. UN-GGIM. http://ggim.un.org/
11. National Development Council. National Geographic Information System. https://ngis.nat.gov.tw/ngis2/
12. World Health Organisation. Dengue and severe dengue. 2018. https://www.who.int/news-room/fact-sheets/detail/dengue-and-severe-dengue. Accessed 13 Sept 2018.
13. Tainan City Government. Geographic Information System for Dengue Prevention and Control. http://dengue.tainan.gov.tw/
14. Tainan City Government. The Centres for Disease Control organised the New Southbound Dengue Fever Prevention and Control Exchange and Collaboration Programme with visiting in Tainan City. https://health.tainan.gov.tw/dengue/page.asp?mainid={361B400D-14D3-4A5C-9E59-6D990B7552C1}
15. Taiwan Centres for Disease Control. The Centres for Disease Control Organised the Professional Training Camp for Dengue Fever Prevention and Control to Promote the New Southbound Dengue Fever Prevention and Control Exchange and Collaboration Programme Together. https://www.cdc.gov.tw/info.aspx?treeid=45DA8E73A81D495D&nowtreeid=1BD193ED6DABAEE6&tid=6E943511256F1EFF
16. National Development Council. Promote the Regional Revitalisation Policy. https://www.ndc.gov.tw/Content_List.aspx?n=78EEEFC1D5A43877&upn=C4DB8C419A82AA5E
17. Ministry of Health and Welfare. New Southbound Pioneer Programme: Medical and Health Collaboration and Industrial Chain Development. 2017. https://dep.mohw.gov.tw/OOIC/cp-3919-40552-119.html?fbclid=IwAR0VLydo90jzVB9zvy5AFC55e7-r3UgT-Suau46h4BrDj6p2UZxGrcsG9MbE. Accessed 27 Dec 2017.
18. Ministry of Health and Welfare, Ministry of Foreign Affairs. Leave No One Behind. https://leavenoonebehind.com.tw/en/index.php?fbclid=IwAR3PQwUEQta0UR1fgy1XPzEIJ_k-xGF13MWsVCMi2eAF1HVVG2p57nSatW0
19. United Nations. Open SDG Data Hub. https://unstats-undesa.opendata.arcgis.com/
20. GOV.UK. Find open data. https://data.gov.uk/
21. National Development Council. Government Open Data Portal. https://data.gov.tw/
22. Taiwan Centres for Disease Control. Taiwan Communicable Disease Control Open Data Portal. https://data.cdc.gov.tw/zh_TW/
23. World Economic Forum. Introduction: The Digital Infrastructure Imperative. http://reports.weforum.org/delivering-digital-infrastructure/introduction-the-digital-infrastructure-imperative/
24. Descant S. Digital Infrastructure Should Be a Part of Any New U.S. Project, Experts Say. 2017. https://www.govtech.com/fs/infrastructure/Digital-Infrastructure-Should-Be-a-Part-of-Any-New-US-Project-Experts-Say.html. Accessed 5 Nov 2017.

25. GOV.UK. Billion pound connectivity boost to make buffering a thing of the past. 2017. https://www.gov.uk/government/news/billion-pound-connectivity-boost-to-make-buffering-a-thing-of-the-past

26. Executive Yuan. Executive Yuan unveils digital infrastructure project. 2017. https://english.ey.gov.tw/News_Content2.aspx?n=8262ED7A25916ABF&sms=DD07AA2ECD4290A6&s=1CC02A30D4D03E44

27. National Health Service. Cyber News Brief. 2018. https://digital.nhs.uk/services/data-security-centre/data-security-centre-latest-news/cyber-news-brief. Accessed 11 May 2018.

28. European Commission. 2018 reform of EU data protection rules. 2018. https://ec.europa.eu/commission/priorities/justice-and-fundamental-rights/data-protection/2018-reform-eu-data-protection-rules_en

29. Executive Yuan. National Centre for Cyber Security Technology. https://www.nccst.nat.gov.tw/

Chapter 19: Telemedicine in India and Its Impact on Public Health

Radha Ramana Murthy Gokula

Introduction

Telemedicine is the application of technological interfaces to facilitate the interaction of a physician and a patient who are in separate geographic locations. Despite the distance, the physician is able to offer services to the patient, often including a differential diagnosis, treatment protocols, and continuous monitoring of the patient's progress. In India, telemedicine has been in practical application for some time and offers great benefits to both healthcare practitioners and patients. Telemedicine has been very instrumental in the field of public health where the health systems serve a large number of patients who would otherwise be impossible to help if they had to see the physician in person. However, the use of telemedicine eliminates this conundrum, and even leverages technological capacity to store information, hence being rendered useful to public health agendas of disease surveillance and monitoring.

Despite the demonstrable benefits, telemedicine is not yet fully adopted in India. The purpose of this technology is to open up healthcare access for the general public who would benefit from the services. In the following sections, the evolution of telemedicine, its progress and barriers, and the impact of this technology on public health are explored in greater detail.

R. R. M. Gokula (✉)
STAYHOME IWILL PC, Toledo, OH, USA

University of Toledo, Maumee, OH, USA
e-mail: rrgokula@gmail.com

© Springer Nature Switzerland AG 2020
P. Murthy, A. Ansehl (eds.), *Technology and Global Public Health*,
https://doi.org/10.1007/978-3-030-46355-7_24

Evolution of Telemedicine in India

India is among the nations that score very low on the dissemination of healthcare services in the underdeveloped regions, such as rural areas, especially with regard to secondary and tertiary healthcare services [1]. However, the introduction of telemedicine has had a significant impact on patients from rural areas because they can receive advice and guidance from healthcare professionals based in the cities without necessarily having to travel to their appointments.

Telemedicine in India has grown significantly during the past two decades, largely from the efforts of both the government and private healthcare facilities. The first introduction of telemedicine in India, as a concept of delivering healthcare in the country, was identified by the government in the year 2000. The government of India formulated the telemedicine initiative in collaboration with the Department of Information Technology, the Indian Space Research Organization, the Ministry of Communication and Technology, and numerous state governmental and medical institutions. The project, which started in the early 2000s and was known as "Apollo," was led by the Department of Information Technology [2]. The initiative led to the birth of Apollo Hospitals, which have undertaken major efforts to oversee the progress of the technology and the dependability of telemedicine in India. The Apollo group of hospitals currently has more than 75 satellite centers throughout the nation that support research and development of telemedicine [2]. The primary goal of these projects has been to convey healthcare to isolated regions of the state as well as teaching paramedical professionals and offering help to healthcare professionals in rural areas.

In the year 2004, the North-Eastern Space Applications Center (NESAC) started a telemedicine project known as ISRO-NEC that uses satellite communication via very small aperture terminals (VSAT) [2]. The objective of ISRO-NEC was to advance interaction between hospitals in the rural areas and specialty tertiary care medical institutions. However, this effort was confined to the northern regions with poor infrastructure. The project was successful and led to the establishment of 25 regional telemedicine centers. In 2005, NESAC started another project in the north-eastern states of the country, called Village Resource Center (VRC), aimed at delivering state-of-art technology to rural areas [2]. Between its initiation and March 2013, the project had treated more than 300,000 patients as a result of successful data management and data transfer. As of today, many private healthcare institutions have recognized the potential of telemedicine in India and continue to successfully implement pilot projects that involve both the government and private enterprises. The success and impact of the Apollo project have propelled telemedicine to the center of medical practice in India.

Current Implementations of Telemedicine in Use in India

Today, telemedicine in India has grown, with a total of 25 operational regional telemedicine points; 47 others are already in the execution phase. One of the significant deployments is the initiative by the NESAC that continues to develop village resource centers (VRCs) in most parts of North India: this is an essential project that brings state-of-art technology to underdeveloped areas. The VRCs offer an array of services ranging from telemedicine, tele-education, and the creation and maintenance of a database on natural resources such as watershed areas and agricultural land and produce. In Tripura, the telemedicine initiatives are executed in 20 hospitals, 17 satellite hospitals, and 3 referrals hospitals. Another example of telemedicine in India is available in the southern parts of the country, the Kerala Oncology Network telemedicine project [3]. The primary goal of this initiative is the early diagnosis of cancer, institution and supervision of treatment, managing the illness, and follow-up services. The broad applications underscore the fact that telemedicine in India is rapidly gaining a reputation as a go-to alternative in healthcare provision and access across the country.

Integration of Telemedicine Technologies in the Communities

Telemedicine in India continues to be launched in various regions of the nation in response to the growing demand and appreciation of the integration of technology into medicine. The continuous tailoring of technologies to address the specific needs of the communities and the growth of community capacity to use the technology are some of the greatest drivers of integration of telemedicine into conventional healthcare in India. The northern states of India have been among the areas benefiting from telemedicine. In the year 2000, the Department of Space (DOS), the Indian Space Research Organization (ISRO), and the North-Eastern Council (NEC) came together to institute the North-Eastern Space Applications Centre (NESAC) aimed at commissioning 72 telemedicine local nodal centers in the northern districts [4]. The aim of this venture has been to link district-level hospitals to specialty tertiary care institutions in and out of the area.

One of the communities that benefit most from the telemedicine initiative is the state of Tripura because it has relatively low infant mortality rates, high female literacy levels, and, in 2012, a low crude birth rate. However, the achievements are not solely attributed to the advent of telemedicine in the region but also to high levels of female literacy and the developed educational system in the community [5].

The Department of Technology acts as the facilitator of telemedicine in India. Current efforts by the department have been focused in the following areas:

1. Development of new technology.
2. Launching of pilot schemes with selected areas of specialty such as oncology and general telemedicine that cover every section of specialization.
3. Initiation of the framework used in building the information technology (IT) framework in healthcare.
4. Development of national standards in technology.

The Centre for Development of Advanced Computing (C-DAC) also participates by developing telemedicine programs that support a variety of related medical fields [6]. Generally, telemedicine programs in India cover teleradiology, teleconsultation, teleophthalmology, tele-ICU (intensive care unit)), teledermatology, telesurgery, telepathology, and telepsychiatry.

Attitudes of Communities Towards Telemedicine

Developing countries such as India experience vast inequality in the distribution of healthcare. Although approximately 75% of Indians have been living in rural areas, more than 75% of the doctors live in the cities, [7] which simply translates to the idea that many Indians who live in rural areas lacked access to healthcare service before the advent of telemedicine in their area. Since the early 2000s, many Indians have developed a positive attitude towards telemedicine because telemedicine has made it possible to retain medical services and doctors in villages that were previously affected by the poor infrastructure [7]. Previously, residents in remote areas would spend much money in transport to city centers to seek healthcare services. As such, some of the areas that have appreciated and embraced telemedicine over time are the rural areas in India. Consequently, many initiatives that began mainly in the northern and southern states of India have been successful. Many people have been receptive to telemedicine in the rural regions because they find it less costly than the previous process, which was both time consuming and expensive, that they must undergo to receive medical attention.

The growing awareness, especially among the younger and middle-aged generations, caused a huge demand for technology-integrated healthcare such as online consultations that help people obtain medical opinions and advice concerning their health conditions [8]. The advent of telemedicine has solved the distance barrier, and many Indians are enjoying the many benefits that come with using this technology. The easy accessibility, affordability, and convenience attract a number of patients who opt for telemedicine and online medical services because they no longer have to wait in long queues for healthcare services. Several factors have resulted in an increase in demand for telemedicine, including increasing awareness of the technology among the younger generation, improved literacy in the rural areas, and a nationwide improvement of technology infrastructure such as satellites and communication systems.

Factors Affecting the Uptake of Telemedicine

The increase in computer literacy has been exponential in India, and the stakeholders in the healthcare services industry are looking towards telemedicine to improve healthcare delivery. However, India has challenges in providing healthcare for all her citizens, especially those that live in the rural areas. The factors that affect the uptake of telemedicine technology can be subdivided into policy factors, political and legal factors, and cultural and demographic factors.

Policy Factors

The government of India became aware of the possibility and potential of using telemedicine as a tool for healthcare delivery in 2000 [2]. The government of India set up a committee including various stakeholders to formulate a set of "Standards and Guidelines for Practice of Telemedicine in India" in 2003. These standards and guidelines were important in the uptake of telemedicine because they could be used to deliver cost-effective solutions, to guide the development and integration of evolving technical innovations, and to optimally leverage existing technologies. The standards and guidelines would also ensure that provision of telemedicine is attainable to all and sustainable [9]. Standards and guidelines also ensure that the standard of healthcare is world class.

The uptake of the technology was also fostered by professional recommendation with governmental support. The National Steering Committee for the 12th Plan (2012–2017) recommended that all district hospitals and primary health centers and subcenters have a connection to telemedicine and be encouraged to have M-health, which is the use of mobile phones to provide healthcare [10]. This practice would ensure that even the most remote parts of the country received healthcare.

The Ministry of Health and Family Welfare in the government of India formed a committee of experts whose job was to develop standards of electronic medical records (EMR) in September 2010 [11]. Electronic Medical Records or Electronic Health Records (EHR) are records of patients' medical data and medical history stored in computer-processable form. These records, which are essential in improving the efficiency of providing healthcare through telemedicine, are stored securely and can only be accessed by authorized persons. Such records make the coordination of healthcare over telemedicine platforms so much easier. Practitioners and institutions, therefore, have an incentive to employ telemedicine.

There is also evident effort to develop sufficient professional capacity for the use of the technology. The National Skills Development Council has formulated guidelines for training healthcare professionals in the use of technology, which has allowed private entities to considering training these professionals [12]. In the coming years, many healthcare professionals conversant with technology will enter the market, thereby significantly improving the adoption of telemedicine.

Legal and Political Factors

Numerous legal factors promote or hinder the adoption of telemedicine in India. Acts such as the Foreign Exchange Management Act of 1999 have enabled direct foreign investment in eHealth and telemedicine in India, a major boost in the uptake of telemedicine as more funds are available to implement new programs and expand the existing ones.

Laws have been enacted to govern eHealth in India. Some of the laws include (1) the Information and Technology Act of 2000, which provides for the protection of patient data. Sensitive data about people are collected and stored by organizations providing healthcare services, including telemedicine. These data must be protected, and doctors cannot use the data without the consent of the patients. (2) The Drugs and Cosmetics Act of 1945 and the Drugs and Cosmetic Rules of 1945 regulate drugs in India in terms of manufacturing and distribution. (3) The Indian Medical Council Act of 1956 and The Indian Medical Council Regulations of 2002 state that only those individuals who have attained a medical degree from colleges that are accredited by the state medical councils can practice medicine in India. Professionals who are involved in telemedicine are no exception and must satisfy this criterion also. (4) The Clinical Establishment Act of 2010 requires all clinical establishments to be registered with the relevant authority, to ensure that these establishments satisfy all the requirements and the minimum standards required. The telemedicine centers also have to conform to this act [13]. These acts and others may present hurdles in the implementation of telemedicine for healthcare delivery but are essential for protecting the welfare of the patients who are, after all, the reason for all this. All these laws create a defined legal framework in which the technology can be implemented.

Local and national politics also impact the practice of telemedicine. The government of India strongly recommends the use of telemedicine. However, in government hospitals, the use of telemedicine is not mandatory and the incentives for implementation are insufficient to encourage the staff to take the initiative [14]. Also, some of the government programs for healthcare education are inefficient for reasons of corruption [14]. Corruption damages the ability of telemedicine to deliver high-quality and efficient healthcare because resources are not deployed efficiently, and this discourages the private sector from becoming involved in telemedicine. Also, telemedicine projects are not lucrative, and therefore they do not get sufficient political attention and support. All these political and regulatory factors have been a hindrance to the adoption of telemedicine in India, and they need attention if the implementation is to be successful.

Cultural and Demographic Factors

The population of India is about 1.3 billion people. This population is very diverse, composed of people from different religions and cultures. Cultural factors have a significant effect on the adoption of telemedicine in India. Telemedicine requires consultation between professionals, but there are some doctors – especially in the rural areas – who may be hesitant to consult their counterparts in the cities [14]. Convincing some of the population that technology is beneficial and that it can be used to deliver healthcare services efficiently is important, and this might require a considerable amount of effort [14]. Some cultures, especially in the south of India, are deeply conservative and may not accept such measures as contraception, family planning, abortion, and other services that are included under the umbrella of telemedicine. This attitude limits the scope of application of this technology.

The number of people who require telemedicine services is large and human capital resources are insufficient. For telemedicine to deliver health services efficiently, professionals from various sectors such as information technology and allied healthcare are required. However, the shortage of professionals is a barrier. The large numbers of patients also bring challenges to recording data. As the government has not fully embraced the digital recording of data, the paper system is still in use, causing inefficiency in the system when handling a large number of patients.

The Impact of Telemedicine on Public Health

The World Health Organization describes telecommunication as the provision of healthcare services in places where the physical distance between the service provider and the patient is significant [15]. The services are provided by very skilled healthcare staff through the use of communications and information technologies for exchanging valid and legitimate information for analysis, treatment, and prevention of illness and injury, research and assessment, and education for healthcare professionals. Telemedicine has brought many benefits to the public health sector worldwide, some of which include easy access to remote areas and reduced waiting time, as well as the reduced costs of transporting patients.

Benefits of Telemedicine

Telemedicine fundamentally joins high-tech electronics, information-communication technology, and related applications in the domain of healthcare provision and also aids in educating healthcare professionals and patients. Telemedicine also has a significant role in the promotion of health, particularly in improving the beliefs, attitudes, and knowledge of the general population.

Telemedicine helps in the prevention of diseases and promotion of health in numerous areas. The associated applications of this technology such as video conferencing, audiovisual aids, and healthcare-associated discussions with doctors can be used to enlighten, educate, and motivate people [15]. Telemedicine also promotes home-care and self-care practices, and relays information to people and their communities and provides access to individuals residing in remote regions. Residents in remote areas can benefit from the self-management of their health issues, which will strengthen healthcare services.

Telecommunication enables individuals to make informed decisions. It establishes communication between the healthcare professionals and patients about diagnosis, treatment, and prevention of illnesses more efficiently, thereby enabling patients to make informed decisions.

It also aids in the emotional support of the patient and peer informational discussion, for example, by internet applications that allow people with specific needs and health conditions to communicate with one another and offer emotional support [16].

Public Health Issues Addressed by Telemedicine in India

Epidemiological Surveillance

Epidemiological surveillance is also known as public health surveillance. It is the constant and methodical gathering, examination, and interpretation of health-associated information that is required for development, implantation, and assessment of healthcare practices [1]. Epidemiological surveillance may provide warning systems for future healthcare emergencies, record the result of an intervention, and follow up on the advancement towards specific goals and monitoring of diseases.

Epidemiological surveillance is strengthened by telemedicine. Observation of disease patterns is essential for early detection of disease outbreaks, incidence, prevalence, morbidity, and mortality rates. In India, disease surveillance was neglected across the healthcare sector until 1997. Telemedicine programs have facilitated disease control in New Delhi where the national center for disease control was established [1]. Some of the diseases under surveillance included fever, meningitis, malaria, and enteric fever.

Telemedicine also aided in epidemiological surveillance with the growth and development of Geographic Information Systems (GIS), which provide one method of learning about healthcare information [1]. Use of GIS technology enables comparison of healthcare expenditures and impacts among geographic regions to develop a perfect system of healthcare provision and to guide policies in healthcare sectors. Telemedicine applications provide insight into the geographic prevalence of a variety of diseases and the overall health status of individuals in different communities. The incorporation of telemedicine and GIS helps to bring changes in the healthcare of rural areas in India. This technology helps us understand how climate, environment, and the transmission of diseases are connected at both regional and national levels.

Disease Prevention and Health Promotion

Telemedicine and information technology are used in India to influence, inform, and motivate populations, individuals, and organizations on health and healthcare-associated topics and issues to help them practice a healthy lifestyle. The diverse applications of telemedicine support and facilitate primary, secondary, and tertiary health financing. They also promote agendas on the prevention of diseases in the impoverished areas of India, which have less infrastructure and limited healthcare services. The North-Eastern Space Application Centre and the Indian Space Research Organization procured support in 47 nodal centers in the states. Apart from the village resource centers, the North-Eastern Council initiative is significant in the dissemination of information and providing changes in healthcare services and practices [17]. Simple quality improvement initiatives assist in delivering and improving vaccination rates in inaccessible, remote areas. Applications such as video conferencing, audiovisuals, and conversations on healthcare-associated issues with pediatricians and other doctors are used to inform and encourage individuals. This initiative offers data to both individuals and large populations, thereby making it easy to access those who reside in remote rural areas [16]. Communication between peers who need emotional support is made simpler by creating a platform where they can communicate with one another and share and give advice, thus getting emotional support.

Notably, suburban Indian communities are also able to share information regarding health services easily by means of telemedicine. Doctors share magnetic resonance imaging (MRI) reports and hospital scans with each other through electronic media, enabling them to learn from one another and provide better and more accurate diagnoses for their patients. Telemedicine also solves the problem of the number of medical specialists in the country; it is much easier and more straightforward to set up a communication infrastructure in both rural and suburban areas than to deploy thousands of health professionals in these areas.

Data Overload

Healthcare in India is one of the most data-demanding and information-driven industries. Large amounts of information from physicians, laboratories, pharmaceuticals, and patients require storing. Telemedicine assists storing data and providing easy access to required information about healthcare services [15]. Patients and healthcare providers can access information concerning services provided and patient records from the internet. The availability of such information and the attendant ease of access helps reduce healthcare problems such as missed diagnosis, violation of patient confidentiality, and inappropriate application of treatment. Obtaining a good internet infrastructure system is an essential boost to medical services. Both rural and urban India are able to store and access their medical information for both doctors and patients.

Decision Support Systems

Telemedicine has increased support to both healthcare providers and consumers. For instance, the consumers can readily access information about various health centers. Consequently, it gives them a more comprehensive choice base. Additionally, data on antibiotic resistance of common organisms is available to doctors.

Enhancing Access to Healthcare Services at a Distance

Telemedicine has done wonders when it comes to providing accessibility of health-care services remotely. Video calls to physicians have significantly reduced time and resources for patient transportation. In rural and suburban India, the necessary infrastructure for such applications was installed and fiber cables put in place for internet connections [15]. Other applications include email services where patients can ask their doctors questions and be advised based on their descriptions of how they feel.

Telemedicine Application to Issues in India

Although the interest in telemedicine in the past 5 years appears to be relatively new, it has been utilized in one way or the other in the past 30 years. In India, the use of telemedicine has revolved around making public health accessible and effi-cient through implementations such as satellite facilities that are cost-effective and convenient for local populations. Some of the areas addressed by telemedicine include epidemiological surveillance, alleviating data overload, enhancing access to healthcare at a distance, and utilization as a decision support system.

Epidemiological Surveillance Application

Epidemiological surveillance is one of the issues addressed by telemedicine in India. Telemedicine has made a reaching contribution in the field of healthcare across India. Presently, most of the utilization of telemedicine has been intensified in therapeutic services. Telemedicine has an enormous role in the area of health promotion, particularly in improving the beliefs, attitudes, and knowledge of the people. The most common reason for the underperformance of public health sys-tems in India is lack of familiarity with prevention of communicable diseases and the erroneous practices and beliefs held by rural populations. Thus, telemedicine has been applied to advancing healthcare programs across the country, offering sup-port to public healthcare systems through an enhanced epidemiological surveillance network set up by the government and health organizations [18]. One such applica-tion is the expansion of geographic information programs used for studying health-care data. Consequently, telemedicine addresses the issue of disease surveillance by providing insight into the geographic distribution of a variety of diseases, disease prevalence rates, and the overall health of entire populations.

Disease Prevention and Health Promotion Application

The healthcare industry and the private sector recognize the potential of telemedicine as a reliable and dependable healthcare relief system in India. The main aim of the telemedicine program is to deliver healthcare services to the most remote parts of India. These services covers a variety of subspecialties such as orthopedics, pediatrics, radiology, neurology, cardiology, HIV, oncology, and dermatology. The program creates a record of patient medical records and healthcare statistics. Telemedicine also facilitates training healthcare professionals in remote areas [18]. There is also evidence supporting the application of telemedicine in primary healthcare in the country. Current experiments in India, such as the use of personal digital assistants used by the rural health workers in the village of Rajasthan, have shown success. Telemedicine has facilitated and supported ingenious ways of utilizing information and communications technology (ICT) to promote and improve health situations of the local people [18]. This scenario proves that telemedicine is useful in the provision of healthcare and disease prevention in remote areas through screening for diseases.

Data Overload Application

The healthcare industry relies heavily on data for decision support. In providing health services, large amounts of data are created from healthcare institutions and other healthcare providers. There is great concern about the storage and access of data, which poses a problem to health officials. India, a country with a population of more than 1.3 billion people, requires vast spaces for healthcare data storage. Telemedicine programs have offset this problem by easing the burden placed on manual systems to record and store data. The inability to store and retrieve data accurately makes the work of healthcare professionals more difficult, with catastrophic health implications for both patients and doctors. India has improved its healthcare system by providing its medical specialists with the real-time right of entry to adequately maintained and updated databases loaded with patient information [17]. Thus, issues of data overload within a hospital are, to a great extent, diminished.

Health at a Distance Application

Telemedicine has dramatically improved functionality in the healthcare industry. By creating consistency and performance capabilities in remote-oriented programs, it creates accessible and reliable medical service for patients in rural and suburban areas. The emphasis of this service has been the improvement of real-time communication and streaming functionalities to provide solutions to the limitations of little or no access to healthcare services in rural and suburban areas.

Conclusion

Even though India continuously makes gigantic economic strides, many of its citizens live in abject poverty, illiteracy, and ill health. The provision of healthcare is one of the significant issues affecting the country. Many Indian citizens are unable to access proper medical services. This problem mainly affects those in rural areas, where there is inadequate infrastructure. Long distances coupled with poor transport modes make it difficult for patients to reach health facilities or for medical practitioners to reach their patients. Another reason for this disparity is the lack of adequately trained medical practitioners. To solve this problem, the government of India has been considering advances in telemedicine. As an advanced form of medical service delivery, telemedicine can help ensure that every Indian citizen, even those in the most remote places, is a beneficiary of high-quality healthcare. Today, several telemedicine centers have been set up all across India. These hubs not only increase accessibility of healthcare but are also economical. Telemedicine comes at a fraction of the cost one would incur at a health facility. In addition, telemedicine eliminates the long journeys and accommodation costs that individuals would have to incur in person-to-person consultations [19].

The government works together with several states and private medical institutions to implement the telemedicine initiative. The Indian Space Research Organization (ISRO) works in conjunction with the Ministry of Communication and Technology, the Department of Information Technology, and several state governments to address the accessibility of telemedicine. These government branches have taken part in the establishment and successful running of projects that implement telemedicine. An example is the establishment of the North Eastern Space Application Center (NESAC). The role of NESAC was to establish 71 telemedicine centers in all the districts of the northeastern region. This region is known for its remoteness and inaccessibility, hence the dire need for telemedicine application.

Another key player in the field of telemedicine in India is the Indo-American Telemedicine Corporation. The organization has been at the forefront of initiatives to introduce telemedicine in rural villages, specifically in Telengana and Andhra Pradesh. It is interested in the integration of HealthCubed systems that will digitize and avail quality and efficient healthcare. The systems are user friendly, providing access to numerous advanced tests and issuing instant results [20]. The telemedicine projects will train personnel, create web portals for patients to interact with healthcare providers, utilize Zoom technology for video conferencing, and keep patient records in an electronic filing system.

IIndo-American Telemedicine Corporation worked with HEALTHCUBED using funding from IDEA Cellular Company to implement telemedicine and integration of the HealthCubed device in primary health centers in both Telangana and Andhra Pradesh. This project successfuly led to the development of social health entrepreneurs, who used digital diagnostics within the public health systems and link patients with doctors, and store patient records in portals that guarantee confidentiality. The steps involved are training in the use of HealthCubed equipment, implementation of the system, evaluation of whether the system is working as planned, and monitoring of the system's outcomes.

In the future, the government seeks to increase telemedicine centers for the accessibility of medical care and education [19]. The Ministry of Health plans to reopen some of the more than 400 telemedicine centers that had been shut down by lack of sustainability. These hubs not only will be used to provide medical services, but they will also be linked to 41 medical colleges, giving students access to mentoring from lecturers in leading institutions. With the ever-increasing advancements in ICT, there is a high likelihood of transforming this vision into reality.

Case Study

In 1997, the Apollo group of hospitals founded a telemedicine program to facilitate the provision of healthcare to people in rural areas. This initiative was called the Apollo Telemarketing Network Foundation (ATNF). The ATNF aimed to provided specialist level medical assistance to people living in rural India. Working with the ISRO, the organization offers services in various medical fields including general consultation, dermatology, cardiology, and radiology [21]. The ANTF aimed to accomplish its task of availing telemedicine services to rural communities by setting up several telemedicine locations. The Apollo Group has been successful in attaining its goals. Currently, it has set up 115 telemedicine centers in India alone and 10 in other countries. These centers succeed in their objectives by offering advice and second opinions to doctors and their patients.

Despite all the success that ATNF boasts today, it has encountered its fair share of challenges in its journey towards the provision of healthcare for all. One such problem is finding doctors who are willing to relocate to the centers set up in rural areas and devote all their time and resources to the betterment of the health of the patients there. Another was the fact that telemedicine is a new concept, and thus some time is needed for patients and practitioners alike to adapt to it. This lag reduced the financial viability of the project. The project also failed to generate the predicted income, leading to a shortage of funds needed to modify the program to fit the outlined business model. Also, there was little financial support from the Indian government. Even though the government possesses a large pool of resources, their utilization of it is unfocused. Such funds should be used to support initiatives such as the telemedicine centers but instead are directed elsewhere.

References

1. Ganapathy K. Telehealth in India: the Apollo contribution and an overview. Apollo Med. 2014;11(3):201–7. https://doi.org/10.1016/j.apme.2014.07.014.
2. Mathur P, Srivastava S, Lalchandani A, Mehta JL. Evolving role of telemedicine in health care delivery in India. Primary Health Care Open Access. 2017;7(1) https://doi.org/10.4172/2167-1079.1000260.
3. Sudhamony S, Nandakumar K, Binu P, Niwas SI. Telemedicine and tele-health services for cancer-care delivery in India. IET Commun. 2008;2(2):231. https://doi.org/10.1049/iet-com:20060701.
4. Government of India. North Eastern-Space Applications Centre (NE-SAC). Department of Indian Space Research Organisation. 2017. Retrieved from https://www.isro.gov.in/about-isro/north-eastern-space-applications-centre-ne-sac. Accessed 10 July 2019.
5. Das I. Infant mortality rate in rural Assam: an empirical analysis. Indian Streams Res J. 2013;2(12)
6. Chandwani RK, Dwivedi YK. Telemedicine in India: current state, challenges and opportunities. Transforming Government: People, Process and Policy. 2015;9(4):393–400. https://doi.org/10.1108/tg-07-2015-0029.
7. Rai J, Acharya R. Evaluation of patient and doctor perception toward the use of telemedicine in Apollo tele health services, India. J Family Med Prim Care. 2016;5(4):798. https://doi.org/10.4103/2249-4863.201174.
8. Álvarez MM, Chanda R, Smith RD. How is telemedicine perceived? A qualitative study of perspectives from the UK and India. Globalization Health. 2011;7(1):17. https://doi.org/10.1186/1744-8603-7-17.
9. Bedi BS. Telemedicine standards: issues and Indian initiatives. The 21st Pacific Science Congress Okinawa. APT Telemedicine Initiative. 2007.
10. Patnaiki S, Patnaik AN. E-health for all – is India ready? Int J Commun Med. 2015;6(4):633–8.
11. Bedi BS. Electronic health record standardization in India. International Conference Transforming Healthcare with IT (THIT), Bengaluru, 2015, pp 6–7.
12. Tata Communication. What will it take to revolutionize E-health in India? 2017. Retrieved from http://www.gloheal.com/glo-blog/2017/04/what-will-it-take-to-revolutionize-e-health-in-india. Accessed 10 July 2019.
13. Nishith Desai Associate. E-health in India: legal, regulatory and tax overview. 2017. p. 7–10. Retrieved from http://www.nishithdesai.com/fileadmin/user_upload/pdfs/Research%20Papers/e-Health-in-India.pdf. Accessed 10 July 2019.
14. Jarosławski S, Saberwal G. In eHealth in India today, the nature of work, the challenges and the finances: an interview-based study. BMC Med Inform Decis Mak. 2014;14(1) https://doi.org/10.1186/1472-6947-14-1.
15. Nair AR, Nair PA. Teledermatology: a possible reality in rural India. Int J Dermatol. 2014;54(3):375–6. https://doi.org/10.1111/ijd.12624.
16. Kanthraj G. A longitudinal study of consistency in diagnostic accuracy of teledermatology tools. Indian J Dermatol Venereol Leprol. 2013;79(5):668. https://doi.org/10.4103/0378-6323.116735.
17. Kalyanpur A, Seshadri S. Teleradiology in India – utilisation, benefits and challenges. Int J Telemed Clin Pract. 2016;1(3):209. https://doi.org/10.1504/ijtmcp.2016.077900.
18. Phalkey RK, Shukla S, Shardul S, et al. Assessment of the core and support functions of the Integrated Disease Surveillance system in Maharashtra, India. BMC Public Health. 2013;13(1) https://doi.org/10.1186/1471-2458-13-575.
19. Kaul R. With 105 centres, govt spreads telemedicine network across country. Hindustantimes 2016.
20. HealthCubed Confidential. HealthCubed ecosystem. A gateway to public health screening. 2017.
21. Sridevi J, Alagarsamy D. A case study on Telemedicine practices implemented with respect to Apollo Hospitals. Int J Appl Environ Sci. 2015;10(1):23–8.

Chapter 20: The Role of Technology in Sustainable Development Goal Performance in Taiwan

Joyce Tsung-Hsi Wang

Introduction

Vibrant night markets, irresistible delicacies, and warm hospitality: these are the first impressions from people who have visited Taiwan. Surrounded by water and covered with high mountains, this relatively small island on the Pacific Ocean boasts its scenery, culture, and diversity. The Portuguese were stunned by Taiwan's exquisite natural scenery 400 years ago, and gave this land the name *Ilha Formosa*, beautiful island, for a place that has spring-like weather all year long. Taiwanese culture is a unique melting pot of historical influences. It is a fusion of indigenous, Chinese, Japanese, and Western cultures. From food to architecture to traditions, the legacy from Taiwan's diverse history can still been seen in Taiwan today.

From being an agriculture-based island, Taiwan has seen a tremendous economic growth in the past decades to a well-industrialized and mature economy. Today, it has developed into a world-class leader in technology [1]. However, in the process of economic development, Taiwan's natural environment has suffered from pollution and other damages. As it is a small island, Taiwan already has limited natural resources and is prone to frequent natural disasters such as typhoons and earthquakes. Though only 1/243 the size of the United States, Taiwan hosts a population over 23 million people, making it one of world's top densely populated places [2]. The urgency for Taiwan to pursue sustainable development for the future generation is even greater than that of other nations [3].

J. T.-H. Wang (✉)
Hsinchu City Public Health Bureau, Taiwan, R.O.C

National Yang-Ming University School of Medicine, Taipei, Taiwan
e-mail: joyce12wang@gmail.com

© Springer Nature Switzerland AG 2020
P. Murthy, A. Ansehl (eds.), *Technology and Global Public Health*,
https://doi.org/10.1007/978-3-030-46355-7_25

United Nations Sustainable Development Goals (SDG)

In September 2015, the United Nation General Assembly unanimously adopted the 2030 Agenda for Sustainable Development that "provides a shared blueprint for peace and prosperity for people and the planet, now and into the future." [3, 4]. The agenda includes 17 Sustainable Development Goals (SDGs) and 169 targets, to stimulate action over the next 15 years in areas of critical importance for people, planet, prosperity, peace, and partnership. Please see the following brief list of the 17 goals [4]:

1. No Poverty
2. Zero Hunger
3. Good Health and Well-being
4. Quality Education
5. Gender Equality
6. Clean Water and Sanitation
7. Affordable and Clean Energy
8. Decent Work and Economic Growth
9. Industry, Innovation and Infrastructure
10. Reduced Inequalities
11. Sustainable Cities and Communities
12. Responsible Consumption and Production
13. Climate Action
14. Life Below Water
15. Life on Land: Protect, restore and promote sustainable use of terrestrial ecosystems
16. Peace, Justice and Strong Institutions
17. Partnerships for the Goals: Strengthen the means of implementation and revitalize the Global partnership for Sustainable Development

SDGs and Taiwan

The ultimate purpose for sustainable development is to fulfill the present day's needs while not endangering the development of future generations [5]. As stated by former Premier of Taiwan Ching-Te Lai, the Taiwanese government pays close attention to sustainable development, because Taiwan has limited natural resources, high dependency on imported energy, and a high population density, causing a huge burden on the environment [6]. From citizens to the government, Sustainable Development is an issue that affects people in every aspect of life, and thus it brings attention to people from individuals to national level. Taiwan heavily emphasizes the importance of SDGs, and the government has been working towards building a sustainable country that could preserve the country's beautiful name of "Formosa." Indeed, for years Taiwan has shown a prideful track record in achieving the SDGs, especially in the areas of Good Health and Well-being (SDG 3) and Gender Equality (SDG 5). This chapter discusses the achievements, the efforts, and the future of Taiwan in pursuing the Sustainable Development Goals.

Taiwan's Achievements in the Sustainable Development Goals

Taiwan's performance in the SDGs presented here in five categories: Economic, Human Rights, Educational, Health, and Environmental [7]. These aspects are taken from the 17 Sustainable Development Goals listed by the United Nations and categorized into five aspects of the SDGs. Taiwan has accomplished top-of-the-world performance in these areas. What has Taiwan achieved regarding promoting a healthy and sustainable country?

Taiwan's SDG Achievements in the Economic Aspect

Inspecting the economic aspect of Taiwan's SDGs includes the following four: No Poverty (SDG 1), Decent Work and Economic Growth (SDG 8), Industry, Innovation, and Infrastructure (SDG 9), and Responsible Consumption and Production (SDG 12).

Since the middle of the past century, Taiwan's economy has shifted from an agricultural-based economy [32% of gross domestic product (GDP) in 1952] to an industry-oriented economy (47% of GDP in 1986 and 52.8% in 2014) [8]. One of the "Four Asian Tigers," Taiwan witnessed a miracle in soaring economy and opportunities in the 1980s. Today, Taiwan is the world's 19th largest economy, based on an export-oriented economy that specializes in production of electronics and machinery [9]. Export goods include semiconductors, petrochemicals, electronics, plastics, and computers. In recent years, the main export partners are neighbors in Asia such as Mainland China (26.3%), Hong Kong (13.7%), and Japan (7%), as well as partners such as the United States (12%) and European Union (8.8%) in the West [10]. Taiwan is home to many leading global brands such as HTC, Acer, Asus, and Giant, as well as such cross-continental corporations as Foxconn and Taiwan Semiconductor Manufacturing Company (TSMC). These corporations and industries, as well as governmental regulation, facilitate the economic aspect of the SDGs in Taiwan.

In line with SDG 1, No Poverty, Taiwan has been actively working to increase the minimum wage. Executive Yuan passed the decision to stipulate the minimum hourly wage raise by 5% effective in October 2016 and minimum monthly wage increase by 5.56% to NT$21,009 (USD$700) effective in January 2017. It was further decided to increase the minimum monthly wage by another 4.72% to NT$22,000 (USD $733) effective in January 2018. The decision is expected to improve workers' lives and protect their rights and interests [3].

In line with SDG 9, Industry, Innovation, and Infrastructure, Taiwan has also been progressing through the Forward-looking Infrastructure Construction Act. In accordance with the act promulgated by presidential decree in July 2017, the act covers a 4-year period for eight major categories of infrastructure, railway projects, water environments, digital infrastructure, urban and rural projects, and human resources infrastructure to nurture talent and boost employment. It is a budget of NT$420 billion allocated to the nation's prosperity. The Health Promotion Administration (HPA) also oversees building a healthy environment through soft and hard infrastructures. In 2017, more than 25% of the 368 rural townships, towns, cities, and districts in Taiwan promoted community health building plans; 432 community safety environment inspections and 14,151 senior living environment safety inspections were conducted. In 2017, there are 121 internationally accredited Health Promoting Schools to foster talents [11]. These statistics shows that Taiwan has been constructing a healthy country through building hospitals and establishing schools.

In line with SDG 8, Decent Work and Economic Growth, Taiwan ranks number 19 in highest GDP per capita around the world. According to the International Monetary Fund (IMF) 2018 release on worldwide national GDP per capita, only 29 countries have a GDP per capita of USD$45,000. Taiwan ranks number 19 with GDP per capita of USD$52,304, surpassing the United Kingdom and France, as well as Japan and Korea [12]. Achieving a strong economy is a foundation to facilitate the resources and opportunities for government and people to achieve other SDGs.

Taiwan's SDG Achievements in the Human Rights Aspect

The Human Rights aspect of SDGs includes the following three: Gender Equality (SDG 5), Reduced Inequalities (SDG 10), and Peace, Justice, and Strong Institutions (SDG 16).

In line with Peace, Justice and Strong Institutions (SDG 16), Taiwan has seen many judicial reforms since 2017. From February to June 2017, The National Conference on Judicial Reform, organized by the Office of the President, adopted more than a hundred resolutions following intensive subcommittee meetings. These resolutions fostered social consensus and set the direction and timetable for judicial reforms. The Ministry of Justice proposed prosecutorial and prison administration reforms, and measures to raise the status and enhance the protection of crime victims [3].

Regarding Gender Equality (SDG 5), Taipei City, the capital of Taiwan, is the most equal in the world. The ranking is according to the Gender Inequality Index (GII) published by the United Nations Development Programme (UNDP) since 2010. The index reflects "the states of gender equality across countries by 5 indicators based on the 3 dimensions of reproductive health, empowerment, and the labor market, which renders five indicators. A lower GII value indicates better quality (0 as very high equality, and 1 as very low equality)." [13]. Taipei received a GII value of 0.027 in 2017, making Taipei the most gender equal country worldwide, surpassing Switzerland (0.039), Denmark (0.040), and Sweden and Netherlands (both 0.044). Taipei leads on a large scale among neighboring such Asian countries as South Korea (0.063), Singapore (0.067), Japan (0.103), and mainland China (0.152) [13].

In addition, the Global Gender Gap Index Report published by the World Economic Forum (WEF) ranks Taipei as the top 2 in Asia, close behind the Philippines. The index annually benchmarks 149 countries on their progress towards gender parity across four thematic dimensions: Economic Participation and Opportunity, Educational Attainment, Health and Survival, and Political Empowerment. Scoring from 0 to 1, the higher the value (i.e., 1), the narrower the gender gap (i.e., total equality), and vice versa. Taipei scored the value of 0.733, ranking 36th in all 149 countries investigated, and 2nd to the Philippines (0.799) in Asia, while still leading among such Asian counterparts as Singapore, Thailand, Vietnam, Indonesia, India, Japan, and South Korea [13].

Government policies and education are crucial in bringing Taiwan's gender equality to the top in Asia and the world. As early as 1996, the Taipei City Committee of Women's Rights Promotion was founded to promote women's rights in governmental and private sectors. The Office for Gender Equality in City Government was also founded in 2014, a pioneering ad hoc project assigned at the local government level.

Taiwan's SDG Achievements in the Educational Aspect

The educational aspect of SDGs covers Quality Education (SDG 4). The education system, consisting of basic elementary education, junior high school, and senior secondary education, is managed by the Ministry of Education in Taiwan. The literacy rate among Taiwanese people aged 15 years and older was 98.5% in 2014. Compared to the rest of the world, students who graduate from the education system in Taiwan achieve some of the highest scores on an international level, especially in mathematics and science. According to the Programme for International Student Assessment (PISA) implemented by the Organization for Economic Cooperation and Development, Taiwan ranks 4th in PISA mathematics and science ranking, while No. 23 in reading, on the global list in 2016 [14]. PISA aims to appraise the efficiency, equity, and quality of school systems worldwide by evaluating the skills and knowledge of 15-year-old students. The ranking not only shows that the children of Taiwan have access to complete free, equitable, and quality primary and secondary education, leading to relevant and effective earning outcomes (SDG 4.1), it also showcases the prestige of Taiwan's education.

Not only does Taiwan impart excellent prestigious higher education, but it also extends education to students from all over the world by providing scholarship programs for international students. According to Taiwan's Voluntary National Review by Executive Yuan (2019), students from developing nations come to Taiwan to enroll in undergraduate, graduate, and PhD programs. "Opportunities are provided for students to receive fair and high-quality education, assisting developing nations in cultivating policy planning, technical and management experts." [3]. Current progress shows that the Taiwan International Cooperation Alliance works with 21 partner universities in Taiwan to provide 35 programs from undergraduate to PhD level. As of 2017, nearly 700 students from 39 countries were studying in Taiwan [3].

Taiwan's SDG Achievements in the Health Aspect

The health aspect of SDGs includes the following three: Zero Hunger (SDG 2), Good Health and Well-Being (SDG 3), and Clean Water and Sanitation (SDG 6).

In December 2016, the Council of Agriculture briefed the then Premier Lin Chuan on the Innovative Agriculture Promotion Program. The Program focuses on building a new agricultural paradigm, establishing agricultural safety systems, and bolstering agricultural marketing capabilities [3]. This plan employs technological innovations to add greater value to agricultural products, safeguard the welfare and income of farmers, and advance resource recycling and the sustainability of the ecosystem and the environment. It is in line with SDG 2, Promoting a large-scale granary project, enhancing food security, and SDG 6, Promoting a farmland cultivation subsidy scheme to ensure agricultural land is used for agricultural purposes, promoting methods of farming that are beneficial to the environment and reduce the use of chemicals.

In line with SDG 3, Good Health and Well-Being, with the National Health Insurance and Health Promotion Administration Taiwan can afford to provide excellent, high-quality, and efficient healthcare, ensuring healthy lives and promoting well-being for all at all ages. Since 1995, Taiwan has constituted a single-payer healthcare system, National Health Insurance (NHI), that covers the full spectrum of essential and high-quality health services, from prevention and treatment to rehabilitation and palliative care; 99.9% of its resident are enrolled in the national healthcare program, regardless of preexisting conditions [15], fulfilling the SDG emphasis on "No One Will Be Left Behind." Comprehensive benefits include inpatient and outpatient care, mental healthcare, prescription drugs, dental care, Chinese medicine, dialysis, and day care for the elderly. In addition, patients in Taiwan can choose their doctors and hospitals freely, in contrast to United States' limited choice of both insurers and providers in the network. All in all, the NHI has seen a satisfactory rate of 85% across Taiwan [11]. Taiwan has long achieved the SDG 3.8 of universal health coverage, including financial risk protection, access to quality essential healthcare services, and access to safe, effective, quality and affordable essential medicines and vaccines for all.

Because of the health insurance and promotion administration policies, from birth to aging to disease prevention, Taiwan has excelled in promoting good health.

From birth, Taiwan's infant mortality rate was 4 per 1000 live births in 2017 [16], already much lower than the targeted 25 per 1000 live births in SDG 3.2.

In line with SDG 3.5 and 3.a and 3.d to strengthen the prevention and treatment of substance abuse such as Tobacco, Taiwan has seen significant results. The smoking rate among junior high school students was less than 4.6% and among senior and vocational high school students fell to less than 9.6% in 2017 [17]. The usage of tobacco by adolescents has been steadily declining since 2004, when the rate was 6.6% in junior high students and 45.2% in high school students. A 60% decrease in middle school students and 40% decrease in high school and vocational students has been seen since the Tobacco Hazard Prevention Act was implemented in 2009 [17]. To reinforce young people's awareness, the "Campus Tobacco Control Implementation Program" emphasized strategies to establish tobacco hazard prevention education, promoting in schools and encouraging colleges to integrate nearby community resources to upgrade teachers' and students' knowledge and skills about tobacco hazard prevention. In addition, the local health department and social resources also promoted, through propaganda events or subsidizing community health creation plans, civil or civil groups to monitor surrounding campus stores, prohibiting tobacco being sold to young adolescents. Early prevention and education successfully reflect the result of decreasing tobacco usage in adults. The smoking rate of adults older than 18 fell from 32.5% in 1990 to 14.5% in 2017, a drop of more than 50% [17].

Taiwan also promoted non-communicable disease prevention, because the leading cause of death in Taiwan is malignant neoplasms. In 2017, the Health Promotion Administration (HPA) pushed for the establishment of 540 diabetes support groups and achieved a 97.8% national coverage rate. Taiwan also achieved a cervical cancer screening rate of 72.5% for women aged 30–69 years, a mammogram screening rate of 39.9 for women aged 45–69 years, and a colorectal cancer screening rate of 41.0% for people aged 50–69 years [18].

Taiwan has spent significant effort in building a Health Promotion Infrastructure, to achieve better health literacy, communication, and surveillance, an important factor to keep the SDG of healthy living on track. In 2017, health literacy had increased regarding various tests, policies, and disease information. Knowledge about cirrhosis and liver cancer, for example, reached 92.4% among people aged 25–64 years [19]. To aid in using diverse channels to disseminate health information, HPA established an official website and 12 other health-themed websites visited by 19,470,000 people in the year 2017 alone [19]. The National Health Interview Survey is conducted annually, with a completion rate of 72.8%. The data gathered are used as references for further planning of citizen health promotion and medical healthcare services and make Taiwan a sustainable country through healthy living.

The healthcare industry has always been a key focus of the nation's policy. The NHI is now widely regarded as one of the best healthcare systems in the world, ranked 14th in *The Economist*'s 2017 Global Access to Healthcare Index, and 9th in the 2018 Health Care Efficiency Index by Bloomberg Finance [20]. Taiwan's healthcare capacity continues to expand with the NHI system and the Health Promotion

Infrastructure designed to allow citizens to fully enjoy the promise of "Good Health and Well-Being" services.

Not only does Taiwan boast in its well-established healthcare system, but Taiwan also has been synonymous with hi-tech manufacturing of chips and components [21]. In recent years Taiwan has been bringing its two assets, health and the technology manufacturing market, into collaboration, merging the two sectors to build digital health. As observed by digital health writer Jon Hoeksma, now the tech market in Taiwan is beginning to target hi-tech medical equipment and disruptive digital health start-ups [21].

Digital health is the "convergence of digital technologies with health, healthcare, living, and society to enhance the efficiency of healthcare delivery and make medicines more personalized and precise." [22]. Many Taiwanese technology and mobile companies are now moving into health, supported by the government. The Taiwanese government provides a diverse range of support to help companies: from innovation clusters, to loans, to support of R&D, export services, and major events to promote key Taiwanese sectors. With governmental support, innovation is on the rise [21]. Brain Age, for instance, is an artificial intelligence developed by the National Taiwan University to interpret magnetic resonance imaging (MRI) scans and spot structural changes in the brain that can enable much earlier detection of dementia, providing physicians and patients an accurate brain age score. Red Spot is another device designed to spot invisible blood in toilet water to aid the early detection of prostate cancer.

As the market is successful in selling to European countries such as Poland, Greece, and Italy, not only does this promote the "Decent Work and Economic Growth" (SDG 8) and "Industry, innovation and Infrastructure" (SDG 9), digital health has brought even more efficiency to the healthcare system in Taiwan. The MediCloud system was launched to enable healthcare providers to query patients' medical records within the NHI system, and the Pharma Cloud system provides prescription drug information to physicians and pharmacists [23]. The Taiwan Minister of Health and Welfare Shih-Chung Chen proudly reports that currently, through digital cloud tools, community-based primary care providers in Taiwan can retrieve test reports, including computed tomography (CT) scans, MRIs, ultrasounds, gastroscopies, colonoscopies, and X-rays and receive prescription information [20]. Thus, digital health technologies have enhanced care services through improving the quality of care, reducing costs, properly matching health services with the locations where services are provided, and lowering the potential risks arising from repeated examinations [23].

Taiwan's hospitals are proving a hotbed for digital health and med tech innovations, and it is clear that Taiwan has much to offer in terms of innovation. Taiwan has learned how to utilize its competitive advantages in information technology and medicine to deliver better care and enhance the health of the overall population [21], very much a response to the goals outlined in the SDGs.

Taiwan's SDG Achievements in the Environmental Aspect

The environmental aspect of the SDGs includes the following five: Affordable Green Energy (SDG 7), Sustainable Cities and Communities (SDG 11), Climate Action (SDG 13), Life Below Water (SDG 14), and Life on Land (SDG 15). As Brookings reporter Simona Grano has noted, "prior to lifting martial law in 1987, Taiwan experienced three decades of rapid industrialization with little or no concern for the environment, and brought forth several problems, which have deteriorated both the quality of life and of the environment. In the past twenty years, Taiwan has seen a surge in environmental organizations, which to a certain degree have enjoyed a remarkable success in fighting polluting industries or affecting environmental policies." [24]. Indeed, the government did heavily push policies and acts to make Taiwan a sustainable and environmental land to live in. The goal is to be in accord with SDGs 14 and 15, to protect, restore, and promote sustainable use of terrestrial and marine ecosystems, sustainably manage forests and the ocean, and halt biodiversity loss.

For Affordable Green Energy (SDG 7), the Health Promotion Administration (HPA) policy for green hospitals is an example. The Administration established a platform to collect and analyze hospital performance in the field of energy conservation, assisting the 174 hospitals in their data on carbon emissions. According to an initial analysis of hospital self-assessment forms, hospital performances in waste reduction, energy efficiency, water conservation, and green buildings were better than average, with an average execution rate of about 88.23–94.73% [19].

For the life below water (SDG 14), the Environmental Protection Administration has implemented a policy to restrict, reduce, and remove plastics by cutting usage at the source and preventing plastic garbage from reaching the ocean. In the first 6 months of 2017, Taiwan removed 192 tons of trash from the sea and seabed. The Marine Pollution Control promotes marine garbage cleanups and marine environment education. Taiwan's river water quality has improved too, drastically since 2001, with the percentage of severely polluted river lengths in 50 Taiwan major rivers dropping from 13.2% to 2.5% in 2016 [3].

For the life on land (SDG 15), acts such as the Wetland Conservation Act in 2015 govern the "planning, conservation, restoration, utilization, and management of wetlands. It is an effort to protect wetlands' natural flood detention function, maintain biodiversity, preserve ecosystem, and ensure that such wetlands are widely used." [25]. Incorporation of good waste management (SDG 11.6) helps protect life on land from pollution; it also helps sustain green cities and communities. Taiwan's recycling rate reached 58% at the end of 2016, and daily per capita garbage collected dropped to 0.364 kg. This is a huge contrast to the recycling rate in 1998, when it was 5.88% and daily garbage collected was 1.135 kg per capita. Once nicknamed "Garbage Island," Taiwan has achieved one of the highest recycling rates in the world [26]. "For a policy like this to work, you have to make each one responsible for his personal consumption. You need waste disposal to sit firmly in the public consciousness," Lai Ying-ying, head of the Taiwan Environmental Protection

Administration's (EPA) waste management department, says. "It's what makes [a] circular economy actually happen." [26].

Taiwan's Efforts in Sustainable Development Goals

Taiwan has gone to great lengths to make the island a sustainable developed country. The sustainable development goals require large project coordination and planning for years. How is Taiwan engaging in accomplishing the SDG agenda?

First, is the Taiwanese central government labeling SDGs with high importance, and taking actions to work? In his 2016 Inaugural address, President Ing Wen Tsai announced that Taiwan is to "bravely chart a different course," which is to build a "New Model for Economic Development" for Taiwan. The administration is to pursue a new economic model for sustainable development based on the core values of innovation, employment, and equitable distribution.

Taiwan also established the National Council for Sustainable Development (NCSD) in August 1997 by Executive Yuan, in response to the UN Earth Summit of 1992. Since then, NCSD has accomplished many documents, including National Sustainable Development Policy Guidelines, the Taiwan Sustainable Development Indicator System, and Taiwan's Declaration on Sustainable Development and the Sustainable Development, in the past 20 years. The council is also responsible for "planning information gathering and analysis, and drafting of the Voluntary National Review." [3]. In 2016, Premier Lin Chuan emphasized that "sustainable development should be the goal of all government policies." [28]. Taiwan is to formulate national goals in accordance with the UN SDGs [27].

The National Sustainable Development Goal Draft was released in 2017. It is based on the United Nations SDGs, with targets and indicators tailored to Taiwan's domestic needs and situations. The UN SDGs provided 17 goals, but Taiwan's National Sustainable Development Goal currently has 18 goals, 138 targets, and 343 indicators [28]. This plan will be an important basis for the government to promote sustainable development across industries and departments. With the draft and policies on the way, Taiwan is on track to reach the SDG goals by 2030 [29].

The Future of Sustainable Development Goals in Taiwan

The Wang Dao Sustainability Index (WDSI) is an index analyzing 74 representative countries and economies in the world to rank them according to "Economic Development," "Environment Protection," and "Social Justice" in the United Nations 1987 Sustainable Development Report. The WDSI has ranked Taiwan No. 36 in the world, just slightly above average and closely after the United States, No. 35 [30]. Taiwan has come a long way in achieving success in many aspects of the SDGs, but there are more aspects to be improved. Taiwan has been and will continue to participate in UN's Sustainable Development Goals fully and enthusiastically.

Areas of Improvement

As stated before, Taiwan is an island with limited natural resources. Unfortunately, at the cost of growth of the economy and industrialization, Taiwan has been suffering from pollution, especially air pollution. Based on the reports by the World Health Organization (WHO), the air quality in Taiwan is generally the worst of all the "Four Asian Tigers." Annual mean greenhouse gas emissions have been increasing each year: greenhouse gas emissions totaled 283.5 million tons CO_2e in 2014. Domestically produced pollution includes industry's factory plants, vehicles such as scooters, and incense from religious rituals. To achieve, to name a few, land and water preservation (SDGs 14 and 15), affordable and clean energy (SDG 7), sustainable cities and communities (SDG 11), and climate watch (SDG 13), air pollution is definitely a large issue that needs to be further addressed. It is an issue that has already seen governmental attention for years but continues to seek action in attaining a green homeland.

Health in All Policies

According to the Director General of Health Promotion Administration Ministry of Health and Welfare, Ying Wei Wang, the goals between SDGs are highly interconnected, in that achieving one goal depends on the other goals. Although a health-related topic only appears once, in SDG 3, it is the core of SDGs. It is especially connected to achieving SDG 1 (poverty), SDG 2 (food, nutrition), SDG 4 (education), SDG 5 (gender equality), SDG 6 (water and environment), and SDG 8 (economic growth). Director General Dr. Wang pointed out that achieving healthy living is not the end goal of the SDG but a strategy or process in achieving all other SDGs. Therefore, Taiwan should present the ideas of "Health in All Policies" when working to bring sustainability in all areas of people's lives.

Global Partnerships

Although still pursuing the 2030 agenda, Taiwan has demonstrated success in achieving the SDGs. From offering scholarships to international students for higher education programs, to joining the International Network of Health Promoting Hospitals (HPH) and becoming the Asian hub for medical networking, Taiwan actively seeks to work with countries across Europe, America, Asia, Africa, and

Oceania. Especially in the health aspect of the SDGs, Taiwan has positioned itself on the global stage as a leader. Based on the success of Taiwan's Universal Health Care System, Taiwan has much to offer to the global community in terms of best practices. Taiwan can share best practices and information on its healthcare advances, disease prevention, and much more. Taiwan will continue to participate in the Sustainable Development Goals, and as the VNR has stated, "calls on the world to work together with Taiwan to actively tackle sustainable development tasks, fulfill responsibilities as members of the international community." [3]

References

1. Taiwan Country Profile. thomaswhite.com. https://www.thomaswhite.com/world-markets/taiwan-asias-technology-hotspot/. Published 2019. Accessed 14 May 2019.
2. Anon. Taiwan population. worldpopulationreview.com. http://worldpopulationreview.com/countries/taiwan-population/. Published 2019. Accessed 20 May 2019.
3. Executive Yuan. Taiwan's voluntary national review: implementation of the UN sustainable development goals. roc-taiwan.org. https://www.roc-taiwan.org/uploads/sites/104/2017/09/Taiwan-VNR.pdf. Published 2019. Accessed 13 May 2019.
4. United Nations. Resolution adopted by the General Assembly on 6 July 2017. undocs.org. https://undocs.org/A/RES/71/313. Published 2017 July 10. Accessed 13 May 2019.
5. Wang TH, et al. 新世代健康戰略4.0: 社區新視野. New Taipei City: Future Career Publishing Corporation (FCPC); 2018.
6. Executive Yuan. 賴揆:2030年為期程　研訂我國永續發展目標. www.ey.gov.tw. http://www.ey.gov.tw/Page/9277F759E41CCD91/b6825d98-73fc-47fb-8f31-8cfe48288114. Published 2018. Accessed 14 May 2019.
7. Why sustainable development goals are important. raptim.org. https://www.raptim.org/why-sustainable-development-goals-are-important/. Published 2016. Accessed 17 May 2019.
8. The story of Taiwan – economy. taiwan.com.au. web.archive.org/web/2010020203213; http://www.taiwan.com.au/Polieco/History/ROC/report04.html. Accessed 14 May 2019.
9. Taiwan GDP annual growth rate 2019. tradingeconomics.com. https://tradingeconomics.com/taiwan/gdp-growth-annual. Published 2019. Accessed 13 May 2019.
10. World Trade Organization. Trade profiles–Chinese Taipei. stat.wto.org. http://stat.wto.org/CountryProfile/WSDBCountryPFView.aspx?Country=TW. Published 2019. Accessed 13 May 2019.
11. Health Promotion Administration, Ministry of Health and Welfare. 2018 annual report of health promotion administration. Taipei City: Health Promotion Administration; 2018.
12. IMF統計:台灣人均GDP 5.23萬美元、全球第19!. Liberty Times. 2018 May 27. https://ec.ltn.com.tw/article/breakingnews/2438837. Accessed 16 May 2019.
13. 12 UN SDGs with a gender perspective poster. Taipei: Taipei City Government Office for Gender Equality; 2019.
14. Taiwan rises to 4th in PISA science rankings. Taiwan Today. 2016 Dec 8. http://taiwantoday.tw/news.php?unit=10&post=105240. Accessed 15 May 2019.
15. Rosenburg E. An American got sick in Taiwan. He came back with a tale of the 'Horrors of Socialized Medicine.' The Washington Post. 2019 Feb 28. www.washingtonpost.com/health/2019/03/01/an-american-got-sick-taiwan-he-came-back-with-tale-horrors-socialized-medicine/?utm_term=.b33fd6199e00. Accessed 17 May 2019.
16. Health Promotion Administration, Ministry of Health and Welfare. 2018 annual report of health promotion administration. Taipei City: Health Promotion Administration; 2018. p. 13–21.

17. Health Promotion Administration, Ministry of Health and Welfare. 2018 annual report of health promotion administration. Taipei City: Health Promotion Administration; 2018. p. 33–53.
18. Health Promotion Administration, Ministry of Health and Welfare. 2018 annual report of health promotion administration. Taipei City: Health Promotion Administration; 2018. p. 82–103.
19. Health Promotion Administration, Ministry of Health and Welfare. 2018 annual report of health promotion administration. Taipei City: Health Promotion Administration; 2018. p. 55–71.
20. Chen SC. Taiwan seeks to share its advances in digital healthcare. The Diplomat. 2019 May 09. https://thediplomat.com/2019/05/taiwan-seeks-to-share-its-advances-in-digital-health-care/. Accessed 4 Oct 2019.
21. Hoeksn J. Taiwan targets digital health and smart tech for exports. Digital Health. 2019 Aug 15. https://www.digitalhealth.net/2019/08/taiwan-targets-digital-health-and-smart-tech-for-exports/. Accessed 4 Oct 2019.
22. Digital Health. Wikipedia. https://en.wikipedia.org/wiki/Digital_health. Accessed 7 Oct 2019.
23. Chen SC. Taiwan's advances in digital healthcare. The Epoch Times. 2019 Apr 25. https://www.theepochtimes.com/taiwans-advances-in-digital-healthcare_2893819.html. Accessed 4 Oct 2019.
24. Grano S. Environmental issues facing Taiwan. brookings.edu. https://www.brookings.edu/opinions/environmental-issues-facing-taiwan/. Published 2018. Accessed 14 May 2019.
25. Executive Yuan. Taiwan's voluntary national review: implementation of the UN sustainable development goals. roc-taiwan.org. https://www.roc-taiwan.org/uploads/sites/104/2017/09/Taiwan-VNR.pdf. Published 2019. Accessed 13 May 2019. p. 12.
26. Rossi M. Taiwan has one of the highest recycling rates in the world. Here's how that happened. Ensia. 2018 Dec 18. https://ensia.com/features/taiwan-recycling-upcycling/. Accessed 10 Mar 2020.
27. 賴揆：在政策中落實永續發展目標. twecoliving.blogspot.com. http://twecoliving.blogspot.com/2016/02/blog-post_1.html. Published 2018 Dec 2018. Accessed 12 May 2019.
28. Executive Yuan. Taiwan's voluntary national review: implementation of the UN sustainable development goals. roc-taiwan.org. https://www.roc-taiwan.org/uploads/sites/104/2017/09/Taiwan-VNR.pdf. Published 2019. Accessed 13 May 2019. p. 6.
29. Executive Yuan. National sustainable development goals draft 我國永續發展目標草案. wix-static.com. https://docs.wixstatic.com/ugd/4aaf0a_6009908481f846aea664e6c2057d99bf.pdf. Published 2019. Accessed 13 May 2019.
30. Liu HH. 全球永續發展指標台灣第36名 美、中落後. Commercial Times. 2018 Dec 6. http://m.ctee.com.tw/livenews/jj/20181206005763-260407. Accessed 16 May 2019.

Chapter 21: Reducing the Burden of Oral Diseases Through Technology

David C. Alexander, Ramon Baez, and Prathip Phantumvanit

Introduction

Oral health and dentistry are seldom considered, for a variety of reasons, to reside in the mainstream of health and medicine. Historically, dentistry has been organized as a profession independent of medicine, and still today dental care providers are educated and trained in dental schools that are usually both physically and administratively outside of the medical school, sometimes not even on the same campus. An outcome of this academic separation is often described by the phrase as 'the mouth being out of the body.' The health professions, policy makers, funding agencies, and society have accepted this dichotomy for too long.

However, in the past decade, there has been an emerging and increasing body of evidence of bidirectional links between poor oral health and numerous remote organs and systemic conditions including diabetes, cardiovascular disease and stroke, pre-term low birthweight babies, and Alzheimer's disease. Interprofessional education and interprofessional collaboration may help 'to place the mouth back in the body' and in so doing enable management of common risk factors for noncommunicable diseases (NCDs), such as sugar, tobacco, alcohol, hygiene, water quality, and health literacy, that will improve both general and oral health. The social determinants for many noncommunicable diseases apply equally to oral diseases.

D. C. Alexander (✉)
New York University, New York, NY, USA

Appolonia Global Health Sciences, Green Brook, NJ, USA
e-mail: david@appoloniaglobalhealth.com

R. Baez
School of Dentistry, University of Texas, San Antonio, TX, USA

P. Phantumvanit
Faculty of Dentistry, Thammasat University, Bangkok, Thailand

© Springer Nature Switzerland AG 2020
P. Murthy, A. Ansehl (eds.), *Technology and Global Public Health*,
https://doi.org/10.1007/978-3-030-46355-7_26

331

Oral diseases are among the most prevalent on the planet. The Global Burden of Disease Studies (GBD) coordinated by the Institute of Health Metrics and Evaluation at the University of Washington and funded by the Bill and Melinda Gates Foundation have monitored diseases and conditions around the globe continually since 1990. The GBD is currently conducted by more than 2300 researchers in 130 countries studying more than 300 diseases and injuries in 195 countries. Recent GBD reports indicate that more than 3.9 billion people suffer oral diseases (age-standardized prevalence, 48.0%). Untreated dental caries in permanent teeth is the single most prevalent disease on the planet, estimated to affect 2.5 billion people (34.1%). Severe chronic periodontal disease affects 538 million people (7.4%) and untreated dental caries in deciduous teeth affects 573 million children (7.8%). Total tooth loss affects 276 million people (4.1%). Oral health has not improved during the 25 years of GBD study, in large part the result of demographic changes, including population increases and aging, with a 64% increase in disability-adjusted life-years 1990–2015 for oral diseases [1].

Over that same 25-year period, technology in dentistry has made tremendous advances. Reparative and aesthetic dentistry have witnessed major strides in digitization and automation, especially in the areas of imaging, CAD/CAM, 3D printing, and materials science. Tooth movement in dentofacial orthopedics and orthodontics has advanced also, through imaging and digitization, and the development of the increasingly popular clear-aligner. Techniques to conceal the wires and brackets for the treatment of many malocclusions that were previously managed by disfiguring wires and cemented stainless steel brackets are now seldom employed.

More durable restorative materials, including some biomaterials, with optical and mechanical properties that are increasingly closer to the natural tooth substances of enamel and dentin, are in widespread use. Where tooth loss has occurred, either through disease-related extractions or trauma, dental implants can be placed, providing a more natural solution with improved aesthetic and functional outcomes over the acrylic removable denture. In cases of severe or total tooth loss, what was a 'removable' denture retained by suction and the cohesion of saliva can now be a 'fixed' denture supported or retained in the mouth with the placement of as few as four osseointegrated implants. Use of lasers of several different wavelengths for cutting both hard and soft tissues, as well as disinfection of inflamed and infected periodontal tissues, is increasing as the evidence base supporting the safety and efficacy of laser devices increases.

Sadly, these strides in technology for restorative and surgical dentistry have largely bypassed the primary and secondary prevention of oral diseases. Contemporary technologies are only accessible where there is access to licensed dentists, and in most situations the consumer must have the ability to pay a significant, if not total, contribution to the cost, as the dichotomy between medicine and dentistry extends to health coverage and reimbursement systems. However, dental diseases are largely preventable and occur through lack of knowledge and health literacy, or adverse and limited choices about everyday behaviors in the bathroom, kitchen, or fast-food outlet. Limited access to services and the everyday underlying behavioral causes of oral diseases mean that preventive efforts by dental professionals are unlikely to have any effect on the overall burden of oral disease: early diagnosis, preventive services, and early intervention are seldom included in primary care.

Dental caries is largely caused by consumption of sugars and periodontal diseases by inadequate oral hygiene. At both the population and individual levels, caries can be prevented by reduced consumption of sugar, especially sugar-sweetened beverages, and use of fluoride agents in community water supplies, milk, and salt, and in oral hygiene products such as toothpastes and oral rinses. Periodontal diseases can be prevented by good oral hygiene habits and effective oral hygiene tools, and by control of other related factors such as tobacco use and glycemic control in diabetes. Little research and development has resulted in any advances in the preventive potential for these common oral diseases. Oral diseases, as many other NCDs, have marked social determinants with social gradients rooted in disparities and inequalities, as well as links to several other systemic conditions. A multisectoral approach is necessary for the control of these highly prevalent and preventable diseases that place an undue burden on society. The "UN Agenda for 2030 – Transforming Our World," outlining the Sustainable Development Goals (SDGs), forms a unique basis for reducing the global burden of oral diseases, as many of the underlying and root causes of oral diseases lie in poverty, hunger and nutrition, education, water and sanitation, and inequalities [2].

Within the SDGs, the focus on Universal Health Coverage (Goal 3.8) and the inclusion of oral diseases and their risk factors offer significant promise for prevention and early intervention, if only policy makers could see beyond the mere 'inconvenience of a few holes in teeth' and understand the significance of the fact that there cannot be general health without oral health – for all the reasons including the common risk factors already cited.

This remainder of this chapter focuses on the prevention of dental caries. In its untreated form, caries is the most ubiquitous disease on the planet. Teeth are at risk to dental caries from the moment they erupt into the oral cavity, as early as 6 months of age, and then remain at risk throughout life. The disease affects the very young and the very old most of all. Thus, in the space of this single chapter the authors have prioritized dental caries in the hope that all health workers can be aware of the risks of dental caries for all people. We include some preventive individual and population approaches to this burden on the global population through understanding the risk factors and determinants and the technologies currently available to all healthcare providers.

Global Situation of Dental Caries: Basic Epidemiology

The prevalence of dental caries is measured using the Decayed, Missing and Filled Teeth Index (DMFT) [3, 4]. DMFT score is the sum of the number of decayed, missing (from caries only), and filled teeth and collectively is often described as a measure of caries experience. The D element represents treatment need, whereas the M and F components represent disease that has been treated, either through extraction and thus tooth loss, or restorative fillings, respectively. The World Health

Organisation (WHO) recommends that national oral health surveys be conducted periodically following standardized methods and criteria. Recommendations are made to include the index ages and age groups of 5, 12, 15, 35–44, and 65–74 years. The age of 12 years is regarded as especially important because it is often the age at which children leave primary school. Therefore, in many countries, 12 years is the last age at which a reliable sample may be obtained easily through the school system. Also, it is likely at this age that all permanent teeth, except third molars, will have erupted into the oral cavity. For these reasons, 12 years of age has been chosen as the global indicator age group for international comparisons and surveillance of disease trends (Fig. 1) [3]. The age group of 35–44 years (mean, 40 years) is the standard group for surveillance of oral health conditions of adults. The full effect of dental caries, the level of severe periodontal involvement, and the general effects of oral healthcare provided can be assessed using data for this age group [3].

According to information available at the WHO Global Oral Health Data Bank, the trends and severity of dental caries vary significantly around the globe. WHO has established the following ranges and categories of DMFT scores (Table 1).

Dental Caries in the Primary Dentition

From the eruption into the oral cavity of the very first tooth around the age of 6 months, tooth surfaces are exposed to the many factors that may encourage demineralization or remineralization. If balance between these opposing processes can be maintained, the teeth will remain healthy and cavitation will not occur. If there is a continual imbalance toward demineralization, then caries will occur. Decay-causing or cariogenic factors, such as transmission of microorganisms (such as *Streptococcus mutans* and *Lactobacillus acidophilus*) from mother or caregivers, sugar from prolonged breastfeeding or bottle feeding, especially at night, and accumulation and maturation of bacterial plaque biofilm on the tooth surfaces and a poor flow of saliva will eventually turn the balance toward demineralization and the establishment of incipient caries lesions. However, remineralizing mechanisms such as calcium and phosphate, and buffering systems, all of which naturally occur in saliva, together with oral hygiene practices involving optimum levels of fluoride ions can shift the balance toward caries prevention and health. Saliva is a supersaturated solution of calcium ions that serves as a reservoir for calcium and phosphate, which through saturation with other calcium-rich foods such as cheese, yogurt, or milk can prevent demineralization. Acids occurring in foods and beverages of the same pH are not equal, depending upon the level of buffering capacity to return to neutral pH, and other factors such as chelation. The citric acid found in many fruit juices not only demineralizes the tooth but does not release the calcium ions back into the immediate tooth environment to allow saturation to be achieved.

Caries in primary dentition is one of the most prevalent diseases presenting as a public health problem, especially in children from families of low socioeconomic status. The disease progresses more rapidly through deciduous teeth as the enamel

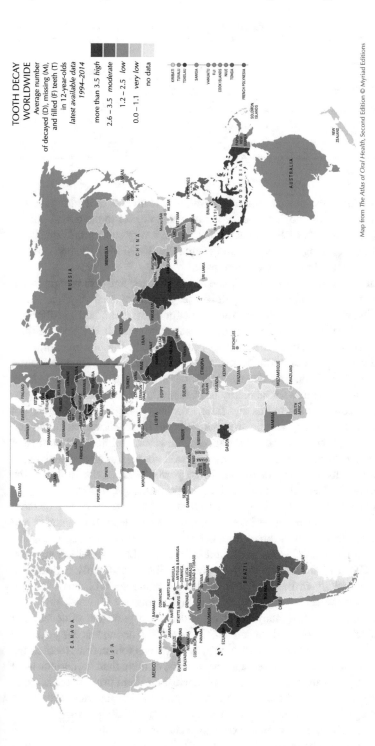

Fig. 1 The global distribution of dental caries in 12-year-old children. (Reproduced with permission from The Challenge of Oral Disease – A Call for Global Action. The Oral Health Atlas, Second Edition, pages 16–17. www.fdiworlddental.org/resources/publications/oral-health-atlas/oral-health-atlas-2015. © Myriad Editions 2015 / www.myriadeditions.com. All rights reserved)

Table 1 Categories and ranges of Decayed, Missing and Filled Teeth Index (DMFT) caries experience for reference ages of children and adults for use in the WHO Global Oral Health Databank

Global Oral Health Databank Category	DMFT score	
	12 years old	35–44 years old
Very low	<1.2	<5.0
Low	1.2–2.6	5.0–8.9
Moderate	2.6–4.4	9.0–13.9
High	>4.4	>13.9

and dentin tend to be less mineralized than permanent teeth and, as deciduous teeth are anatomically smaller, the distance for the disease to travel to the dental pulp is much less. Both these factors lead to acute pulpitis in a very short timeframe, with the symptom of throbbing dental pain and eventually pulpal necrosis and abscess formation, accompanied by chronic dental pain.

All 20 primary teeth usually erupt by the age of 2 years, and will remain in the oral cavity until 6–10 years of age before the permanent teeth replace them. Therefore, primary teeth are critically important for mastication and nutrition, as well as for speech development and to maintain adequate space in the jaws for their permanent successors. Premature loss of a primary tooth, through extraction or trauma, often leads to loss of adequate space to accommodate the permanent tooth, resulting in a malocclusion and increased risk of further oral disease. A healthy primary dentition is essential for a healthy permanent dentition, a fact often misunderstood or overcome by the myths and fallacies. Thus, the primary teeth are not considered important as they will be shed naturally, so if prevention has failed and disease is apparent, there is no need for concern. However, children with untreated dental caries will experience pain, may not eat as well nor gain as an adequate nutrition as children with a healthy dentition. To be perfectly clear, the health of the primary dentition is essential for the health of the permanent dentition.

Early childhood caries (ECC) are characterized by the presence of one or more teeth affected by severe carious lesions or with white spot lesions in anterior and posterior primary teeth, extraordinary loss of teeth from caries, or filled tooth surfaces in affected teeth. ECC is mostly found in young children under the age of 6 years [5]. ECC can be found even in very young children with early exposure to sugar intake, especially in the first year of life [6] and even with breastfeeding beyond 12 months, especially at night and with high frequency [7].

ECC prevalence varies in many countries and is most prevalent in developing countries, especially in Asia [8]. Severe ECC (S-ECC) is defined as early smooth surface caries in children under 3 years of age, or more than four carious teeth at age 3 years, or more than five carious teeth at age 4 years, or more than six carious teeth at age 5 years [9]. However, epidemiological data for caries in primary teeth, especially at a very young age such as 3 years, are not commonly reported. Many surveys focus on age 12 years and older for various reasons including avoidance of the primary dentition and the convenience of using schools as the site of examination. This gap only serves to strengthen the myths and fallacies that the primary dentition is of no value to longer-term health.

Table 2 Caries status in primary teeth in some Asian countries

Country	Age (years)	Prevalence (%)	Year
Japan	3	24.4	2005
Nepal	5–6	57.5	2004
Thailand	5	78.5	2012
Malaysia	5	76.2	2005
Mongolia	3–5	87.8	2007
Vietnam	6–8	92.2	2007
Cambodia	6	93.1	2011
Laos	5	96.1	2010
Philippines	6	97.1	2006

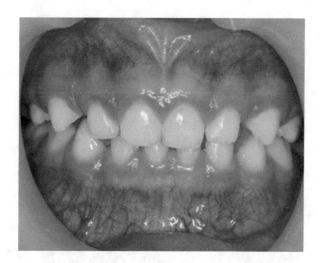

Fig. 2 Deciduous dentition: healthy and caries-free

Table 2 shows the prevalence of dental caries in children aged 3–8 years in a selection of Asian nations. In Japan less than one quarter of three-year-olds exhibit the disease, whereas for the Philippines the extent of the disease is ubiquitous among 6-year-olds (Figs. 2, 3, and 4).

Primary Prevention for Early Childhood Caries

The early prevention for ECC should commence as soon as the first tooth erupts into the oral cavity and is therefore exposed to the challenges of the oral environment. Routine cleansing with a soft cloth or appropriately sized 'baby' toothbrush is indicated, with a light smear amount of fluoride toothpaste. The appropriate amount of

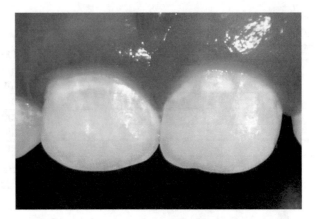

Fig. 3 Deciduous dentition: upper central incisors showing white-spot lesions before cavitation. These lesions are reversible. Optimal time for prevention to avoid destruction of the dentition showing the early warning signs before cavitation and destruction. (Used with permission from Dr. Norman Tinanoff, University of Maryland, Baltimore College of Dentistry, USA)

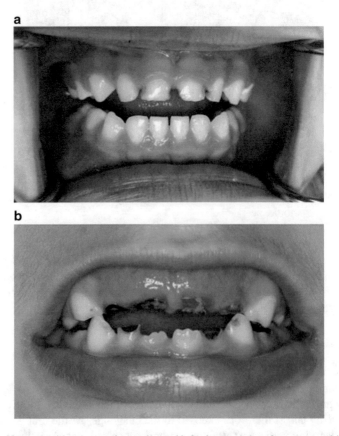

Fig. 4 Deciduous dentition: severe destruction and infection (top); hopeless case requiring extraction, too late for preventive intervention (bottom). (Used with permission from Dr. Norman Tinanoff, University of Maryland, Baltimore College of Dentistry, USA)

fluoride from toothpaste can shift the balance toward prevention. However, the most important for primary prevention for ECC is to avoid all sugar-containing foods and drinks during the first few years of life [6]. The World Health Organisation has issued guidelines for sugar consumption, especially in young children, to prevent not only early obesity but also early childhood caries as well [10]. Even high-frequency or nocturnal breastfeeding can also increase the risk for ECC [7]. No sugar should be added to baby food, milk, or fruit juice. These items contain naturally occurring sugars that may present a lesser risk of decay if used judiciously, that is, primarily at meal times and not continuously throughout the day. At bedtime, bottles or sippy cups should be filled only with water. During sleep, saliva flow decreases and thus its protective power of remineralization, buffering of acids, and flushing the mouth clear of sugars, is diminished. At nighttime the natural sugars in milk (lactose) and juices (fructose, glucose) are converted to acids by the biofilm and can initiate carious lesions and cavities.

Tooth brushing with an appropriate amount of fluoride toothpaste is another important factor for primary prevention of ECC. It has been recommended [11] that toddlers and infants aged 6–24 months should use a 'smear' amount of fluoride toothpaste, and thereafter at age 2–6 years should use a 'pea-sized bead' of fluoride toothpaste, or apply an amount of fluoride toothpaste across the width of the tooth-brush. This amount will effectively prevent caries, as well as avoid side effects such as white flecks and mottling of tooth enamel. To allow the fluoride to bind to sites on the enamel or dentin surface, the toothbrushing should extend to 2 min, and the mouth should not be rinsed on completion. Some mechanically powered brushes now have in-built timers to aid adherence to the 2-min brushing time. It is important for the brush to reach all teeth, especially those hard to reach at the back of the mouth, ensuring not only removal of the cariogenic biofilm but also distribution and uptake of fluoride.

Good oral hygiene, including twice-daily brushing and once-daily between-teeth-cleaning, together with any necessary dental care for parents and other care-givers, will reduce the transmission of decay-causing microorganisms from adult to child. Nothing should be placed in the infant's mouth that has been placed in an adult's mouth, including pacifiers, spoons or other food utensils, and toothbrushes, which can all act as carriers to transfer cariogenic microorganisms.

Secondary Prevention of Early Childhood Caries

Detection or diagnosis of early lesions of ECC is the key for secondary prevention. The early sign of caries is the 'white spot' lesion at the enamel surface under deposits of plaque biofilm. However, these early lesions can still be reversed or arrested, because although demineralization is marked, there is no cavitation and the enamel matrix remains intact, enabling remineralization to occur if the environment is favorable. A favorable environment is one that is not exposed to sugar, is frequently exposed to fluoride, and is free of any accumulations of plaque biofilm.

Fluoride varnish is a relatively high concentration (5%) preventive agent that can be easily applied by dental professionals and other healthcare workers to control early carious lesions effectively, especially those on the smooth tooth surfaces. Fluoride varnish can be applied once every 3–6 months, depending on the severity of the carious lesions, during the dental checkup or other health visit. Application of fluoride varnish should be augmented with twice-daily toothbrushing with fluoride toothpaste, especially aiming for dental plaque removal at the tooth surfaces, together with sugar control.

Dental caries also occur in the pits and fissures of the teeth. Pit and fissure sealants, typically a resin or glass-ionomer cement that can be flowed onto susceptible tooth surfaces, can also provide secondary prevention because the deep pits and fissures (anatomically too narrow to be reached by a toothbrush bristle) are prone to accumulation of plaque, which may lead to caries if sugar is present in the diet. Glass ionomer cements are the material of choice for pit and fissure sealing as they release low concentrations of fluoride over a long duration and are more practical, being less technique sensitive to the challenges of moisture control in children.

Silver diamine fluoride (SDF) (38%) is a highly effective secondary preventive agent. It has a high cariostatic action from fluoride, and the high silver content also inhibits the microorganisms and plaque accumulation in the carious lesions. The silver ion in SDF can also stain the carious lesions, which can become an aesthetic issue, especially in the anterior teeth where dentin caries progression is most effective stopped by SDF. SDF is a valuable tool for arresting the caries process when restorative dentistry is not possible. Use of SDF has recently been endorsed by the American Academy of Pediatric Dentistry as a caries preventive agent [12].

Tertiary Prevention for Early Childhood Caries

In cases where carious lesions progress into the dentine and become an open frank cavity, then restoration might be the only choice for tertiary prevention for ECC. To restore function of the teeth for mastication the open frank cavity should be filled. This procedure removes the softened carious material from the cavity and restores the tooth to an adequate contour and function by placing restorative material. This procedure will also reduce the burden of cariogenic microorganisms being carried in the saliva from the open lesion to other sites in the oral cavity, reducing the opportunity for recolonization. Conventional dental restoration using the "drill and fill" technique with occasional local anesthetic injection is not well accepted and unfriendly to most children through fear of pain and sensitivity. In the past decades, minimal intervention techniques in dentistry have been developed to conserve natural tooth tissue and minimize the pain and discomfort, and thus need for local anesthetic, of conventional restorative procedures. In the atraumatic restorative technique (ART), carious tissue is removed with only hand instruments (no drilling) and the excavated cavity is restored with glass ionomer cements [13]. More recently, the simplified modified atraumatic restorative technique (SMART) has been further developed for young children using only partial caries removal and encapsulated glass ionomer cements [14]. SMART is well accepted even by children 2–3 years old because there is no need for local anesthetic injection, no cutting with the drill, and only minimal intervention, therefore causing no pain. This minimal intervention concept of partial and selective caries removal necessitates only removal of soft dentin and is recommended even for deep cavities [15]. SMART has been introduced in a number of developing countries in Asia to provide care for children onsite in child daycare centers or kindergartens rather than clinics and hospitals.

Case Study

Thailand

Thailand is a developing country located in Southeast Asia with a population of approximately 68 million. The caries prevalence in primary teeth is high whereas in that in permanent teeth is much lower. The Thai government provides universal health coverage, including oral healthcare, through the facilities of the Ministry of Public Health. About half the total number of dentists serve at the public hospitals throughout the country, supported by dental nurses (therapists) at all levels of healthcare facilities. At the district level there are about four to eight public dentists at each district hospital, with a number of dental nurses stationed at subdistrict health centers looking after the oral health of the nearby population.

Since 2012, Thailand had passed legislation banning sugar-added infant formula in the market, which was the appropriate upstream policy level for both childhood obesity and caries primary prevention [16]. Additionally, in August 2017 new legislation was passed to charge higher taxation rates for sugar-containing beverages or soda drinks.

A national campaign for toothbrushing to commence as soon as the first primary tooth eruption (at around 6 months of age) has been launched throughout the country and is supported by training targeted toward mothers and caregivers for proper toothbrushing with the appropriate amount of fluoride toothpaste (a 'smear').

Early caries detection takes place when the children visit the well-child clinic for vaccinations at health centers or hospitals. Children are examined by dental nurses or public dentists. Fluoride varnish applications on white spot carious lesions are routine procedures, especially at the grassroots level for secondary prevention. Interprofessional collaboration with nurses, pediatricians, and public health workers is necessary for holistic healthcare, including oral health, of the children.

At 3–5 years of age, young children attend local day-care centers or kindergartens under the supervision of trained nannies or teachers. Dental nurses then conduct regular dental examinations for early caries detection in each semester. Toothbrushing techniques with fluoride toothpaste are reinforced, and simple sugar-control dietary education is introduced. Recently some trained dental nurses also

Table 3 Case study: Primary teeth caries control activities in Thailand

When	What	Where	Who	How
0–6 months	Diet counseling (sugar avoidance) Early oral examinations, toothbrushing with fluoride toothpaste	Home visit	Parents and caregivers Health workers, dental nurses	Advocacy training, community
6 months–3 years, vaccination	Diet counseling (sugar avoidance) Early checkup Toothbrushing with fluoride toothpaste Fluoride varnish Glass ionomer sealants	Health center	Parents and caregivers Health workers, dental nurses	Advocacy training, community, evaluation
3–5 years	Diet counseling (sugar avoidance) Early checkup Toothbrushing with fluoride toothpaste Fluoride varnish Glass Ionomer sealants SMART Sweet-enough	Day-care center or pre-school or kindergarten	Parents and caregivers Health-workers, dental nurses, teachers, nannies, dentists	Advocacy training, community, curriculum evaluation, impact

offer SMART preventive restorations as tertiary preventive measures for cavitated carious lesions. SMART procedures are conducted at the day-care centers or kindergartens as a field rather than in-clinic practice (Table 3).

Dental Caries in the Permanent Dentition

The permanent dentition begins with appearance in the mouth of the first permanent molars at about 6 years of age, followed by lower incisors, maxillary incisors, canines, premolars, and second and third molars. The latter usually appear between 18 and 21 years although eruption age varies considerably among individuals.

The caries process in the permanent dentition has the same pathophysiology as in the primary dentition, but the treatment options differ. The first tissue affected is the dental enamel. Demineralization, frequently observed as a white-spot lesion, is often followed by destruction of matrix structure with the consequent formation of a cavity. If the lesion is not treated, the lesion progresses into the dentin, the tissue immediately underneath enamel. If left untreated the lesion progresses and will reach the dental pulp, which includes nerve tissues and blood vessels. The pulp tissues become inflamed (pulpitis), the main symptom of which is throbbing pain as the hard dental tissues surrounding the pulp chamber are unyielding to the increased edema and resulting pressure. Pulpal necrosis ensues and typically leads to formation of a dental abscess. Depending upon the location of the tooth involved, infection can spread through the fascial planes and may compromise the airway. The simple treatment for a necrotic pulp or abscess is tooth extraction. If skilled care is available in a dental clinic, extraction can be avoided, and the tooth saved through a root canal filling, in which the necrotic pulp tissues are removed, the surfaces of the pulp chamber debrided, and the space filled with inert material such as gutta-percha.

Dental caries are often observed in individuals who lack adequate oral hygiene and consume excess sugars. Location of teeth, as well as certain foods and drinks, particularly those containing free sugars, suboptimal exposure to fluorides, younger and older age, and insufficient saliva have been identified as contributing risk factors for dental caries occurrence. According to the WHO, worldwide 60–90% of school children and nearly 100% of adults have dental cavities, often leading to pain and discomfort. Both dental cavities and chronic inflammatory periodontal disease are major causes of tooth loss. Complete loss of natural teeth is widespread and particularly affects older people [1]. Globally, about 30% of people aged 65–74 years have no natural teeth [17].

Dental caries can affect anyone with teeth regardless of age, race, or country of origin. However, it is known that those who belong to disadvantaged population groups are more severely affected, as dental diseases are rooted in adverse social determinants. Unfortunately, oral health has not received the attention it deserves within health policies, and individuals around the world are exposed to needless pain and suffering, devastating complications to individual well-being with consequential financial and social costs, in addition to a diminishing of quality of life and ultimately a burden to society.

Oral Health Promotion and Disease Prevention

Health promotion is the core foundation that enables people to increase control over their own health by addressing the determinants. The WHO identifies three key elements of health promotion: (1) good governance, (2) health literacy, and (3) healthy cities [18]. Adopting these principles to the promotion of oral health and prevention of dental diseases is no different from any other aspect of total health, and reducing common risk factors will help address multiple conditions. The WHO Global Oral Health program developed guidelines for establishing oral health promotion initiatives in schools [19]. Schools are an efficient and effective way to reach many children together with their families and community members, and it is well accepted that what is learned in school influences people's lives. Further, children who are receptive develop good habits that will have a long-lasting impact. Schools also can offer a supportive environment, for example, provision of safe water and sanitation, which are essential for tooth brushing. If schools do not have such facilities, oral health advocates can promote their establishment. Opportunities to include daily tooth brushing (with fluoride toothpaste) with handwashing programs should be considered and require little additional logistical and supervisory support. Schools are a safe physical environment where trauma risk can be reduced and proper emergency decisions made if necessary. School policies on healthy diet can be implemented in terms of healthier foods and reduced sugar consumption. Schools may be the only place for children at high risk to access dental care.

In summary, it is important that individuals make the commitment to optimize their oral health because oral health has an intimate relationship with general health and well-being. Practices that can be adopted or strengthened and are fundamental for proper oral health include oral hygiene, proper nutrition with emphasis on sugar control, regular physical exercise, and avoidance of risk habits.

Oral Hygiene Brush twice a day with a dentifrice containing fluoride, and perform interdental cleaning at least once a day (the proximal surfaces of adjacent teeth to which tooth brushes cannot reach. Clean the tongue, inspect all oral tissues (become familiar with normal appearance and detect any changes in color or consistency), and visit the oral health professional at least twice a year.

Proper Nutrition Eat well-balanced meals, avoid excess sugar and carbohydrates, avoid excess intake of fatty foods, eat fruits and vegetables, and include fibrous foods in the diet. If snacking between meals, eat fruits and avoid candy. Be familiar with the food pyramid and use it as a guide.

Regular Exercise Exercise regularly daily or at least three times a week. Regular exercise helps eliminate calories. It can help lower cholesterol by lowering the low-density lipids (LDL), increasing high-density lipids (HDL), and lowering triglycerides, which help reduce risk of cardiovascular disease.

Avoidance of Risk Factors (Behavior) Avoid use of tobacco products, excessive use of alcohol, drinking high sugar-containing beverages, consumption of sugary foods, consumption of foods containing saturated fats, and using the teeth for holding objects or cutting.

Changing behavior is difficult because it is the result of interaction of what we believe and how we feel [20]. It is important to remember that usually the information about the risk is not enough to change unhealthy behavior. However, it has also been recognized that people's beliefs are not based simply on what they are told to believe, and there is evidence that health behaviors can be influenced by health promotion techniques at the population level. However, a significant proportion of patients with health problems do not achieve behavior change and even fewer maintain these changes.

Community Approaches Available for Dental Caries Prevention

Water Fluoridation

More than 70 years of scientific research has consistently shown that an optimal level of fluoride in community water is safe and effective in preventing tooth decay by at least 25% in both children and adults [21]. The overwhelming weight of scientific evidence indicates that fluoridation of community water supplies is both safe and effective [22].

However, it is important to know that a limitation is that water fluoridation requires a well-established centralized piped water distribution system and that implementation of fluoridation schemes require support of the top health authorities and of the government (laws, decrees, regulations, budget allocation) and support to the agency executing the fluoridation program. In addition, equipment must be adapted to local conditions and the needs of the water network. It must be efficacious, safe and precise in all climatic conditions, and should be of a standard type recognized as satisfactory and for which maintenance is also easily provided. The practical aspects of water fluoridation are that almost by definition water fluoridation is a procedure for use in countries with a fair level of economic development. Key considerations include these:

There is a municipal supply reaching a reasonable number of homes.

People drink water from the main municipal supply rather than the water from individual wells, bottled water, and rainwater tanks.

Suitable equipment is available in a treatment plant or pumping station. A supply of a suitable fluoride chemical is assured.

There are workers in the water treatment plant able to maintain the system and keep adequate records. There is sufficient money available for the initial installation and running costs.

The level of dental caries must be sufficiently high, or the risk of increasing prevalence of caries sufficiently grave, to justify the investment.

Cost of installation for one unit varies between approximately $5,000 and $50,000. In the US, approximate cost has been estimated at $0.50 per person per year. A calculation of costs can be estimated by multiplying the cost of equipment and installation plus 1 year of chemicals divided by the number of people to be served Water fluoridation is used in more than 25 countries around the world [23].

Salt Fluoridation

The first studies of the effect on dental caries of fluoride added to alimentary salt were carried out from around 1965 to 1985 in Switzerland, Hungary, and Colombia and proved this to be as effective as water fluoridation; the number of teeth affected by caries was reduced by approximately 50% [24].

Fluoridated salt has been on sale in Switzerland since 1955, and by 1967 three quarters of domestic salt sold in Switzerland was fluoridated at 90 mg F^- kg salt. However, Marthaler et al. [25, 26] concluded that the caries-preventive effectiveness of 250 mg F^- kg salt used in the Swiss Canton of Vaud was greater than the reduction of approximately 25% observed following the addition of 90 mg F^- kg salt in other Swiss cantons [27].

During the 1990s further reports appeared from countries where salt fluoridation has been implemented [28–31], and recently studies have been published that demonstrate the persistence of the caries-protective effect into adulthood [32, 33]. The full potential of salt fluoridation, at least equivalent to water fluoridation, is reached when most of the salt for human consumption is fluoridated. It is important to distribute fluoridated salt through channels used by low socioeconomic groups and communities; in these strata, caries is highest and dental caries treatment often unaffordable or neglected [34].

The effectiveness of salt fluoridation has been demonstrated in various countries with a caries percentage decline of 80% when all salt for human consumption is fluoridated. Salt fluoridation is ideal for countries or regions with few water systems and in which salt production and distribution can be controlled. Addition of fluoride to salt is technically possible in salt refineries but is not feasible in cases of preferred use of "crude salt." Fluoridated salt, when feasible, can easily reach the entire population even in remote areas at very little cost. The concentration of fluoride in salt used around the world ranges from 200 to 350 mg/kg, with an optimal concentration of about 250 mg/kg [27]. One concern expressed is that promotion of the dental benefits of fluoridated salt would be unacceptable and contradictory to public health messages that encourage the reduction of consumption of salt and thus decrease the risk of hypertension. However, populations are not encouraged to consume more salt to improve their dental health; rather, the "automatic" or passive effect of fluoridated salt is accepted. In other words, people do not need to change their usual behavior to benefit. Indeed, reduced consumption of salt could and should be encouraged and, where this is successful, the concentration of fluoride in salt could simply be increased appropriately.

Milk Fluoridation

Milk fluoridation, as an alternative vehicle for automatic population-directed administration of fluoride, began in Switzerland approximately 58 years ago. In 1988 the first community-based scheme was introduced in Bulgaria and reached some 15,000 children. By 2000 this figure had increased to 114,000 children as programs were introduced in four other countries. More recently, there has been further expansion, particularly in Thailand and Chile, and there are now 800,000 children in the Russian Federation, Chile, United Kingdom, Thailand, and the Republic of Macedonia participating in the international programme [35]. The interested reader would benefit from consulting the booklet on milk fluoridation for dental caries prevention published by the World Health Organisation in 2009 [35]. In most cases the viability and sustainability of a program is likely to depend on the availability of a suitable milk supply.

Fluoride-Containing Toothpastes

Probably the most widespread and significant vehicle used for fluoride has been toothpastes. Introduced in the late 1960s and early 1970s, their rapid increase in market share was remarkable. The consensus view from high-income countries was that the introduction of fluoride-containing toothpastes was the single factor most responsible for the massive reduction in dental caries seen in many countries during the 1970s and 1980s [36]. Furthermore, of the various vehicles for fluoride, toothpaste has been the most rigorously evaluated. Marinho et al. [37] included 74 randomized, controlled clinical trials of good quality in their systematic review of fluoride toothpastes. However, an important limitation is that the effectiveness of these toothpastes depends upon the behavior of the individual and the family in purchasing and regularly using the products. Studies have shown that use of toothpaste containing fluoride are not uniform and is less likely among underprivileged groups [38, 39]. The fall in the incidence of dental caries after the introduction of fluoride into toothpaste formulations, although seen in all social classes, was particularly noticeable in higher social classes; consequently, a very marked social class gradient exists in many countries.

In countries where persons brush their teeth daily, dentifrices are a useful vehicle for applying topical fluoride to the dentition. It could be the only lifelong vehicle for providing fluoride to teeth. It is important to note that children 3–5 years of age may swallow considerable amounts of fluoride from dentifrices, thus, only a very small amount of toothpaste, such as a smear on a small toothbrush, should be used by young children, and close supervision during brushing is essential. Swallowing fluoride-containing dentifrice has the potential of causing enamel fluorosis. According to Professor T.M. Marthaler, topical fluoride can almost fully prevent caries on smooth surfaces; it is strongly effective on approximal surfaces and least effective on pits and fissures.

WHO Policy on Use of Fluoride for Prevention of Dental Caries

The WHO policy on effective use of fluoride is reflected in four World Health Assembly Resolutions:

WHA22.30 (1969) and WHA28.64 (1975) on fluoridation and dental health
WHA31.50 (1978) on fluoride for prevention of dental caries; and the most recent
   WHA60.17 (2007): *Oral Health: Action Plan for Promotion and Integrated Disease Prevention*

The 2007 Resolution urges Member States to ensure that populations benefit from appropriate use of fluoride [39], and the statement reads as follows:

> (4) for those countries without access to optimal levels of fluoride, and which have not yet established systematic fluoridation programmes, to consider the development and implementation of fluoridation programmes, giving priority to equitable strategies such as the automatic administration of fluoride, for example, in drinking-water, salt or milk, and to the provision of affordable fluoride toothpaste

The WHO Oral Health Program continues to emphasize the importance of public health approaches to the effective use of fluorides for the prevention of dental caries, and the Program is involved with support, guidance, and practical assistance to several countries [40].

Accordingly, people should be encouraged to brush their teeth twice daily with effective fluoride-containing toothpaste, that is, fluoride recommended at the level of 1500 parts per million (ppm). It is worth noting that "topical" fluorides such as toothpaste can also have a "systemic" effect when they are inadvertently ingested by young children. Dispensing a smear or pea-sized amount of toothpaste, encouraging parents to supervise tooth brushing by their young children, and the use of toothpastes containing less fluoride by young children are approaches to ameliorating this problem. Countries may recommend toothpastes with low concentration of fluoride, that is, 500 ppm or less, specifically for such young age groups (1–3 years of age).

Where the incidence and prevalence of dental caries in the community is high to moderate, or where there are firm indications that the incidence of caries is increasing, an additional source of fluoride (water, salt, or milk) should be considered. Where the country (or area of the country) has a moderate level of economic and technological development, a municipal water supply reaching a large population, trained water engineers, and favorable public opinion, water fluoridation using fluoride at a concentration of 0.5–1 mg/l (dependent upon climate) is the method of choice [41, 42].

In cooperation with the WHO Collaborating Centre for Community Oral Health Programs and Research at the School of Dentistry, University of Copenhagen, a project to assess whether countries in various regions of the world have implemented the World Health Assembly Resolution WHA 60.17 *Action Plan for Promotion and Integrated Disease Prevention*, and to identify possible barriers that countries may have faced, is being conducted at the present time. Information gained will assist in developing proper courses of action and strengthening strategies in place for optimizing oral health and preventing disease.

Aiming to Optimize Oral Health

Adequate oral health promotion and disease prevention strategies are conducive to improving the oral health of the community. However, it is critical to mention that there should be a favorable environment and that this includes not only the external environment but the healthcare systems as well. Healthcare systems are indispensable for promoting, improving, and maintaining the health of the population of any country. It is important also to recognize that in developed countries healthcare systems may be well structured and are designed based on research data obtained within the country, whereas in developing countries health services may be considerably limited in structure, scope, and obviously in resources. Further, in developed countries systems may have clinics or hospitals that are supported by health professionals from various specialties that allow their cooperation to benefit the patient and may be equipped with the latest technical facilities. In developing countries, health services may be directed to provide emergency care only, or health services may be directed to provide emergency care only or interventions of conditions that may be present in certain age groups of people.

Oral health services in developed countries may offer both preventive and curative procedures based on public and private systems with advanced oral care health systems that primarily provide curative services to patients. Most systems are based on demand for care, and private dental practitioners provide patients with sophisticated oral healthcare including high technologies in oral rehabilitation (implantology, CAD/CAM, digital X-rays, lasers, new diagnostic tools) with or without third-party payment schemes [43].

In oral health service systems in developed countries, the curative treatment of oral disease is extremely costly and is a significant economic burden for many industrialized countries, with 5–10% of public health expenditure related to oral health. It is known that there are, however, major disparities in oral healthcare depending on the country and the regions within that country which may be linked to the socioeconomic status, race or ethnicity, age, gender, or state of general health of the patient [42].

Attributes of an Ideal Oral Healthcare System

Key attributes for an ideal oral healthcare system would include the following:

Integration with the rest of the healthcare system
Emphasis on health promotion and disease prevention
Monitoring of population oral health status and needs
Be evidence-based; effective; cost-effective; sustainable; equitable; universal coverage; comprehensive; ethical
Inclusion of continuous quality assessment and assurance
Culturally competent
Empowering communities and individuals to create conditions conducive to health [36]

Do oral health systems in developing countries meet these criteria? Probably not. Although some countries have adopted effective strategies for dental caries prevention, little has been done in terms of health promotion to modify risk factors that can contribute to the prevention, for example, of periodontal disease. It is clear that financial resources are of paramount importance for sustaining any health system [44].

World Health Organisation Recommendations

WHO recommendations include building capacity in oral healthcare systems directed toward disease prevention and primary healthcare. Special emphasis should be placed on meeting the needs of disadvantaged and poor populations. The oral health system should be organized to target prevention, early diagnosis, and intervention. The provision of treatment and rehabilitation should be managed according to the needs of the population and the resources available. Primary healthcare workers, specially trained in oral disease preventive care, could provide essential care. Training programs for primary health workers already working in rural areas can improve both access to professional care and the accuracy of oral health messages. Medical practitioners could and should have an important role in the promotion of oral health. Surveillance should be considered as an essential component of any public health program infrastructure. Some developing, as well as developed, countries lack oral health policies. Thus, it would be appropriate for health administrators to promote inclusion of oral health in the national health plan and to design adequate oral health strategies that consider promotion and disease prevention activities.

Conclusion

Oral diseases are some of the most prevalent diseases on the planet, affecting more than 3.9 billion people [1]. Untreated dental caries in permanent teeth are the single most prevalent disease worldwide, affecting more than 2.4 billion people. Severe chronic inflammatory periodontal disease is associated with a number of systemic conditions including diabetes, cardiovascular diseases, pre-term low birth weight babies, and Alzheimer's disease. Reduction in the inflammatory burden and the associated dental plaque biofilm may reduce contributing risk factors for these NCDs.

Noting that oral diseases are preventable through addressing common NCD risk factors of sugar, tobacco, alcohol, and clean water, primary care could provide early intervention for at-risk communities. Oral diseases are a neglected issue, rarely seen as a priority in health policy [45]. Commonly, dental care is excluded from primary care. Universal Health Coverage and primary care should include the following as a minimum:

1. Access to community and individually delivered fluoride and other remineralizing agents
2. Reductions in sugars, especially sugar-sweetened beverages
3. Routine oral healthcare to relieve pain and restore function through inclusion in primary care

There is no health without oral health. General health is compromised until the global oral health burden is addressed, *leaving no one behind.*

References

1. Kassebaum NJ, Smith AGC, Bernabe E, et al. Global, regional, and national prevalence, incidence, and disability-adjusted life years for oral conditions for 195 countries, 1990–2015: a systematic analysis for the global burden of diseases, injuries, and risk factors. J Dent Res. 2017;96(4):380–7.
2. United Nations. Sustainable Development Goals http://www.undp.org/content/undp/en/home/sustainable-development-goals.html. Accessed 29 May 2018.
3. Petersen PE, Baez RJ. World Health Organization. Oral health surveys. Basic methods. 5th ed. Geneva: World Health Organization; 2013.
4. Petersen PE, Burgeois B, Ogawa H, Estupinan-Day S, Ndiaje C. The global burden of oral diseases and risks to oral health. WHO policy and practice. Bull World Health Organ. 2005;83:661–9.

5. The Joint Task Force (JTF). The steering group for ICD-11 version for Mortality and Morbidity Statistics (ICD-11-MMS). ICD-11 Beta Draft (Mortality and Morbidity Statistics). http://apps.who.int/classifications/icd11/browse/f/en#http%3a%2f%2fid.who.int%2ficd%2fentity%2f1112319601. Accessed 10 Apr 2017.

6. Chaffee BW, Feldens CA, Rodrigues PH, Vítolo MR. Feeding practices in infancy associated with caries incidence in early childhood. Community Dent Oral Epidemiol. 2015;43(4):338–48.

7. Duangthip D, Gao SS, Lo EC, Chu CH. Early childhood caries among 5- to 6-year-old children in Southeast Asia. Int Dent J. 2016;67(2):98–106. https://doi.org/10.1111/idj.12261.

8. Tham R, Bowatte G, Dharmage SC, et al. Breastfeeding and the risk of dental caries: a systematic review and meta-analysis. Acta Paediatr. 2015;104(467):62–84.

9. American Academy of Pediatric Dentistry. Definition of Early Childhood Caries (ECC). 2008. Available from: http://www.aapd.org/assets/1/7/D_ECC.pdf

10. World Health Organization. Sugars intake for adults and children guideline. 2015. http://www.who.int/nutrition/publications/guidelines/sugars_intake/en/

11. Zero DT, Marinho VC, Phantumvanit P. Effective use of self-care fluoride administration in Asia. Adv Dent Res. 2012;24(1):16–21.

12. American Academy of Pediatric Dentistry. Silver diamine fluoride management of dental 177 caries: chairside guide. Pediatr Dent. 2017;39(6):special issue.

13. Raggio DP, Hesse D, Lenzi TL, Guglielmi CA, Braga MM. Is atraumatic restorative treatment an option for restoring occlusoproximal caries lesions in primary teeth? A systematic review and meta-analysis. Int J Paediatr Dent. 2013;23(6):435–43.

14. Phantumvanit P. SMART preventive restoration for primary dentition. J Int Oral Health. 2012;8:v.

15. Schwendicke F, Frencken JE, Bjørndal L, et al. Managing carious lesions: consensus recommendations on carious tissue removal. Adv Dent Res. 2016;28(2):58–67.

16. Government of Thailand. Thai Health Promotion. Sweet Enough Campaign. Thai Health Promotion. 2012.

17. World Health Organization. http://www.who.int/mediacentre/factsheets/fs318/en/. Fact sheet N°318 April 2012.

18. World Health Organization. https://www.who.int/features/qa/health-promotion/en/. Online Q&A August 2016.

19. Kwan S, Petersen PE. WHO Information series on school health document eleven. Oral Health Promotion: An Essential Element of a Health-Promoting School, WHO Global Oral Health Programme, Department of Noncommunicable Diseases Prevention and Health Promotion, World Health Organization, Geneva. WHO/NMH/NPH/ORH/School/03.3. 2003.

20. Bundy C. Changing behavior: using motivational interviewing techniques. J R Soc Med. 2004;97(suppl 44):43–7.

21. American Dental Association. Fluoridation Facts. Available at: http://www.ada.org/en/public-programs/advocating-for-the-public/fluoride-and-fluoridation/fluoridation-facts

22. American Dental Association. http://www.ada.org/consumer/fluoride/facts/saf/13-22.html

23. O'Mullane DM, Baez RJ, Jones S, Lennon MA, Rugg-Gunn AJ, Whelton H, Whitford GM. Fluoride and oral health. Community Dent Health. 2016;33:1–31.

24. Marthaler TM, Petersen PE. Salt fluoridation – an alternative in automatic prevention of dental caries. Int Dent J. 2005;55:351–8.

25. Marthaler TM, et al. Frecuence globales de la caries dentaire dans le canton of Vaud, apres fluoruration par comprimes a la fluoruration de sal alimentaire [Global frequency of dental caries in the canton of Vaud after changing from fluoride tablets to salt fluoridation]. Schweiz Mschr Zahnheilk. 1977;87:147–58.

26. Marthaler TM, et al. Caries preventive salt fluoridation. Caries Res. 1978;12(suppl 1):15–21.

27. Marthaler TM, Schenardi C. Inhibition of caries in children after 5 1/2 years use of fluoridated table salt. Helv Odont Acta. 1962;6:1–6.

28. Salas MT, Solorzano S. La fluorudracion de la sal en Costa Rica y su impacto en la caries dental. Fluoruración al Día. 1994;4:13–9.

29. Stephen KW, McPherson LMD, Gorzo I, et al. Effet of fluoridated salt intake in infancy: a blind caries and fluorosis study in 8th grade Hungarian pupils. Community Dent Oral Epidemiol. 1999;27:210–5.
30. Estupinan SR, Baez RJ, Horowitz H, et al. Salt fluoridation and dental caries in Jamaica. Community Dent Oral Epidemiol. 2001;29:247–52.
31. Warpeha R, Beltran-Aguilar E, Baez R. Methodological and biological factors explaining the reduction in dental caries in Jamaican school-children between 1984 and 1995. Pan Am J Public Health. 2001;10:37–44.
32. Mengini GD, Marthaler TM, Steiner M, et al. Caries Pravalanz and gingicale Enzündug Bein rekruted in Jahre 1985 Einfluss der Vorveugung. Schweiz Monatsschr Zahnmed. 1991;101:1119–26.
33. Radnai M, Fazekas A. Caries prevalence in adults seven years after previous exposure to fluoride in domestic salt. Acta Med Dent. 1999;4:163–6.
34. Petersen PE. Society and oral health. In: Pine C, editor. Community oral health. London: Butterworth and Heinemann; 1966.
35. Banoczy J, Petersen PE, Rugg-Gunn A. Milk fluoridation for the prevention of dental caries. World Health Organization, Geneva. 2009. Available at: http://whqlibdoc.who.int/publications/2009/9789241547758_eng.pdf
36. Bratthall D, Hansel-Petersson G, Sundberg H. Reasons for the caries decline: what do the experts believe? Eur J Oral Sci. 1996;104:416–22.
37. Marinho VCC, Higgins JPT, Logan S, Sheiham A. Fluoride toothpastes for preventing dental caries in children and adolescents (Cochrane Review). The Cochrane Library. Wiley, Chichester. 2004. Available from: http://www.update-software.com/abstracts/ab002278.htm
38. Mansbridge JN, Brown MD. Changes in dental caries prevalence in Edinburgh children over three decades. Community Dent Health. 1985;2:3–13.
39. Steele J, Lader D. Children's dental health in the United Kingdom, 2003. Social factors and oral health in children. Office for National Statistics, London. 2004. Available from: http://www.statistics.gov.uk/cci/nugget.asp?id=1000
40. Petersen PE. World Health Organization global policy for improvement of oral health: World Health Assembly 2007. Int Dent J. 2008;58:115–21.
41. World Health Organization Expert Committee on Oral Health Status and Fluoride Use. Fluorides and oral health. WHO Technical Report Series No. 846. World Health Organization, Geneva. 1994.
42. Petersen PE, Baez RJ, Lennon MA. Community-oriented administration of fluoride for the prevention of dental caries: a summary of the current situation in Asia. Published by http://www.sagepublications.com. On behalf of International and American Associations for Dental Research, January 18, 2012.
43. Kandelman D, Arpin S, Baez RJ, Baehni P, Petersen PE. Oral health care systems in developing and developed countries. Periodontology 2000. 2012;60:98–109.
44. Tomar SL, Cohen LK. Attributes of an ideal oral health care system. J Public Health Dent. 2010;70(suppl 1):S6–S14.
45. Benzian H, Hobdell M, Holmgren C, et al. Political priority of global oral health: an analysis of reasons for international neglect. Int Dent J. 2011;61:124–30.

Chapter 22: Future and Impact of Rehabilitation Robotics on Post-stroke Care and Recovery

Anindo Roy and Prasad Mavuduri

Introduction

The advent of robotics and artificial intelligence (AI) has been the harbinger to many advances across many industries, and especially the health sector from diagnosis to hospital care to recovery. AI is leading to many discoveries in this sector including drug development, medical research, hospital care, insurance, and many other areas. The success of these inventions is dependent on how well they address the cost-effectiveness and accessibility issues in healthcare. I am very proud to introduce one such invention, which is not only addressing these issues at the business level but is also "life-changing" for some stroke victims. Dr. Anindo Roy has pioneered the development of modular ankle exoskeletons ("AnkleBot") for recovering stroke victims to "relearn" walking. According to Dr. Roy: "Majority of stroke survivors have persistent mobility deficits as the current treatments are not effective, contributing to more than 70% of patients sustaining a fall within 6 months, leading to hip or wrist fractures. These disabling consequences of stroke not only limit participation in community life but also set the stage for a sedentary lifestyle."

A. Roy (✉)
Department of Neurology, University of Maryland School of Medicine, Baltimore, MD, USA

Next Step Robotics Inc, Baltimore, MD, USA
e-mail: aroy1975@umd.edu

P. Mavuduri
Global Health Information Systems, Bowers & Wilkins, San Francisco, CA, USA

Chairman & President (Non-profit Board) AIBDP, San Francisco, CA, USA

© Springer Nature Switzerland AG 2020
P. Murthy, A. Ansehl (eds.), *Technology and Global Public Health*,
https://doi.org/10.1007/978-3-030-46355-7_27

Etiology and Scope of the Problem

Neurological injury to the brain is a life-changing event that impacts more people globally than maternal disorders, conflicts and terrorism, and natural disasters combined (Fig. 1) [3]. In particular, disability from stroke, the most prevalent among neurological disorders [4], is a rising global issue, driven by aging trends and westernized lifestyles across the planet. Although stroke remains the leading cause of serious disability in the U.S. with nearly 850,000 new cases per year and nearly 5 million stroke survivors [5], prevalence in low- and middle-income countries has risen to now exceed that of developed nations, contributing to loss of more than 113 million disability-adjusted life-years worldwide [6]. About 50% of stroke survivors have persistent mobility deficits [7], particularly hemiparetic gait with ankle weakness including foot-drop defined by dorsiflexion deficits, which impairs walking efficiency and balance and greatly increases the risk of fall [8]. These deficits limit functional mobility, contributing to more than 70% of stroke survivors sustaining a fall within 6 months, leading to hip and wrist fractures [9–12]. Hence, the

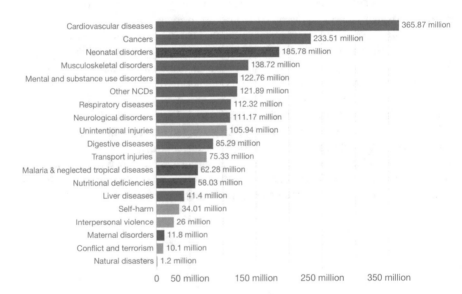

Fig. 1 Burden of disease by cause, in the world, 2017. Shown is the total disease burden, measured in disability-adjusted life-years (DALYs) by subcategories of disease or injury. DALYs are used to measure total burden of disease, from both years of life lost and years lived with a disability. One DALY equals one lost year of healthy life. (Reproduced from Global Burden of Disease Collaborative Network. Global Burden of Disease Study 2016 (GBD 2016) Results. Seattle, United States: Institute for Health Metrics and Evaluation (IHME), 2017; https://ourworldindata.org/grapher/burden-of-disease-by-cause, licensed under the terms of the Creative Commons Attribution License (https://creativecommons.org/licenses/by/4.0/deed.en_US))

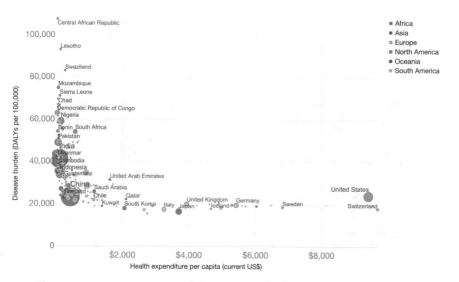

Fig. 2 Disease burden versus health expenditure per capita, 2014. Shown is total disease burden from all causes, measured as the number of DALYs per 100,000 individuals, versus health expenditure per capita (measured in US$). (Reproduced from Global Burden of Disease Collaborative Network. Global Burden of Disease Study 2017 (GBD 2017) Results. Seattle, United States: Institute for Health Metrics and Evaluation (IHME), 2018; https://ourworldindata.org/grapher/disease-burden-vs-health-expenditure-per-capita, licensed under the terms of the Creative Commons Attribution License (https://creativecommons.org/licenses/by/4.0/deed.en_US))

disabling consequences of stroke not only limit participation in community life but also set the stage for a sedentary lifestyle that reinforces learned nonuse toward further declines in mobility and balance functions. Despite its prevalence, disabling consequences, and long-term economic burden, the health expenditure per capita on the treatment and therapy for persons with neurological injuries is minimal, especially in low- to middle-income countries (Fig. 2). This lack leads to a "vicious cycle," one in which the patient develops secondary medical problems for lack of mobility (e.g., metabolic syndrome), further imposing an ongoing burden on the healthcare system.

Robotic Therapy: A Promising Solution?

Best care now consists of ankle–foot orthoses (AFO), functional electrical stimulation (FES), and canes and other "assistive devices" that do not address the underlying neuromotor deficits (Fig. 3, right) [13–20]. Although AFOs do offer some

3000 B.C.   **2019 A.D.**

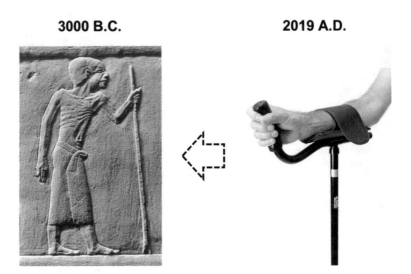

Fig. 3 Left: Depiction of a stick employed as a walking aid in ancient Egypt. The person por-
trayed in the hieroglyph is accurately shown with osteoarthritic disease that includes a bunion of
the first metatarsophalangeal joint of his front foot, impeding normal gait. (Source: Loebl WY,
Nunn JF (1997). Staffs as walking aids in ancient Egypt and Palestine. J R Soc Med 90:453. doi:
https://doi.org/10.1177/014107689709000811. Reprinted with permission from SAGE
Publishing). Right: Modern-day hand-held mobility crutch. (Reproduced from Wikimedia
Commons; photograph by Henrik Smith, 2017. https://en.wikipedia.org/wiki/Crutch#/media/
File:Platform-crutch.jpg, licensed under the terms of the Creative Commons Attribution License
(https://creativecommons.org/licenses/by/4.0/deed.en))

biomechanical benefits, such as preventing foot drop while worn, they do not treat
or improve foot drop deficits in the long-term [18, 20]. The same holds true for
computerized functional electrical stimulation (e.g., WalkAide, L300) [8] and
implantable microstimulators (BIONs) that stimulate the deep peroneal nerve and
tibialis anterior muscle to dorsiflex during swing. Indeed, AFOs, crutches, and such
nerve stimulation devices may, in fact, enforce disuse, biomechanically inefficient
compensatory strategies, and constrain activity-dependent plasticity that is crucial
for recovery [13–20]. Clearly, crutches and foot orthoses have been around since the
time of ancient Egyptians (Fig. 3, left). Now, we can do better for individuals with
mobility disabilities.

Robot-aided therapy has emerged as a promising approach to enhance recovery
and to extend structured task-practice, while reducing therapist labor and cost.
Robotics can also enable precise measures that can be leveraged to optimize therapy, as an alternative to more subjective clinical benchmarks. In particular, arm
robotics that provides assistance "as-needed" has proven most effective in chronic
stroke and has altered national care standards [1, 2]. VA cooperative studies show
impedance-controlled arm robotics can improve arm function [21], even years after
stroke, which has led to changes in best care standards [1, 2]. Yet, lower-extremity
(LE) robotics for stroke remains controversial, with the consensus that current

technologies are inferior to usual care, or even deleterious [1, 2]. Indeed, most LE robots for stroke have ignored the ankle as an actuated joint for motor learning, despite its critical role in gait and balance. Thus, commercially available LE robots primarily deliver pre-programmed multi-joint movement patterning, without therapeutically addressing the ankle, leaving little or no room for natural limb dynamics that is essential for motor learning. Motion and/or force-controlled leg robots also cannot dynamically tailor assistance to match deficits across differing levels of joint engagement, modulate timing or magnitude of robotics support based on step-by-step variability, or "adapt" across each patient's learning profile.

Despite the advances in our understanding of neuroplasticity and motor learning post stroke, now being leveraged with the use of robotics technology to change the natural history of stroke recovery, in terms of clinical translation the greatest advances have been made with the use of upper-extremity (UE) robotics, which have been tested for efficacy in multi-site trials [21]. In contrast, the implementation of lower-extremity (LE) robotics to promote locomotor relearning through massed practice has been more recent and presents unique challenges by virtue of the complex dynamics of gait, including the coordination of both legs and the multisegmental balance control inherent to upright locomotion. Early applications of robotics to UE therapy were chiefly directed at whole arm movements that are largely defined by end-effector trajectories, as when reaching with the entire shoulder–elbow–wrist complex to contact a target [22–25]. More recently, a multimodular approach has been advocated to apply therapy at the individual joints to address specific deficits or to promote a sequential approach [26]. Development of LE robotics has followed a similar pattern. The first large-scale efforts were aimed at re-creating the essentials of task-oriented treadmill training with partial body weight support (PBWS), emphasizing the consistency of gait-like stepping patterns that could be repeated for long periods without relying on therapists to assist with the stepping actions [27–29]. More recently, we have moved into modular LE robotics, using novel human–robot interaction control systems to optimize motor learning and customize these approaches to deficit profiles and clinical setting [30–33]. In concert with these engineering advances are studies of cortical neurophysiology that may provide insights into the mechanisms of activity-dependent plasticity and their optimal delivery to mediate motor learning and improve functional outcomes [34, 35].

Treadmill Locomotor Training: What Do Robots Leverage?

As prelude to LE robotics, the advent of treadmill training for gait rehabilitation after stroke was largely predicated on results from various spinalized cat models that showed locomotor patterning could be elicited without supraspinal inputs to the fore- and hindlimbs [36, 37]. Pioneering studies in persons with spinal cord injuries and stroke sought to test whether humans might benefit from treadmill as a stimulus for gait patterning and did show that it was possible to train severely impaired patients with varying degrees of partial body weight supported (PBWS) treadmill training [38–41]. Evidence of improved walking function was observed, and efforts to discern whether the treadmill approach yields meaningful gains in function are ongoing. A variant of the PBWS treadmill method has been to focus less on gait patterning and assisted stepping and more on the aerobic exercise aspect of effortful walking. In chronic stroke, this approach provides a locomotor stimulus with massed practice and has shown marked improvements in cardiovascular fitness and floor walking velocity, along with functional magnetic resonance imaging changes in paretic leg activation [42, 43]. These findings provide evidence that, even years after a disabling stroke, locomotor improvements with treadmill training activate appropriate areas of the brain, suggesting mechanisms of neuroplasticity. Other promising approaches include the use of a split-belt treadmill, which aims to induce motor adaptations that carry over to more symmetrical stepping patterns when transferred to overground walking [44, 45]. Still, there remain questions about the impact of treadmill compared to more generic locomotor activities such as home walking and exercise programs, which appear just as effective for mediating improvements in independent mobility outcomes [46]. Moreover, the issues of whether these approaches improve the biomechanical quality of gait and dynamic balance are not settled.

Innovations in Robotics for Locomotor Training

The promise of using the driving stimulus of the treadmill to train locomotor patterning has motivated major innovations in the area of powered gait orthoses and other robotic gait trainers. Recent advances in therapeutic robotics have led to several devices specific to the lower extremity (LE), including those for ankle rehabilitation. The Lokomat (similar to others, e.g., LOPES) is one of the first widely used LE robots, designed as a bilateral computerized gait orthosis used in conjunction with PBWS during treadmill walking (Fig. 4) [27]. It mainly guides the hips and knees through preprogrammed kinematics but does not provide active assistance at the ankle: foot drop is counteracted by a spring-loaded mechanism to support dorsiflexion during the swing phase of gait. This patterned locomotor training has produced positive effects on self-selected gait speed but has not shown an advantage compared to an equal dose intensity of standard physical therapy [47, 48]. The footplate activated Gait Trainer I is another device that evokes a physiological stepping pattern by moving the feet symmetrically as the patient stands on two moving foot supports [28, 29]. This design too has shown benefits, but the absence of a true swing phase and ground impact may be limitations when transferring to overground walking [49]. Another device is the active AFO (AAFO), which is a novel actuated ankle system placed in parallel with a human ankle that allows dorsi-plantarflexion [50]. The AAFO consists of a series of elastic actuators attached posterior to a conventional AFO, and a motor system modulates orthotic joint impedance based on position and force sensory information. The "Rutgers Ankle" orthopedic

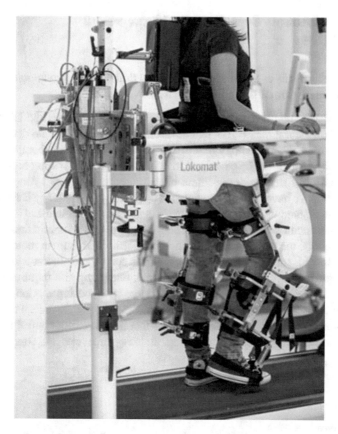

Fig. 4 Person undergoing robotic gait therapy using the Lokomat (Hocoma AG, Switzerland). (Source: © 2018 IEEE. Reprinted, with permission, from Tsangaridis P, Obwegeser D, Maggioni S, Riener R, Marchal-Crespo L. Visual and Haptic Error Modulating Controllers for Robotic Gait Training. 2018 7th IEEE International Conference on Biomedical Robotics and Biomechatronics (Biorob), Enschede, 2018, figure 1, p. 1051. Some modifications to the photo were made. doi: https://doi.org/10.1109/BIOROB.2018.8488011)

rehabilitation interface is yet another ankle rehabilitation device, consisting of a computer-controlled robotic platform that measures foot position and orientation [51]. The system uses double-acting pneumatic cylinders, linear potentiometers, and a six-degree-of-freedom (6-DOF) force sensor. It provides resistive forces and torques on the patient's foot, in response to virtual reality-based exercises. The robotic gait trainer (RGT) is another ankle exoskeleton that employs muscle rubber actuators, but has limited range of motion (ROM) in both the sagittal and frontal planes [52]. Another innovation has been to elaborate on the treadmill approach by introducing robotic actuators that interface with the pelvic girdle to promote weight shifts and multi-planar rotations which affect stepping as the patient walks. There are potential benefits from using robotics in gait training after stroke, but we have much to learn about specific interventions. Among the unknowns is whether targeting specific joint deficits will impact whole task functions such as gait and balance.

Why Have Robots Been Largely Unsuccessful for Gait Recovery?

Our experience leads us to believe that there are three factors attributable to the lack of clinical translation of LE robots for gait recovery:

1. *Efficacy*: We submit that the contrasting effectiveness of UE and LE therapies arises from neural factors, not technological factors. Although no doubt it might be improved, the technology deployed to date for locomotor therapy is elegant and sophisticated. Unfortunately, it may be misguided, providing highly repeatable control of rhythmic movement but ultimately doing the wrong thing. The technology we have deployed to date for upper-extremity therapy is firmly based on an understanding of how UE behavior is neurally controlled and derived from decades of neuroscience research. The limitations of LE robotic therapy lie not in the robotic technology but in its incompatibility with human motor neuroscience. Most LE robots impose motion, which is contrary to our knowledge of how neuroplasticity occurs (Fig. 5). For example, relearning gait requires the manifestation of passive gravito-inertial dynamics: by imposing motion, the robots suppress this mechanism and prevent room for voluntary practice, a central tenet of motor learning. Further, we also know that human motor control is based on dynamic 'building blocks,' including at least three classes: submovements,

Fig. 5 Model of a human–robot interaction for lower limb rehabilitation robots. Most contemporary robots impose motion rather than promote voluntary movement practice, while at the same time also not learning from human performance and recovery to adjust their own behaviors

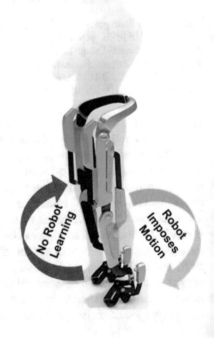

oscillations, and mechanical impedances. Stereotyped submovements are evident in the earliest actions of persons recovering after stroke. Reorganization of these submovements, as during robot-assisted arm reaching, quantifies the progress of recovery. Conversely, learning based on rhythmic performance (e.g., arm reaching) transfers poorly to discrete actions (e.g., walking). Current LE robot controllers are not customized to the inherent discrete nature of the task, which partly accounts for the surprising difficulty of robot-aided locomotor rehabilitation, as is evidenced by a plethora of clinical evidence that show a lack of superiority of current LE robots over usual care, that is, physical therapy (PT) (e.g., Lokomat) [48]. Finally, current LE robots are not conformant with cooperative control – that is, an architecture in which the robot learns from human performance to dynamically modulate its own behavior, much like the human entrains to the robot to better their performance (Fig. 5).

2. *Cost*: Current LE robots are prohibitively expensive, ranging from $80,000 to $200,000. This price point makes them beyond the reach of most PT clinics and rehabilitation hospitals in the industrialized nations, let alone LMI countries. In terms of billable therapy, directly from a patient or from an insurance company, considering a typical daily throughput of patients, it would take years for a PT clinic or rehabilitation hospital to recover the cost of the device.

3. *User Buy-In*: LE robots have, for most part, been developed in "isolation" by engineers without little or no buy-in from end users such as physical therapists, biomechanists, neuroscientists, and neurologists. Consequently, the operational features are often misaligned with the therapeutic target(s). For example, contemporary motor learning dictates task-specific voluntary practice to leverage neuroplasticity, which requires robot controllers to be designed such that the device dynamically interacts with the patient, providing assistance only when the patient is unable to complete the task or part of the task. In contrast, traditional motion- or force-based controllers deployed in most contemporary LE robots for gait therapy impose motion learning with little or no room for voluntary practice. Such established tenets of motor learning need to be taken into account by engineers during the conceptualization, development, and prototyping process by working alongside therapists and movement scientists.

We propose a new conceptual model for the development and testing of rehabilitation robotics, taking the aforementioned factors into account (Fig. 6). We believe that proving efficacy *before* dissemination or commercialization; lowering cost through additive manufacturing including 3D printing and using smart materials; and obtaining user input throughout the product life cycle, are essential for a successful translational pathway. Conversely, continually obtaining end-user feedback *after* dissemination to refine device features is vital for a refinement model. We have successfully applied this model toward a new class of exoskeletons for gait and mobility recovery after stroke and other neurological injury.

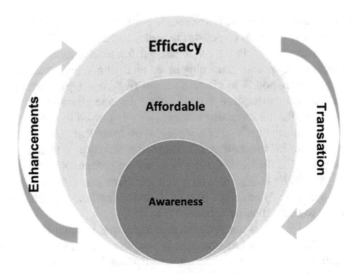

Fig. 6 A refined conceptual model for development and translation of rehabilitation robotics. Key factors such as efficacy, cost, and awareness are sequentially taken into account during translation whereas client feedback from field testing is taken into account for product refinements

Current Innovations: The "AnkleBot": A New Class of Robotic Device

Over the past few years our group has pioneered a modular ankle robot ("AnkleBot") that translates upper-extremity (UE) arm robotics technology to gait rehabilitation in stroke (Fig. 7) [53]. The AnkleBot is designed to deliver therapy in seated, over-ground, treadmill, and supine positions [54]. The device mediates ankle motor learning through mechanisms of neuroplasticity to improve independent mobility function after stroke. The paretic ankle was targeted because it is the site of major biomechanical contributions to normal gait and to the sensorimotor control of balance [55]. In particular, the generation of mechanical power through the paretic ankle is severely impaired after stroke [56–59]. Reduced propulsive impulses during the paretic stance phase of hemiparetic gait may also reflect this ankle power deficit [58, 59] and contribute to interlimb asymmetry. Important for gait safety after stroke are ankle dorsiflexion, eversion deficits, and spasticity that contribute to foot drop and falls [8, 9]. Hence, improving paretic ankle contributions to the biomechanics of walking could benefit gait velocity, reduce fall risk, and reduce increased demands at the nonparetic limb, making it a logical focus for robotic intervention.

A fundamental conceptual question in stroke neuromotor rehabilitation is whether to emphasize task-specific gait pattern training or modular and joint-specific mass training aimed at specific stroke impairments. Two clinical trials, each consisting of 6-week seated robot training, were conducted to determine initial feasibility for using the AnkleBot in extended training in individuals with chronic

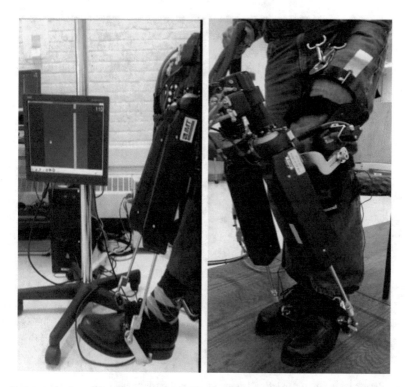

Fig. 7 A two-degree-of-freedom, modular ankle exoskeleton designed to improve ankle function in persons with neurological injuries. Two key therapeutic applications of the robot: seated, computer video-interfaced training (left); overground, robot-assisted gait therapy (right). Key components of the robot include a customized orthopedic shoe and a knee brace that is worn by the subject and secured with quick connectors and a strap attached over the bridge of the subject's foot. The robotic hardware includes two brushless DC motors that drive a pair of linear actuators, which are connected to the shoe using ball joints. A rotary encoder is used to commutate the motor and a linear incremental encoder inside the traction estimates angle. Other peripherals include a potentiometer mounted laterally on the knee to estimate knee angle and a shoulder strap to optionally support the weight of the subject. (Source: United States Patent and Trademark Office. Photo credit: Anindo Roy)

stroke [30, 31]. Subjects with chronic stroke, who had completed conventional therapy, and had persistent LE hemiparesis with at least minimal ankle activation in both DF and PF directions, participated in the study. Training protocol consisted of playing a videogame that required repetitive movements of the paretic ankle to move a screen cursor "up or down" to pass through "gates" that approached across the screen at different vertical levels (Fig. 8). Gate locations were individualized for each subject based on their voluntary range of motion. Improved voluntary control of the paralyzed ankle was indicated by changes at 6 weeks in several metrics of performance and the quality of unassisted ankle pointing movements on the videogame task. Surprisingly, these benefits at the ankle translated into faster and more symmetrical independent walking [30, 31].

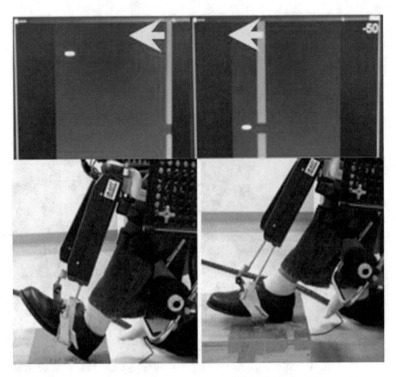

Fig. 8 Person undergoing AnkleBot therapy in a seated position while playing a videogame that is adjusted to individual ankle deficits. (Photo credit: Anindo Roy)

The transition from nonambulatory robotic therapy to treadmill and overground gait training requires new control systems to address task-specific challenges. One clinical concern is the impact of the device mass. Early clinical studies have shown that the AnkleBot mass does not significantly alter the hemiparetic gait pattern [60]. Another concern is safely and effectively controlling the dynamic interaction between the stroke client's leg and floor, which is challenging, because interaction with unknown "objects" (human in-loop) can destabilize the integrated system, a phenomenon known as contact instability. Another concern is the inherently pronounced stride-to-stride variability present in the gait patterns of neurologically disabled persons. To address these challenges, a novel control algorithm was developed that utilizes insole footswitches to detect the timing of key gait events (e.g., toe-off) [61, 62]. This device enables linking the timing of robotic assistance precisely to the manifestation of specific functional deficits (e.g., foot drop), often each patient's predominant gait deficit. For example, it is possible to deliver plantar-flexion torque during late stance into early swing phase; dorsiflex the ankle to assist foot clearance in mid-swing and if needed; or orient the foot for proper landing (Fig. 9, right). These features have enabled the integration of AnkleBot into treadmill-based training (Fig. 9, left) by rendering this device capable of addressing patient needs across a continuum of deficit severity and stroke recovery profiles.

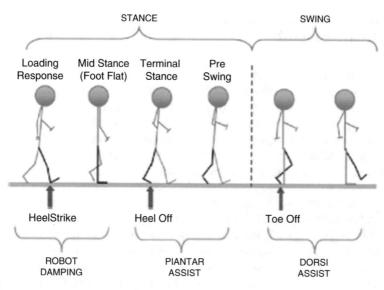

Fig. 9 Adaptive system for precise timing of robotic support to key gait events. (Source: © 2013 IEEE. Reprinted, with permission, from Roy A, Krebs HI, Barton J E, Macko RF, Forrester LW. Anklebot-assisted locomotor training after stroke: a novel deficit-adjusted control approach. 2013 IEEE International Conference on Robotics and Automation, Karlsruhe, 2013, Figure 1, p. 2176. doi: https://doi.org/10.1109/ICRA.2013.6630869)

What Is the Clinical Evidence?

We recently completed the first clinical study of AnkleBot integrated treadmill exercise (TMR) showing that 18 sessions in 6 weeks reversed foot drop and normalized foot landing (heel-first), enabling safer and more independent walking, even years after the stroke [63]. These benefits collectively contributed to reduced reliance on assistive devices and increased daily free-living ambulatory activity, even 6 weeks after training ceases in adults with chronic stroke disability. Additionally, TMR roughly doubled the estimated ambulatory workload capacity per session, with higher self-selected training speed and walking duration even as robotic support was "weaned down" when patients took over more of the work of walking. Collectively, these benefits translated into an 85% self-reduction in previously prescribed AFO and/or assistive device use, which was an unexpected and unprecedented observation that we did not have on our outcome wish list. Generally, such ankle deficits in chronic stroke are considered immutable. Our two decades of task-oriented exercise research without robotics in chronic hemiparesis have not demonstrated as substantial an impact on assistive device usage. Furthermore, the fact that the benefits fully persisted 6 weeks after training was completed suggests incorporation of increased paretic ankle function and mobility training into the free-living environment. Importantly, all our clinical trials report high client satisfaction, a desire to continue training, and an absence of study-related adverse events [30, 31, 60, 63].

Overground Robot-Assisted Mobility Therapy: The Gold Standard

Although the AnkleBot offers the first evidence-based solution for ankle hemiparesis and foot drop, it has several major limitations. As are most contemporary LE robots, the device is heavy (>7 lb), wire-tethered to a bulky electrical computer panel, and prohibitively expensive ($130,000), albeit efficacious. Hence, it can only be used in research settings, as it lacks the operational autonomy for training overground gait and mobility activities that are an essential focus of PT practice, preventing us from realizing the full promise afforded by the AnkleBot. To address these limitations, we recently produced and tested an untethered (battery-operated, on-board computer control) and lightweight (3D-printed carbon fiber components) ankle robot prototype (AMBLE) with equivalent motion–force functionality as the AnkleBot. AMBLE's main enhancement from its predecessor is its autonomy and low mass (<4 lb) through battery power, on-board computer, and single-axis design, while retaining the technical features necessary for neuromotor recovery (highly back-drivable hardware, assist as-needed, adaptive timing stimulus) (Fig. 10). In addition, the AMBLE has in-built machine learning capabilities that afford dynamic auto-adjustment and shaping of robot behavior (e.g., device assistance) based on evolving trends of human performance. In a cohort of five chronic stroke subjects with clinically assessed foot drop, pilot tests were conducted with the AMBLE to

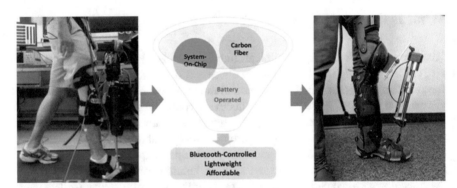

Fig. 10 Left: Person undergoing Anklebot-assisted treadmill therapy. (Reprinted from Ahn J, Hogan N (2012) Walking Is Not Like Reaching: Evidence from Periodic Mechanical Perturbations. PLoS ONE 7(3): e31767. Some modifications to the photo were made. https://doi.org/10.1371/journal.pone.0031767, licensed under the terms of the Creative Commons Attribution License (https://creativecommons.org/licenses/by/4.0/)). Center: Developmental transition from the tethered Anklebot to produce portable exoskeletal technology, including embedded electronics, lightweight materials, and battery power. Right: An untethered ankle exoskeleton (AMBLE). (Used with permission from NextStep Robotics, Inc.)

assess user fit, comfort, and efficacy under both unactuated and actuated conditions during 30-ft walk tests. Users expressed high level of satisfaction with respect to fit and comfort (absence of skin irritations/abrasions). Within a single session, overground gait speed increased and resulted in higher heel-first foot strikes, providing initial evidence of safety treatment (unpublished data).

Conclusions

1. *Modular Ankle Robotics*: Clinical testing of a novel ankle exoskeletal technologies, such as the AnkleBot, has lent support to the idea of using a joint-specific modular approach as a therapeutic modality for hemiparetic stroke. Use of the seated approach has answered initial questions about the potential for augmenting traditional task-specific therapies, and may prove to be a valuable enhancement of early interventions by providing a platform to address underlying impairments in the realm of motor control [30, 31]. Additional work is needed to establish the optimal timing for modular robotics treatment across the spectrum of motor recovery after stroke, beginning with the inpatient rehabilitation hospital setting through the outpatient phase of clinical follow-up care. The modular AnkleBot offers a means to probe the effectiveness of early intensive robotic training for promoting neural plasticity associated with motor learning and whether this will increase the prospects for long-term improvements in mobility and balance functions. The integration of the AnkleBot into actual task-oriented gait training has proven efficacious, giving clinicians the ability to focus on specific paretic side deficits, such as foot drop, improper ankle–foot orientation at foot strike, or weak propulsion in late stance [60]. The ability to provide overground gait and mobility training has been realized through an engineering successor of the AnkleBot, an untethered ankle exoskeleton called AMBLE, which is currently undergoing clinical testing.

2. *Spectrum of Recovery*: Rehabilitation robotics have tremendous potential to change the quality of life for persons living with neurological injuries such as stroke, while decreasing the public health and economic burden of neurological disease at the macro level. For this to occur, however, policymakers need to consider adoption of effective robotic solutions into their healthcare systems. For developers, the caveat is to develop the "right" technology and deploy it at the "right" time period of recovery with the "appropriate" therapeutic modality (Fig. 11).

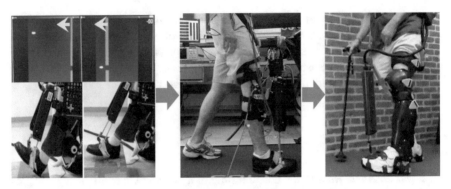

Fig. 11 Left: Life cycle of rehabilitation robots such as the Anklebot being deployed as part of sequential therapeutic modalities based on the clinical needs (ambulatory levels) and recovery stages. Seated: Videogame robotic therapy for severely impaired, non-ambulatory stroke patients. (Photo credit: Anindo Roy). Center: Treadmill-based robotic therapy for stroke patients with mild-to-moderate ambulatory capacity. (Reprinted from Ahn J, Hogan N (2012) Walking Is Not Like Reaching: Evidence from Periodic Mechanical Perturbations. PLoS ONE 7(3):e31767. Some modifications to the photo were made. https://doi.org/10.1371/journal.pone.0031767, licensed under the terms of the Creative Commons Attribution License (https://creativecommons.org/licenses/by/4.0/)). Right: Portable robotic gait and mobility therapy for stroke patients capable of ambulating with assistive aids such as canes. (Used with permission from NextStep Robotics, Inc.)

For example, in the instance of the AnkleBot, providing proprioceptive stimulus to the ankle in a seated condition is the appropriate modality during the early phases of stroke recovery [30, 31], which has shown durable benefits in walking and balance function at the time of discharge. Similarly, for patients who are capable of limited ambulation, AnkleBot-assisted treadmill training provides a safe and effective environment, allowing most chronic stroke patients to partly regain their functional independence as evidenced by discarding assistive devices [63]. As ambulatory capacity and function increase, untethered exoskeletons such as AMBLE may be used in conjunction with robotic harness systems with adaptive body weight support (e.g., ZeroG) to further increase recovery. Finally, robotic devices such as AMBLE should be deployed for unsupported overground therapy to transition persons from limited community to full community ambulators.

3. *Bench-To-Bedside Model*: In conclusion, our decades-long experience with the design and clinical testing of LE robots has identified many pitfalls, as well as solutions. At the heart of successful commercialization should be an evidence-based solution (Fig. 12), which necessitates taking input from clinicians before and during engineering conceptualization and development, followed by clinical trials to demonstrate safety and comparative efficacy. This trial may be followed by commercialization, but in a manner such that end-user inputs are continually obtained to further refine and advance operational features of the device and user interface toward better ergonomics and ease of use.

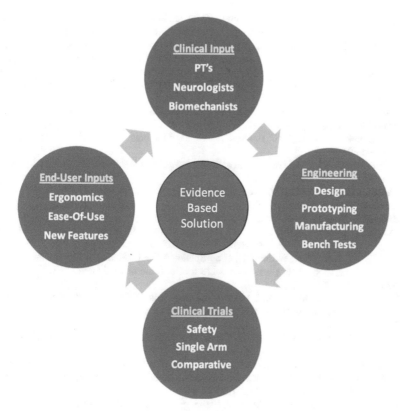

Fig. 12 A new development model for rehabilitation robotics centered around evidence-based science. The model necessitates a sequence of clinically identifying the injury, engineering the solution, conducting clinical trials, and continually obtaining end-user inputs after deployment

References

1. Bates B, Glasberg J, Hughes K, Katz R, et al. VA/DOD clinical practice guideline for the management of stroke. J Rehabil Res Dev. 2010;47(9):1–43.
2. Miller EL, Murray L, Richards L, et al. Comprehensive overview of nursing and interdisciplinary rehabilitation care of the stroke patient: a scientific statement from the American Heart Association. Stroke. 2010;41(10):2402–48.
3. Global Burden of Disease Collaborative Network. Global Burden of Disease Study 2017 (GBD 2017) results. Seattle: Institute for Health Metrics and Evaluation (IHME); 2018. http://www.healthdata.org/gbd
4. Gooch CL, Pracht E, Borenstein AR. The burden of neurological disease in the United States: a summary report and call to action. Ann Neurol. 2017;81(4):479–84.
5. Heart disease and stroke statistics—2012 update. American Heart Association. http://www.americanheart.org/statistics
6. GBD 2016 DALYs and HALE Collaborators. Global, regional, and national disability-adjusted life-years (DALYs) for 333 diseases and injuries and healthy life expectancy (HALE) for 195 countries and territories, 1990–2016: a systematic analysis for the Global Burden of Disease Study 2016. Lancet. 2017;16(390(10100)):1260–344.

7. Jorgensen HS, Nakayama H, Raaschou HO, et al. Recovery of walking function in stroke patients: the Copenhagen Stroke Study. Arch Phys Med Rehabil. 1995;76(1):27–32.

8. Bosch PR, Harris JE, Wing K, American Congress of Rehabilitation Medicine (ACRM) Stroke Movement Interventions Subcommittee. Review of therapeutic electrical stimulation for dorsiflexion assist and orthotic substitution. From the American Congress of Rehabilitation Medicine Stroke Movement Interventions Subcommittee. Arch Phys Med Rehabil. 2014;95(2):390–6.

9. Forster A, Young J. Incidence and consequences of falls due to stroke: a systematic inquiry. BMJ. 1995;311(6997):83–6.

10. Ramnemark A, Nyberg L, Borssen B, et al. Fractures after stroke. Osteoporos Int. 1998;8(1):92–5.

11. Dennis MS, Lo KM, McDowall M, et al. Fractures after stroke: frequency, types, and associations. Stroke. 2002;33(3):728–34.

12. Kanis J, Oden A, Johnell O. Acute and long-term increase in fracture risk after hospitalization for stroke. Stroke. 2001;32(3):702–6.

13. Bethoux F, Rogers HL, Nolan J, et al. Long-term follow-up to a randomized controlled trial comparing peroneal nerve functional electrical stimulation to an ankle-foot orthosis for patients with chronic stroke. Neurorehabil Neural Repair. 2015;29(10):911–22.

14. Sheffler LR, Bailey SN, Wilson RD, et al. Spatiotemporal, kinematic, and kinetic effects of a peroneal nerve stimulator versus an ankle foot orthosis in hemiparetic gait. Neurorehabil Neural Repair. 2013;27(5):403–10.

15. Ring H, Treger I, Gruendlinger L, et al. Neuroprosthesis for footdrop compared with an ankle-foot orthosis: effects on postural control during walking. J Stroke Cerebrovasc Dis. 2009;18(1):41–7.

16. Kluding PM, Dunning K, O'Dell MW, et al. Foot drop stimulation versus ankle foot orthosis after stroke: 30-week outcomes. Stroke. 2013;44(6):1660–9.

17. Everaert DG, Stein RB, Abrams GM, et al. Effect of a foot-drop stimulator and ankle-foot orthosis on walking performance after stroke: a multicenter randomized controlled trial. Neurorehabil Neural Repair. 2013;27(7):579–91.

18. Nair PM, Rooney KL, Kautz SA, et al. Stepping with an ankle foot orthosis re-examined: a mechanical perspective for clinical decision making. Clin Biomech. 2010;25(6):618–22.

19. Burdett RG, Borello-France D, Blatchly C, et al. Gait comparison of subjects with hemiplegia walking unbraced, with ankle-foot orthosis, and with air-stirrup brace. Phys Ther. 1988;68(8):1197–203.

20. Radtka SA, Oliveira GB, Lindstrom KE, et al. The kinematic and kinetic effects of solid, hinged, and no ankle-foot orthoses on stair locomotion in healthy adults. Gait Posture. 2006;24(2):211–8.

21. Lo AC, Guarino PD, Richards LG, et al. Robot-assisted therapy for long-term upper-limb impairment after stroke. N Engl J Med. 2011;362:1772–83.

22. Krebs HI, Hogan N, Aisen ML, et al. Robot-aided neurorehabilitation. IEEE Trans Rehabil Eng. 1998;6(1):75–87.

23. Krebs HI, Volpe BT, Williams D, et al. Robot-aided neurorehabilitation: a robot for wrist rehabilitation. IEEE Trans Neural Syst Rehabil Eng. 2007;15(3):327–35.

24. Lum PS, Burgar CG, Kenney DE, et al. Quantification of force abnormalities during passive and active-assisted upper-limb reaching movements in post-stroke hemiparesis. IEEE Trans Biomed Eng. 1999;46(6):652–62.

25. Reinkensmeyer DJ, Dewald JP, Rymer WZ. Guidance-based quantification of arm impairment following brain injury: a pilot study. IEEE Trans Rehabil Eng. 1999;7(1):1–11.

26. Krebs HI, Volpe BT, Lynch D, et al. Stroke rehabilitation: an argument in favor of a robotic gym. In: Proceedings of the 9th international conference on rehabilitation robotics (USA), Chicago, USA; 2005. p. 219–22.

27. Colombo G, Joerg M, Schreier R, et al. Treadmill training of paraplegic patients using a robotic orthosis. J Rehabil Res Dev. 2000;37(6):693–700.

28. Hesse S, Uhlenbrock D. A mechanized gait trainer for restoration of gait. J Rehabil Res Dev. 2000;37(6):701–8.
29. Schmidt H, Sorowka D, Hesse S, et al. Development of a robotic walking simulator for gait rehabilitation. Biomed Tech (Berl). 2003;48(10):281–6.
30. Forrester LW, Roy A, Krebs HI, et al. Ankle training with a robotic device improves hemiparetic gait after a stroke. Neurorehabil Neural Repair. 2011;25(4):369–77.
31. Forrester LW, Roy A, Krywonis A, et al. Modular ankle robotics training in early sub-acute stroke: a randomized controlled pilot study. Neurorehabil Neural Repair. 2014;28(7):678–87.
32. Roy A, Forrester LW, Macko RF. Short-term ankle motor performance with ankle robotics training in chronic hemiparetic stroke. J Rehabil Res Dev. 2011;48(4):417–30.
33. Roy A, Krebs HI, Patterson SL, et al. Measurement of passive ankle stiffness in subjects with chronic hemiparesis using a novel ankle robot. J Neurophysiol. 2011;105(5):2132–49.
34. Goodman RN, Rietschel JC, Roy A, et al. Increased reward in ankle robotics training enhances motor control and cortical efficiency in stroke. J Rehabil Res Dev. 2014;51(2):213–28.
35. Halsband U, Lange RK. Motor learning in man: a review of functional and clinical studies. J Physiol. 2006;99(4-6):414–24.
36. Grillner S. Locomotion in vertebrates: central mechanisms and reflex interaction. Physiol Rev. 1975;55(2):247–304.
37. Grillner S, Wallen P. Central pattern generators for locomotion, with special reference to vertebrates. Annu Rev Neurosci. 1985;8:233–61.
38. Barbeau H, Visintin M. Optimal outcomes obtained with body-weight support combined with treadmill training in stroke subjects. Arch Phys Med Rehabil. 2003;84(10):1458–65.
39. Hassid E, Rose D, Commisarow J, et al. Improved gait symmetry in hemiparetic stroke patients induced during body weight-supported treadmill stepping. Neurorehabil Neural Repair. 1997;11:21–6.
40. Hesse S, Bertelt C, Jahnke MT, et al. Treadmill training with partial body weight support compared with physiotherapy in nonambulatory hemiparetic patients. Stroke. 1995;26(6):976–81.
41. Hesse S, Bertelt C, Schaffrin A, et al. Restoration of gait in nonambulatory hemiparetic patients by treadmill training with partial body-weight support. Arch Phys Med Rehabil. 1994;75(1):1087–93.
42. Luft AR, Macko RF, Forrester LW, et al. Treadmill exercise activates subcortical neural networks and improves walking after stroke: a randomized controlled trial. Stroke. 2008;39(12):3341–50.
43. Macko RF, Ivey FM, Forrester LW, et al. Treadmill exercise rehabilitation improves ambulatory function and cardiovascular fitness in patients with chronic stroke: a randomized, controlled trial. Stroke. 2005;36(10):2206–11.
44. Reisman DS, Wityk R, Silver K, et al. Locomotor adaptation on a split-belt treadmill can improve walking post-stroke. Brain. 2007;130(pt 7):1861–72.
45. Reisman DS, Wityk R, Silver K, et al. Split-belt treadmill adaptation transfers to overground walking in persons poststroke. Neurorehabil Neural Repair. 2009;23(7):735–47.
46. Duncan PW, Sullivan KJ, Behrman AL, et al. Body-weight–supported treadmill rehabilitation after stroke. N Engl J Med. 2011;364:2026–36.
47. Hornby TG, Campbell DD, Kahn JH, et al. Enhanced gait-related improvements after therapist-versus robotic-assisted locomotor training in subjects with chronic stroke: a randomized controlled study. Stroke. 2008;39(6):1786–92.
48. Westlake KP, Patten C. Pilot study of Lokomat versus manual-assisted treadmill training for locomotor recovery post- stroke. J Neuroeng Rehabil. 2009;6:18.
49. Schmidt H, Werner C, Bernhardt R, et al. Gait rehabilitation machines based on programmable footplates. J Neuroeng Rehabil. 2007;4:2.
50. Blaya JA, Herr H. Adaptive control of a variable-impedance ankle-foot orthosis to assist drop-foot gait. IEEE Trans Neural Syst Rehabil Eng. 2004;12(1):24–31.
51. Girone M, Burdea G, Bouzit M, et al. A Stewart platform-based system for ankle telerehabilitation. Auton Robot. 2010;10(2):203–12.

52. Bharadwaj K, Sugar TG, Koeneman JB, et al. Design of a robotic gait trainer using spring over muscle actuators for ankle stroke rehabilitation. ASME Trans Biomech Eng. 2005;127(6):1009–13.
53. Roy A, Krebs HI, Williams DJ, et al. Robot-aided neurorehabilitation: a robot for ankle rehabilitation. IEEE Trans Robot. 2009;25(3):569–82.
54. Forrester LW, Roy A, Goodman RN, et al. Clinical application of a modular ankle robot for stroke rehabilitation. NeuroRehabilitation. 2013;33(1):85–97.
55. Neptune RR, Kautz SA, Zajac FE. Contributions of the individual ankle plantar flexors to support, forward progression and swing initiation during walking. J Biomech. 2001;34(11):1387–98.
56. Olney SJ, Richards C. Hemiparetic gait following stroke. Part I: characteristics. Gait Posture. 1996;4(2):136–48.
57. Bowden MG, Balasubramanian CK, Neptune RR, et al. Anterior-posterior ground reaction forces as a measure of paretic leg contribution in hemiparetic walking. Stroke. 2006;37(3):872–6.
58. Olney SJ, Griffin MP, Monga TN, et al. Work and power in gait of stroke patients. Arch Phys Med Rehabil. 1991;72(5):309–14.
59. Gerston L, Orr W. External work of walking in hemiparetic patients. Scand J Rehabil. 1997;3(1):85–6.
60. Khanna I, Roy A, Rodgers MM, et al. Effects of unilateral robotic limb loading on gait characteristics in subjects with chronic stroke. J Neuroeng Rehabil. 2010;7:23.
61. Roy A, Krebs HI, Barton JE, et al. Anklebot-assisted locomotor training after stroke: a novel deficit-adjusted control approach. 2013 IEEE International Conference on Robotics and Automation, Karlsruhe; 2013. p. 2175–82. https://doi.org/10.1109/ICRA.2013.6630869.
62. Roy A, Forrester LW, Macko F. Method and apparatus for providing deficit-adjusted adaptive assistance during movement phases of an impaired joint. US Patent 9,943,459. Issued: April 17, 2018.
63. Forrester LW, Roy A, Hafer-Macko C, et al. Task-specific ankle robotics gait training after stroke: a randomized pilot study. J Neuroeng Rehabil. 2016;13(1):51.
64. Loebl WY, Nunn JF. Staffs as walking aids in ancient Egypt and Palestine. J R Soc Med. 1997;90:450–4. https://doi.org/10.1177/014107689709000811.
65. Tsangaridis P, Obwegeser D, Maggioni S, Riener R, Marchal-Crespo L. Visual and haptic error modulating controllers for robotic gait training. 2018 7th IEEE International Conference on Biomedical Robotics and Biomechatronics (Biorob), Enschede; 2018. p. 1050–55. https://doi.org/10.1109/BIOROB.2018.8488011.
66. Ahn J, Hogan N. Walking is not like reaching: evidence from periodic mechanical perturbations. PLoS One 2012;7(3):e31767. https://doi.org/10.1371/journal.pone.0031767. Accessed 15 Mar 2020.

Correction to: Health Transformation in Saudi Arabia via Connected Health Technologies

Hebah ElGibreen

Correction to:
Chapter 10 in: P. Murthy, A. Ansehl (eds.),
Technology and Global Public Health,
https://doi.org/10.1007/978-3-030-46355-7_10

The chapter was inadvertently published with middle name included in the author's name as "Hebah Abdul Aziz ElGibreen" instead of "Hebah ElGibreen".

The author's name has been corrected by removing the middle name "Abdul Aziz" in "Hebah Abdul Aziz ElGibreen". The name has been updated as "Hebah ElGibreen".

The updated online version of the chapter can be found at
https://doi.org/10.1007/978-3-030-46355-7_10

Epilogue

Padmini Murthy and Amy Ansehl

A pervasive theme throughout the book *Technology and Global Public Health* is the capacity of the global community to ensure healthy lives for the population and to determine the degree to which countries will be able to meet the targets of the 17 Sustainable Development Goals of the United Nations, with a focus on SDG 3, which is "Ensure healthy lives and promote well-being for all at all ages." The degree to which countries fully support utilization of technology enables global access to healthcare-related innovations in their rural and urban populations. In this sense, technology builds a bridge that links diverse populations which are spread out over vast geographic spaces to health information and advances. Interoperability between networks and platforms, as discussed and emphasized by several authors in their chapters, is both a necessity and a vital component of information exchange between systems. Therefore, if systems cannot communicate with each other in an efficient, effective, and secure manner, the transfer of information will be inhibited. We have learned in the Chap. 8 "Law, Technology and Public Health" that in the United States of America that there is currently no uniform legal approach to regulating telehealth, which is obviously a challenge to the growth of telehealth technology and communication. As the author states, recent reports to the United States Congress have reaffirmed there is great potential to access healthcare using telehealth technology, which can yield better outcomes and cost savings and promote universal healthcare. Telehealth is clearly increasing at a very fast rate and in quality. Interoperability and reliability are key factors that must be integrated into the widespread dissemination of telehealth services.

The concept of connected health is crucial in providing populations with the ability to open innovative communication channels over diverse and disparate geographic regions. Furthermore, successful interoperability of connected health means it must be integrated with digital devices, electronic health records, and mobile

P. Murthy · A. Ansehl
School of Health Sciences and Practice, New York Medical College, Valhalla, NY, USA

© Springer Nature Switzerland AG 2020
P. Murthy, A. Ansehl (eds.), *Technology and Global Public Health*,
https://doi.org/10.1007/978-3-030-46355-7

devices, which is captured under the mHealth umbrella so that smartphones and tablets are synchronous. Countries have developed several realization programs to enhance connectivity and cost savings. These realization programs described in the book use technology and its regulation to transform the delivery of information and healthcare services. An important finding is the necessity of building an infrastructure and integrating research to ensure success and sustainability. Data science is needed to analyze metrics and overcome gaps and cost inefficiencies. Policies are needed to support easy-to-use and connected healthcare services. Other authors emphasize the importance of creating enhanced professional teams to deliver healthcare services. They view technology-enabled teams as a key strategy to meet the targets of the Sustainable Development Goals. There has been a major system change from a healthcare system based on individual practitioners to one based on large healthcare networks or systems. Technology is needed to promote and protect internal and external communications in a large healthcare system. The concept of health systems strengthening is essential to maximize outcomes. The book further emphasizes that we must move from a donor-based system to a healthcare system perspective. Healthcare systems are made up of teams and these teams need to be supported with continuous quality education, human resources management, certification standards, and supporting professional associations. The use of technology promotes and fulfills the right of every global citizen to ensure they have access to healthcare information and services. Many examples in the book highlight that technology is a cost-effective way of reaching the healthcare providers within a healthcare system by providing them with knowledge, skills, and secure platforms so they can facilitate the global actions of healthcare information and services provided.

The Chap. 15 on the "Worldwide Digital Divide and Access to Healthcare Technology" discusses the notable digital divide that exists globally, causing significant disparities between populations that have access to reliable telecommunications and those which do not have reliable access to technology. This difference has a direct negative impact on countries and access of their populations to healthcare information and services, so that populations have become underserved and faced significant health-related disparities up to now.

Risk stratification is an important concept in health systems and delivery of services. The many technology-based tools that facilitate risk stratification include data mining, epidemiology and surveillance, healthcare system-based electronic medical records, personal health records, and decision support tools that enable both patients and providers to communicate and identify risks of disease, outbreaks of disease over vast geographic areas, and improved healthcare status. The utilization of risk stratification technology allows patients to be categorized using demographic and medical conditions, analyzing the potential severity of the disease. The costs of connectivity are a significant barrier to adoption, and both public and private sectors must think both innovatively and strategically to mitigate these costs because global connectivity is omnipotent and important.

The Chap. 6 "Simple Technology for Menstrual Hygiene Management: A Case Study from Northern Ethiopia" illustrates how technology fosters social enterprise to help women manage an essential component of their physiology. The authors of this chapter explain the struggles many women have with coping with monthly menstrual hygiene. These struggles culminate in decreased quality of life and lost days of productivity from school or work. Lack of access to and expenses associated with procurement of sanitary pads for women are factors contributing to lack of menstrual supplies for women and girls in many parts of the world. Additionally, the authors discuss the negative impact on the environment from using the traditional pads. Interestingly, very little had changed in the management of menstrual hygiene until an Ethiopian woman and chemical engineer became an innovator for the purpose of improving the lives of her countrywomen. The innovation described in this chapter is the development of a recyclable and more cost- and time-efficient sanitary pad. In addition, from a waste management perspective this innovation avoids environmental contamination. The innovator now has a government patent, and the product is being sourced and developed locally in Northern Ethiopia by local workers. This is a great example of entrepreneurship and social enterprise creating economic and environmental sustainability and improving the lives of many women.

In the Chap. 9 "mHealth for Better Quality of Life, Healthier Lifestyles and More Meaningful Lives," mHealth is described as part of the division of eHealth services, emphasizing its value in the dissemination of health-related information that can be analyzed and utilized to inform the delivery of healthcare in low-resource settings. As we learn in this chapter, mHealth can be delivered in a multitude of ways including short messaging services, multimedia messaging services, video conferences, health applications, and software installed in mobile devices. These tools can be highly efficient for surveillance, community outreach, wearable technology, and health campaigns. As a result of technology, which is the driver behind mHealth, we now have more robust systems to identify and manage infectious diseases which can cause global pandemics such as SARS, H1N1, Zika, Ebola, and COVID-19. We now have borderless technologies for people to identify self-care strategies to manage chronic diseases such as diabetes, HIV, cancer, and cardiovascular disease. However, as the authors describe there is still need for global integration, adoption, and a generalized scaling up of healthcare services. Future research studies are needed to identify the gold standard mHealth technologies and ensure high-quality, cost-effective, equitable delivery to reduce health disparities.

Technology has a significant role in the prevention, identification, monitoring, and management of disasters. We learn in the Chap. 17 "Global Public Health Disaster Management and Technology" of the four reactionary stages: preparedness, response, recovery, and mitigation. In every phase there is a need for technology to capture and communicate information and data. Technology enables important strategies in disaster preparedness that include modeling and simulation, virtual reality simulation, and disaster response. Recovery and information dissemination, early warning systems, cloud repository services, mHealth, and social media platforms are also vital to communications in a disaster scenario.

The Chap. 14 "Trafficking, Technology, and Public Health: The Malignant Malady of Modern Slavery" details the major public health problem known as human trafficking and modern slavery (HTMS). Technology, which can be harnessed for so much good in expanding the human right to access healthcare, can also be weaponized and exploited by traffickers of human beings. Why? Because those who traffic in human beings use social media as a way to identify and abuse unknowing people. Population management and survivor engagement strategies using social media have unfortunately lagged behind. Also, using technology through social media is a very effective way to promote awareness of the scope of the human trafficking problem to create informed partnership. Community capacity building to build resistance through grassroots coalitions that can be linked worldwide through technology is another important strategy. A recent survey described by the author demonstrates that victims of trafficking do engage with the medical community while they are being trafficked. Unfortunately, most of the victims are hesitant or feel ashamed to confide in their healthcare provider. Clearly, continuing education for healthcare providers to address this global public health challenge and use the internet and training modules that can being transmitted rapidly and reliably are greatly needed to combat the huge trafficking crisis.

"Technology and the Practice of Health Education in Conflict Zones" (Chap. 7) describes how during times of crisis in a country there is a negative impact on access to education, the collateral damage and safety rendering it almost impossible for its population to continue their education. It is relevant to note that access to education is impacted at all levels from primary to advanced secondary. Reports have shown that there is a major need for medical education in conflict zones. Examples include the conflict in Syria where there were physician shortages before the conflict and now also after the conflict. With access to medical education being limited, these shortages are more severe, which negatively impacts the delivery of healthcare services to patients. Other barriers include cultural, language, financial, lack of human resources, safety, gender-based violence, and legal. Technology can be used effectively to overcome or reduce many of these barriers. For example, e-learning platforms that can be delivered to smartphones, tablets, and other mHealth tools can minimize barriers of cost, safety, culture, and language and improve overall access to education. This aid is particularly ideal in conflict zones where it is far too dangerous and life risking to travel to a school. The online education examples detailed in the chapter offer evidence-based examples of technology-driven healthcare education to medical students that was effective in the Middle East. Some of the barriers described that adversely impact online education are lack of access to electricity, or a slow internet connection, interoperability of smartphones with a particular platform, and in some places the cost of internet access. There continues to be a high need to prioritize increasing the number of on-line education programs to train medical students. Through the development of partnerships, this may be a promising strategy to share and enhance existing resources to promote access and quality education in conflict zones.

In the Chap. 18 "Employing Data Science Technologies Towards Shaping a Sustainably Healthy Future: The Efforts in Contemporary Taiwan" we learn about the value of big data and the field of data science as it contributes to the health status of populations globally. We are living in times of great population shifts, and we are at the forefront of a dramatic increase in the older population. Diseases from which people years ago would frequently die at a faster rate and an earlier age are now becoming chronic diseases, such as cancer and AIDS. Data science and the tremendous growth that we have achieved in analyzing and applying the evidence from the data present unparallel opportunities to intervene at the population health level globally to increase access to healthcare information and services and in the conservation of resources. Geographic Information Systems are widely employed to identify, prevent, and track data trends among healthcare systems and private and public industries. Data science is useful in monitoring progress toward the achievement of the Sustainable Development Goals. Cybersecurity is a critical component in any data science system and the dissemination of information to partners.

The reflections and the chapters from numerous distinguished authors in their respective fields all emphasize the significance of technology to fulfill the potential of the Sustainable Development Goals worldwide. The ever-increasing achievement of technological advances presents new opportunities and challenges to globalize a health equity paradigm for all people.

We hope you have enjoyed this literary journey as much as we did while working to craft this collage of innovative writing, which encompasses impactful and insightful new technologies that make a major difference at grassroots levels globally.

Index

© Springer Nature Switzerland AG 2020
P. Murthy, A. Ansehl (eds.), *Technology and Global Public Health*,
https://doi.org/10.1007/978-3-030-46355-7

Printed in the United States
by Baker & Taylor Publisher Services